THE CLEVELAND CLINIC
INTERNAL MEDICINE CASE REVIEWS

THE CLEVELAND CLINIC
INTERNAL MEDICINE CASE REVIEWS

Editors-in-Chief

DAVID L. LONGWORTH, M.D.

Chairman, Department of Medicine
Baystate Medical Center
Springfield, Massachusetts
Deputy Chairman, Department of Medicine
Tufts University School of Medicine
Boston, Massachusetts

JAMES K. STOLLER, M.D., M.S.

Vice Chairman, Division of Medicine
Associate Chief of Staff
and
Head, Section of Respiratory Therapy
Department of Pulmonary and Critical Care Medicine
The Cleveland Clinic Foundation
Cleveland, Ohio

Co-Editors

DAVID M. CASEY, M.D.

Assistant Professor
Department of Medicine
University of Connecticut School of Medicine
Farmington, Connecticut
Attending Physician
Division of General Medicine and Geriatrics
New Britain General Hospital
New Britain, Connecticut

JOHN K. JEWELL, M.D.

Associate Staff
Department of General Internal Medicine
The Cleveland Clinic Foundation
Cleveland, Ohio

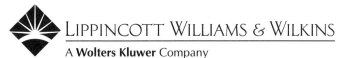

LIPPINCOTT WILLIAMS & WILKINS
A **Wolters Kluwer** Company
Philadelphia • Baltimore • New York • London
Buenos Aires • Hong Kong • Sydney • Tokyo

Acquisitions Editors: Rich Winters, Danette Knopp
Developmental Editor: Karen Carter
Production Editor: Jonathan Geffner
Manufacturing Manager: Colin J. Warnock
Cover Designer: Christine Jenny
Compositor: Lippincott Williams & Wilkins Desktop Division
Printer: Edwards Brothers

Library of Congress Cataloging-in-Publication Data

The Cleveland Clinic internal medicine case reviews / editors-in-chief, David L.
   Longworth, James K. Stoller ; co-editors, David M. Casey, John K. Jewell.
      p. ; cm.
   Includes bibliographical references.
   ISBN 0-7817-4266-8
      1. Internal medicine—Case studies. I. Longworth, David L. II. Cleveland Clinic
Foundation.
   [DNLM: 1. Internal Medicine—Case Report. 2. Internal Medicine—Examination
Questions. 3. Diagnosis, Differential—Case Report. 4. Diagnosis,
Differential—Examination Questions. WB 18.2 C6352 2003]
RC66.C595 2003
616'.0076—dc21
                                                                    2003040044

Care has been taken to confirm the accuracy of the information presented and to describe generally accepted practices. However, the authors, editors, and publisher are not responsible for errors or omissions or for any consequences from application of the information in this book and make no warranty, expressed or implied, with respect to the currency, completeness, or accuracy of the contents of the publication. Application of this information in a particular situation remains the professional responsibility of the practitioner.

The authors, editors, and publisher have exerted every effort to ensure that drug selection and dosage set forth in this text are in accordance with current recommendations and practice at the time of publication. However, in view of ongoing research, changes in government regulations, and the constant flow of information relating to drug therapy and drug reactions, the reader is urged to check the package insert for each drug for any change in indications and dosage and for added warnings and precautions. This is particularly important when the recommended agent is a new or infrequently employed drug.

Some drugs and medical devices presented in this publication have Food and Drug Administration (FDA) clearance for limited use in restricted research settings. It is the responsibility of the health care provider to ascertain the FDA status of each drug or device planned for use in their clinical practice.

10 9 8 7 6 5 4 3 2 1

CONTENTS

EDITORS' NOTE

The Cleveland Clinic Internal Medicine Case Reviews has been compiled from resources and references that are felt to be reliable and has been edited to ensure the highest degree of medical accuracy. This book, however, should serve as an educational guide and is not meant as a substitute for clinical training or continuing medical education. Individual patient care should not be based solely on information contained in this book. Clinicians should individualize patient care based on current literature and clinical practice guidelines.

CONTRIBUTING AUTHORS

Cynthia C. Abacan, M.D.   Resident, Internal Medicine Residency Program, The Cleveland Clinic Foundation, Cleveland, Ohio

Ahmed K. Abdel Latif, M.D.   Resident, Internal Medicine Residency Program, The Cleveland Clinic Foundation, Cleveland, Ohio

Rony M. Abou-Jawde, M.D.   Resident, Internal Medicine Residency Program, The Cleveland Clinic Foundation, Cleveland, Ohio

Ahmed A. Absi, M.D.   Resident, Internal Medicine Residency Program, The Cleveland Clinic Foundation, Cleveland, Ohio

Ronald Adams, M.D.   Staff, Department of Internal Medicine, Ohio Permanente Medical Group, Cleveland, Ohio

Roderick Adams, M.D.   University of Minnesota, Minneapolis, Minnesota

Feyrouz T. Al-Ashkar, M.D.   Resident, Internal Medicine Residency Program, The Cleveland Clinic Foundation, Cleveland, Ohio

Mohammed Alghoul, M.D.   Resident, Internal Medicine Residency Program, The Cleveland Clinic Foundation, Cleveland, Ohio

Eyad Al-Hattab, M.D.   Resident, Internal Medicine Residency Program, The Cleveland Clinic Foundation, Cleveland, Ohio

Amjad AlMahameed, M.D.   Staff, Section of Vascular Medicine, Department of Cardiovascular Medicine, The Cleveland Clinic Foundation, Cleveland, Ohio

Soufian AlMahameed, M.D.   Resident, Internal Medicine Residency Program, The Cleveland Clinic Foundation, Cleveland, Ohio

Anil Asgaonkar, M.D.   Resident, Internal Medicine Residency Program, The Cleveland Clinic Foundation, Cleveland, Ohio

Ashish Atreja, M.D., M.P.H.   Resident, Internal Medicine Residency Program, The Cleveland Clinic Foundation, Cleveland, Ohio

Robin K. Avery, M.D.   Staff Physician, Department of Infectious Diseases, The Cleveland Clinic Foundation, Cleveland, Ohio

May Azem, M.D.   Resident, Internal Medicine Residency Program, The Cleveland Clinic Foundation, Cleveland, Ohio

Sarkis B. Baghdasarian, M.D.   Resident, Internal Medicine Residency Program, The Cleveland Clinic Foundation, Cleveland, Ohio

Christopher T. Bajzer, M.D.   Associate Director, Carotid and Peripheral Intervention, Department of Cardiovascular Medicine, The Cleveland Clinic Foundation, Cleveland, Ohio

Timir S. Baman   Pennsylvania State University School of Medicine, Hershey, Pennsylvania

Michael Baytion, M.S., M.D.   The Cleveland Clinic Foundation; The Ohio State University School of Medicine, Cleveland, Ohio

Susan M. Begelman, M.D., R.V.T.   Associate Medical Director, Noninvasive Vascular Laboratory, Section of Vascular Medicine, Department of Cardiovascular Medicine, The Cleveland Clinic Foundation, Cleveland, Ohio

Yasser M. Bhat, M.D.   Resident, Internal Medicine Residency Program, The Cleveland Clinic Foundation, Cleveland, Ohio

M. Fernanda Bonilla, M.D.   International Scholar, International Center, The Cleveland Clinic Foundation, Cleveland, Ohio

Gabriel Bou Merhi, M.D.   Resident, Internal Medicine Residency Program, The Cleveland Clinic Foundation, Cleveland, Ohio

Johannes Brechtken, M.D.   Resident, Internal Medicine Residency Program, The Cleveland Clinic Foundation, Cleveland, Ohio

Suzanne M. Breckenridge, M.D.   Resident, Internal Medicine Residency Program, The Cleveland Clinic Foundation, Cleveland, Ohio

Daniel J. Brotman, M.D.   Associate Staff, Department of General Internal Medicine, The Cleveland Clinic Foundation, Cleveland, Ohio; Assistant Clinical Professor, Department of Medicine, Pennsylvania State University, Hershey, Pennsylvania

Aaron Brzezinski, M.D.   Staff Gastroenterologist, Inflammatory Bowel Disease Center, Department of Gastroenterology, The Cleveland Clinic Foundation, Cleveland, Ohio

William D. Carey, M.D.   Staff Hepatologist, Department of Gastroenterology and Hepatology, The Cleveland Clinic Foundation; Professor, Department of Medicine, Ohio State University, Cleveland, Ohio

Teresa L. Carman, M.D.   Clinical Associate, Department of Cardiovascular Medicine, The Cleveland Clinic Foundation, Cleveland, Ohio

David M. Casey, M.D.   Assistant Professor of Medicine, University of Connecticut School of Medicine, Farmington, Connecticut; Attending Physician, Division of General Medicine and Geriatrics, New Britain General Hospital, New Britain, Connecticut

Derrick C. Cetin, D.O.   Staff, Department of General Internal Medicine, The Cleveland Clinic Foundation, Westlake, Ohio

Jeffrey T. Chapman, M.D.   Associate Staff, Department of Pulmonary and Critical Care Medicine, The Cleveland Clinic Foundation, Cleveland, Ohio

Toni Choueiri, M.D.   Resident, Internal Medicine Residency Program, The Cleveland Clinic Foundation, Cleveland, Ohio

Darwin L. Conwell, M.D.   Staff Physician, Department of Gastroenterology, The Cleveland Clinic Foundation, Cleveland, Ohio

Natalie G. Correia, D.O., M.A.   Associate Director, Internal Medicine Residency Program, Department of General Internal Medicine, Section of Hospital Medicine, The Cleveland Clinic Foundation, Cleveland, Ohio; Clinical Associate Professor, Department of Medicine, Milton S. Hershey Medical School, Pennsylvania State University, Hershey, Pennsylvania

Shadi N. Daoud, M.D.   Resident, Internal Medicine Residency Program, The Cleveland Clinic Foundation, Cleveland, Ohio

Michael B. Davidson, D.O.   Resident, Internal Medicine Residency Program, The Cleveland Clinic Foundation, Cleveland, Ohio

Rohtashav Dhir, M.B.B.S., M.P.H.   Resident, Internal Medicine Residency Program, The Cleveland Clinic Foundation, Cleveland, Ohio

Raed Dweik, M.D.   Staff Physician, Department of Pulmonary and Critical Care Medicine, The Cleveland Clinic Foundation, Cleveland, Ohio

Yaser Abu El-Sameed, M.D.   Resident, Internal Medicine Residency Program, The Cleveland Clinic Foundation, Cleveland, Ohio

Richard A. Fatica, M.D.   Associate Staff, Department of Nephrology and Hypertension, The Cleveland Clinic Foundation, Cleveland, Ohio

Fetnat Fouad-Tarazi, M.D.   Staff, Department of Cardiology (Cardiovascular Medicine), Head (Medical Director) of Syncope Clinic, Department of Cardiovascular Medicine, The Cleveland Clinic Foundation, Cleveland, Ohio

Benjamin J. Freda, D.O.   Resident, Internal Medicine Residency Program, The Cleveland Clinic Foundation, Cleveland, Ohio

Shaun D. Frost, M.D.   Staff, Section of Hospital Medicine, The Cleveland Clinic Foundation, Cleveland, Ohio; Clinical Assistant Professor, Department of Medicine, Pennsylvania State University College of Medicine, Hershey, Pennsylvania

Anthony Furlan, M.D.   Head, Section of Stroke, Department of Neurology, The Cleveland Clinic Foundation, Cleveland, Ohio

Sasan Ghaffari, M.D.   Associate Director, Internal Medicine Residency Program, Staff Cardiologist, Department of Cardiology, The Cleveland Clinic Foundation, Cleveland, Ohio

Mohammed S. Ghanamah, M.D.   Resident, Internal Medicine Residency Program, The Cleveland Clinic Foundation, Cleveland, Ohio

John P. Girod, D.O.   Resident, Internal Medicine Residency Program, The Cleveland Clinic Foundation, Cleveland, Ohio

Sibyll Goetze, M.D.   Resident, Internal Medicine Residency Program, The Cleveland Clinic Foundation, Cleveland, Ohio

Andres A. Gonzalez, M.D.   Resident, Department of Neurology, Georgetown University Hospital, Washington, DC

Jason M. Guardino, D.O., M.S.   Resident, Internal Medicine Residency Program, The Cleveland Clinic Foundation, Cleveland, Ohio

David V. Gugliotti, M.D.   Associate Staff, Department of General Internal Medicine, The Cleveland Clinic Foundation, Cleveland, Ohio

Basuki K. Gunawan, M.D. Liver Fellow, Department of Hepatology/Hepatology, University of Southern California, Los Angeles, California; Liver Fellow, Department of Hepatology, Rancho Los Amigos Medical Center, Downey, California

Ritesh Gupta, M.D. Resident, Internal Medicine Residency Program, The Cleveland Clinic Foundation, Cleveland, Ohio

Amir H. Hamrahian, M.D. Clinical Associate, Department of Endocrinology, Diabetes and Metabolism, The Cleveland Clinic Foundation; Adjunct Assistant Professor, Department of Medicine, Case Western Reserve University, Cleveland, Ohio

John Kevin Hix, M.D. Fellow, Department of Nephrology and Hypertension, The Cleveland Clinic Foundation, Cleveland, Ohio

Byron J. Hoogwerf, M.D. Professor of Endocrinology, Department of Internal Medicine, The Cleveland Clinic Foundation Health Services Center of the Ohio State University; Staff Physician, Department of Endocrinology, The Cleveland Clinic Foundation, Cleveland, Ohio

Jason G. Hurbanek The Cleveland Clinic Foundation; The Ohio State University School of Medicine, Cleveland, Ohio

J. Harry Isaacson, M.D. Vice Chairman, Department of General Internal Medicine, The Cleveland Clinic Foundation; Clinical Associate Professor, Department of Internal Medicine, Ohio State University, Cleveland, Ohio

Saleh A. Ismail, M.D. Resident, Internal Medicine Residency Program, The Cleveland Clinic Foundation, Cleveland, Ohio

Jesse T. Jacob, M.D. Resident, Internal Medicine Residency Program, The Cleveland Clinic Foundation, Cleveland, Ohio

Amir K. Jaffer, M.D. Medical Director, The IMPACT (Internal Medicine Preoperative Assessment Consultation and Treatment) Center and the Anticoagulation Clinic, Department of General Internal Medicine, The Cleveland Clinic Foundation, Cleveland, Ohio; Clinical Assistant Professor, Department of Medicine, Milton S. Hershey Medical College, Pennsylvania State University, Hershey, Pennsylvania

Lara E. Jeha, M.D. Resident, Department of Neurology, The Cleveland Clinic Foundation, Cleveland, Ohio

Allen Jeremias, M.D. Clinical Fellow in Medicine, Department of Internal Medicine, Harvard Medical School; Fellow, Division of Cardiology, Beth Israel Deaconess Hospital, Boston, Massachusetts

Chelif Junor, M.D. Resident, Internal Medicine Residency Program, The Cleveland Clinic Foundation, Cleveland, Ohio

Anne Kanderian, M.D. Resident, Internal Medicine Residency Program, The Cleveland Clinic Foundation, Cleveland, Ohio

Katherine Keith, M.D. Chief Resident, Department of Internal Medicine/Pediatrics, The Cleveland Clinic Foundation, Cleveland, Ohio

Thomas F. Keys, M.D. Interim Chairman, Department of Infectious Disease, The Cleveland Clinic Foundation, Cleveland, Ohio; Clinical Professor, Department of Medicine, Milton S. Hershery Medical Center, Pennsylvania State College of Medicine, Hershey, Pennsylvania

Gazala N. Khan, M.D. Resident, Department of Internal Medicine, The Cleveland Clinic Foundation, Cleveland, Ohio; Resident Physician, Department of Internal Medicine, University of Michigan Medical Center, Ann Arbor, Michigan

Richard S. Lang, M.D., M.P.H. Chairman, Department of General Internal Medicine, The Cleveland Clinic Foundation, Cleveland, Ohio

Steven P. LaRosa, M.D. Associate Staff Physician, Department of Infectious Diseases, The Cleveland Clinic Foundation, Cleveland, Ohio

Martin E. Lascano, M.D. Resident, Internal Medicine Residency Program, The Cleveland Clinic Foundation, Cleveland, Ohio

Rita Shi-Ming Lee, M.D. Clinical Associate, Department of Internal Medicine, The Cleveland Clinic Foundation, Cleveland, Ohio

Michael J. Lee, M.D. Resident, Internal Medicine Residency Program, The Cleveland Clinic Foundation, Cleveland, Ohio

Michael B. Lehman, M.D. Resident, Division of Pathology and Laboratory Medicine, The Cleveland Clinic Foundation, Cleveland, Ohio

Anthony K. Leung, D.O. Resident, Internal Medicine Residency Program, The Cleveland Clinic Foundation, Cleveland, Ohio

Sabba Maqbool, M.D. Resident, Internal Medicine Residency Program, The Cleveland Clinic Foundation, Cleveland, Ohio

Angela M. Marschalk, M.D. Fellow, Department of Infectious Disease, The Cleveland Clinic Foundation, Cleveland, Ohio

Mark E. Mayer, M.D. Clerkship Director in Internal Medicine, Department of Internal Medicine, The Cleveland Clinic Foundation, Cleveland, Ohio; Clinical Professor, Department of Internal Medicine, Pennsylvania State University College of Medicine, Hershey, Pennsylvania

Peter J. Mazzone, M.D., M.P.H. Associate Staff, Department of Pulmonary and Critical Care Medicine, The Cleveland Clinic Foundation, Cleveland, Ohio

Tarek Mekhail, M.D., M.Sc. Staff, Department of Hematology and Medical Oncology, Taussig Cancer Center, The Cleveland Clinic Foundation, Cleveland, Ohio

Frank Michota, M.D. Section Head, Hospital Medicine, Department of General Internal Medicine, The Cleveland Clinic Foundation; Assistant Professor, Department of Medicine, The Ohio State University, Cleveland, Ohio

Kevin J. Mikielski, D.O. Resident, Internal Medicine Residency Program, The Cleveland Clinic Foundation, Cleveland, Ohio

Alejandro Morales, M.D. Nephrology Fellow, Renal Unit, Massachusetts General Hospital, Boston, Massachusetts

Christian Nasr, M.D. Associate Staff, Department of Endocrinology, The Cleveland Clinic Foundation, Cleveland, Ohio

Saul Nurko, M.D. Staff Physician, Department of Nephrology and Hypertension, The Cleveland Clinic Foundation, Cleveland, Ohio

Armando Philip S. Paez, M.D. Resident, Internal Medicine Residency Program, The Cleveland Clinic Foundation, Cleveland, Ohio

Robert M. Palmer, M.D., M.P.H. Head, Section of Geriatric Medicine, Department of General Internal Medicine, The Cleveland Clinic Foundation, Cleveland, Ohio

W. Frank Peacock IV, M.D. Director, Emergency Department Clinical Operations, Department of Emergency Medicine, The Cleveland Clinic Foundation; Associate Professor, Department of Emergency Medicine, The Ohio State University, Cleveland, Ohio

Robert J. Pelley, M.D. Staff Physician, Department of Hematology and Medical Oncology, The Cleveland Clinic Foundation, Cleveland, Ohio

James C. Pile, M.D. Staff Physician, Department of General Internal Medicine, Section of Hospital Medicine, The Cleveland Clinic Foundation, Cleveland, Ohio; Clinical Assistant Professor, Department of Medicine, Pennsylvania State University, Hershey, Pennsylvania

Jonathan A. Rapp Internal Medicine Residency Program, The Cleveland Clinic Foundation; Ohio State University College of Medicine and Public Health, Cleveland, Ohio

Susan J. Rehm, M.D. Staff Physician, Associate Chief of Staff, Department of Infectious Diseases, The Cleveland Clinic Foundation, Cleveland, Ohio

Curtis M. Rimmerman, M.D., M.B.A. Gus P. Karos Chair in Clinical Cardiovascular Medicine, Head, Section of Clinical Cardiology, Department of Cardiovascular Medicine, The Cleveland Clinic Foundation, Cleveland, Ohio

Jose Rafael Romero, M.D. Resident, Internal Medicine Residency Program, The Cleveland Clinic Foundation, Cleveland, Ohio

Mark Everett Rose, M.D. Clinical Associate, Division of Internal Medicine, The Cleveland Clinic Foundation, Cleveland, Ohio

Mark A. Roth, M.D. Staff, Division of Medicine, The Cleveland Clinic Foundation; Senior Clinical Instructor, Department of Medicine, Case Western Reserve University College of Medicine, Cleveland, Ohio

Bindu Sangani, M.D., M.P.H. Associate Staff, Department of Internal Medicine, The Cleveland Clinic Foundation, Cleveland, Ohio

Steven K. Schmitt, M.D. Staff Physician, Department of Infectious Diseases, The Cleveland Clinic Foundation, Cleveland, Ohio

Martin J. Schreiber, Jr., M.D. Staff, Department of Hypertension and Nephrology, The Cleveland Clinic Foundation, Cleveland, Ohio

Todd Schwedt, M.D. Resident, Department of Neurology, The Cleveland Clinic Foundation, Cleveland, Ohio

Bridget P. Sinnott, M.D. Resident, Internal Medicine Residency Program, The Cleveland Clinic Foundation, Cleveland, Ohio

Firas Z. Sioufi, M.D. Resident, Internal Medicine Residency Program, The Cleveland Clinic Foundation, Cleveland, Ohio; Resident, Department of Neurology, University of Pittsburgh, Pittsburgh, Pennsylvania

Mario Skugor, M.D. Clinical Associate, Department of Endocrinology, Diabetes and Metabolism, The Cleveland Clinic Foundation, Cleveland, Ohio

Matthew G. Smith, M.D. Resident, Department of Family Medicine, Bayfront Medical Center, St. Petersburg, Florida

Gordan Srkalovic, M.D., Ph.D. Associate Staff, Department of Hematology and Medical Oncology, The Cleveland Clinic Foundation, Cleveland, Ohio

Tyler Stevens, M.D.   Fellow, Department of Gastroenterology and Hepatology, The Cleveland Clinic Foundation, Cleveland, Ohio

James K. Stoller, M.D., M.S.   Vice Chairman, Division of Medicine, Associate Chief of Staff, Head, Section of Respiratory Therapy, Department of Pulmonary and Critical Care Medicine, The Cleveland Clinic Foundation, Cleveland, Ohio

Khalid Tabbarah, M.D.   Resident, Department of Neurology, Duke University Medical Center, Durham, North Carolina

Olympia A. Tachopoulou, M.D.   Fellow, Department of Infectious Diseases, The Cleveland Clinic Foundation, Cleveland, Ohio

Khaldoun G. Tarakji, M.D.   Resident, Internal Medicine Residency Program, The Cleveland Clinic Foundation, Cleveland, Ohio

Snehal G. Thakkar, M.D.   Resident, Internal Medicine Residency Program, The Cleveland Clinic Foundation, Cleveland, Ohio

J. Walton Tomford, M.D.   Staff Physician, Department of Infectious Diseases, The Cleveland Clinic Foundation; Assistant Professor of Medicine, Department of Internal Medicine, Ohio State University, Cleveland, Ohio

Bryan E. Tsao, M.D.   Associate Staff, Department of Neuromuscular Disorders and Neurology, The Cleveland Clinic Foundation, Cleveland, Ohio

Elisa Tso, M.D.   Fellow, Department of Hematology and Oncology, The Cleveland Clinic Foundation–Taussig Cancer Center, Cleveland, Ohio

Andrea Wang-Gillam, M.D., Ph.D.   Resident, Department of Internal Medicine, University of Arkansas School of Medicine; Department of Internal Medicine, University Hospital of Arkansas, Little Rock, Arkansas

Joel Weisblat, M.D.   Staff, Department of General Internal Medicine, The Cleveland Clinic Foundation, Solon, Ohio

Bruce Wilkoff, M.D.   Director of Cardiac Pacing and Tachyarrhythmia Devices, Staff Physician, Department of Cardiovascular Medicine, The Cleveland Clinic Foundation, Cleveland, Ohio

Alan Wong, M.D.   Resident, Internal Medicine Residency Program, The Cleveland Clinic Foundation, Cleveland, Ohio

PREFACE

The impetus for this first edition of *The Cleveland Clinic Internal Medicine Case Reviews* is the ongoing challenge that we face as clinicians to provide superb, expert care to our patients. With the increasing emphasis on evidence-based medicine and an ever-expanding pool of information, internists must work diligently to remain current in order to provide high-quality patient care. In a small way, we hope this book will assist busy clinicians in achieving this goal.

Like *The Cleveland Clinic Intensive Review of Internal Medicine*, this book is an outgrowth and companion text of the Cleveland Clinic Intensive Review of Internal Medicine Symposium. The Symposium is a six-day course that has been offered annually since 1989 and is designed for physicians preparing for certification examinations in internal medicine and for those seeking a comprehensive review of the field. A consistent and important feature of the Symposium has been a series of cases displayed on posters throughout the exhibit hall. Designed for review by clinicians attending the Symposium, these clinical vignettes have been enthusiastically received as valuable teaching instruments. The success of these vignettes has engendered our vision for a book like *The Cleveland Clinic Internal Medicine Case Reviews*, in which we present a series of short but, we believe, instructive cases in a standard, question-based format.

As with the Symposium itself, this book reflects an ongoing desire to convey our enthusiasm and passion to master the broad range of disorders that comprise internal medicine. We strive to achieve this goal through a series of case vignettes of patients cared for by the housestaff of the Cleveland Clinic Foundation Internal Medicine Residency Program. Importantly, residents in our program are the primary authors of every vignette in this book. In this regard, the book represents not only our attempt to collect relevant information but also an effort to showcase the substantial talents and scholarly energy of our medical housestaff. We hope that readers will agree that this book embodies the commitment of the Cleveland Clinic and, more specifically, the Internal Medicine Residency Program to academic excellence and continued scholarship.

In organizing *The Cleveland Clinic Internal Medicine Case Reviews*, we have designed each vignette to demonstrate specific teaching points pertinent to a topic of inter-est to those caring for patients with medical problems. While the book is expressly focused and not exhaustive, cases were solicited from the housestaff to ensure adequate representation of all areas of internal medicine. Importantly, we have explicitly avoided assembling a compendium of unusual cases that only physicians working at tertiary care centers will encounter. Rather, we believe that the case presentations detailed in the book will appeal to an audience of medical students, medical residents, general internists, subspecialists, and family practitioners who practice in both inpatient and outpatient settings. Moreover, while the vignettes are designed to be thought provoking and informative, they are not meant to serve as a comprehensive review of a particular subject.

We have found, through the years of the Symposium, that physicians learn best in a case-based format. Therefore, using a format similar to the Internal Medicine Board Review Series in the *Cleveland Clinic Journal of Medicine*, we begin each vignette with a brief case presentation, followed by a series of three to five multiple choice questions. Most of these questions focus on differential diagnosis and management. Following each question is a discussion of the pertinent teaching points. Most of the vignettes also include photographs of relevant radiographs, electrocardiograms, echocardiograms, histologic specimens, or skin findings, which are designed to help reinforce the relevant teaching points of each vignette. Each case also includes a list of selected references.

As editors, we owe an enormous debt of gratitude to many people at the Cleveland Clinic Foundation who have supported this project. Without the support, dedication, and desire of the outstanding housestaff in our Internal Medicine Residency Program, this project would have remained simply an interesting idea. The residents' commitment to identifying good teaching cases, submitting quality vignettes, and acquiring interesting photographs allowed this book to take shape in a timely and efficient fashion. We are honored to have worked with them on creating this book. We are also deeply indebted to our colleagues at the Cleveland Clinic Foundation, who have supported and encouraged the housestaff in the preparation of these vignettes. Their critiques and editing of the vignettes have added immeasurably to the overall quality of the vignettes.

Equal gratitude goes to our colleagues at Lippincott Williams & Wilkins for their willingness to embrace the concept of this book and their attention to detail in its preparation. Specifically, we thank Richard Winters, Sonya Seigafuse, and Karen Carter, without whose constant involvement and expertise the book would remain our dream alone. We are grateful to our families, who indulged and supported us throughout the entire process of creating this book.

Finally, we are grateful to the patients who always make clinical medicine such a fascinating and educational experience. Our patients truly are the best teachers, and without them a book such as this one would not be possible.

As editors, we take tremendous pride in the content of this book. While striving for perfection in the book, we accept sole responsibility for any errors or shortcomings. We hope that these vignettes enrich your knowledge of internal medicine and stimulate your desire for continued learning.

David L. Longworth, M.D.
James K. Stoller, M.D., M.S.
David M. Casey, M.D.
John K. Jewell, M.D.

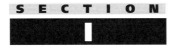
CARDIOVASCULAR DISEASE

1

A 32-YEAR-OLD WOMAN WITH ISCHEMIA OF THE LEFT FOOT AND RIGHT FIFTH FINGER

JOSE RAFAEL ROMERO
JOHN KEVIN HIX
JAMES C. PILE
TERESA L. CARMAN

CASE PRESENTATION

A 32-year-old woman was transferred to our institution for further evaluation of abrupt onset of left foot pain. The patient described the pain as moderately severe, nonradiating, and worse with movement. The patient denied any preceding trauma or injury. Shortly after the onset of pain, the patient developed bluish discoloration of the tips of all toes of her left foot. Two days after the pain developed, she was admitted to an outside hospital because of worsening pain, progressive discoloration, and development of similar color changes and pain in the right fifth finger. The patient denied weight loss, appetite changes, fever, chills, rash, history of Raynaud phenomenon, chest pain, shortness of breath, syncope, or claudication.

Her medical history was relevant for a right-lower-extremity deep venous thrombosis (DVT) 4 years earlier, which was treated with heparin, followed by warfarin therapy for approximately 2 years. She also had a 1-year history of a right calf ulcer, which was being treated with bacitracin ointment. A stage II serous ovarian carcinoma with serosal involvement of the uterus and fallopian tubes was diagnosed 2 months before presentation. The patient underwent a total hysterectomy and bilateral salpingo-oophorectomy. Upon presentation, she had completed one cycle of chemotherapy with paclitaxel and carboplatin (Paraplatin). The patient had never been pregnant. She was single and sexually active. She was not using any form of contraception. She had a 40-pack-year smoking history, having quit 2 months before presentation with the use of a nicotine patch. Her family history was not contributory.

Physical examination revealed an uncomfortable 32-year-old woman with pain in her left foot. Her blood pressure was 104/60 mm Hg; heart rate, 104 beats per minute; respiratory rate, 20 breaths per minute; pulse oximetry, 93% on room air; and temperature, 37.1°C. Examination of the head and neck was unremarkable; no carotid bruits were noted. Lung and cardiac examinations were normal. Abdominal examination revealed a well-healed, midline infraumbilical surgical scar, with the examination otherwise normal. Examination of the extremities was limited by pain but did demonstrate cyanosis, decreased temperature, and hyperesthesia in the distal portion of the left toes and in the middle and distal phalanges of the right fifth finger (Fig. 1.1). Left femoral and popliteal pulses were diminished, and left posterior tibialis and dorsalis pedis pulses were absent. The left ulnar pulse was diminished. The remainder of the upper-extremity pulses were normal. The Allen test revealed decreased perfusion through the left ulnar artery. An ulcer in the right lower extremity was tender to palpation, with a fibrous and necrotic base, irregular and elevated borders, and clear exudates (Fig. 1.2).

QUESTIONS/DISCUSSION

Which of the following is a potential cause of this patient's symptoms?

A. Embolism
B. Vasculitis
C. Thromboangiitis obliterans (Buerger disease)
D. Hypercoagulable syndrome
E. All of the above

This patient presented with findings suggestive of occlusion in multiple vascular territories. Classic findings of large artery occlusion include pain, pulselessness, pallor, paresthesias, and paralysis. However, occlusions in small vessels, such as those that perfuse the digits, frequently present with cyanosis. Clinicians need to make every effort to determine

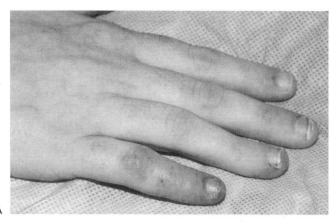 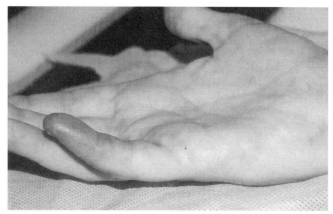

A   B

FIGURE 1.1. Photographs of the right hand **(A)** demonstrating discoloration of the middle and distal phalanx of the fifth digit as well as **(B)** livedo reticularis on the palm.

the mechanism of vascular occlusion in order to provide proper treatment. All the causes of vascular occlusion previously listed need to be considered in this patient.

Embolism is the most frequent cause of acute limb ischemia, accounting for approximately 80% of cases (1). Emboli may originate from either cardiac or other vascular sources. The heart is the source in about 80% of embolic cases (2). Conditions associated with cardiac emboli include atrial fibrillation, myocardial infarction, endocarditis, valvular disease, and presence of prosthetic valves. A surface echocardiogram should be performed initially to search for a cardiac condition that predisposes to embolic disease. A transesophageal echocardiogram (TEE) is frequently needed to evaluate further for a cardiac source. Atheroscle-

rotic plaques or aneurysms are the source of artery-to-artery embolization in about 20% of cases. Atheroembolism most frequently follows vascular instrumentation such as arterial catheterization; however, it also may occur spontaneously, as in the blue toe syndrome (3).

Vasculitis may also be associated with vascular occlusion in the limbs. Depending on the type of vasculitis, small, medium, or large arteries may be affected. Polyarteritis nodosa, giant cell arteritis, Takayasu arteritis, leukocytoclastic vasculitis, Behçet disease, polyangiitis overlap syndrome, and Kawasaki disease are among the vasculitides known to produce limb ischemia (4–10). Systemic vasculitis may be associated with other medical conditions, most notably, connective-tissue diseases such as systemic sclerosis and systemic lupus erythematosus (11). Clinical findings in this patient are most consistent with a vasculitis potentially affecting small or medium-sized vessels, since her symptoms involve the distal extremities. However, the apparent lack of systemic symptoms or multiorgan involvement makes vasculitis less likely.

Thromboangiitis obliterans (Buerger disease) affects small and medium-sized arteries, veins, and lymphatic vessels. Although classically seen in young males, the incidence of Buerger disease is increasing in women. The cause of the disease is unknown, but tobacco plays a pivotal role in the initiation and progression of the disease. Inflammatory thrombi form in affected vessels. Patients with Buerger disease most frequently develop disease in the vessels of the hands, arms, legs, and feet, although the disease may affect other vascular structures. Arteriography shows involvement of small and medium-sized vessels, more severe distal involvement, segmental occlusive lesions, and collateral formation ("corkscrew collaterals"). Other causes of vascular occlusion need to be excluded before diagnosing Buerger disease. Unfortunately, there is no definitive therapy for the disease. The only effective measure to prevent disease progression is cessation of smoking and the use of all nicotine-containing products (12).

Hypercoagulability describes an increased tendency toward thrombosis that can result from acquired or inherited

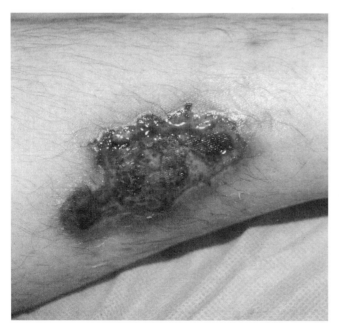

FIGURE 1.2. Photograph of the right calf ulcer with irregular borders and a fibrous, necrotic base.

TABLE 1.1. CAUSES OF HYPERCOAGULABILITY

C	Protein **C** deficiency
A	**A**ntiphospholipid antibody syndrome
L	Factor V **L**eiden
M	**M**alignancy
S	Protein **S** deficiency
H	**H**yperhomocysteinemia
A	**A**ntithrombin deficiency
P	**P**rothrombin G20210A mutation
E	Factor **E**ight (VIII) elevation
S	**S**ticky platelet syndrome

Adapted from Thomas RH. Hypercoagulability sndromes. *Arch Intern Med* 2001;161:2433–2439.

conditions. Patients with an unexplained thrombosis at an early age, usually before age 50 (13), recurrent thrombotic events, thrombosis in unusual sites (mesenteric vessels, dural venous sinuses, or thoracic venous system), massive thrombosis, a family history of thrombotic events, recurrent spontaneous abortion, or warfarin-associated skin necrosis should undergo an evaluation for hypercoagulability. A useful mnemonic to remember common causes of hypercoagulability is *CALM SHAPES* (Table 1.1) (14). Identification of the

specific hypercoagulable disorder is important to provide appropriate treatment for the appropriate duration.

Hospital Course. Before transfer to our institution, initial testing included a normal complete blood count with differential, prothrombin time, and partial thromboplastin time. An electrocardiogram (ECG) was normal. A transthoracic echocardiogram revealed left ventricular ejection fraction of 50% to 55%, normal-sized chambers, normal valves, and no evidence of thrombus. An arteriogram revealed a normal aortic arch and unremarkable subclavian and axillary arteries. The radial and interosseous arteries were patent. Mild distal dilatation of the left ulnar artery was noted. There was occlusion of the lateral digital artery of the fifth digit and faint filling of the fourth digit in the right hand. In the left foot, the dorsalis pedis artery was occluded below the ankle, the posterior tibial artery was diminutive, and the lateral and medial plantar arteries were not visualized. The arcuate artery was not continuous. There was occlusion of the deep plantar branch feeding the left fifth toe, and the plantar branch to the great toe was diminutive (Fig. 1.3). The remainder of the vasculature,

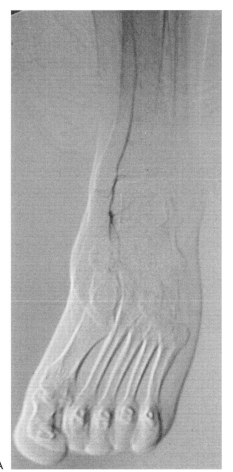 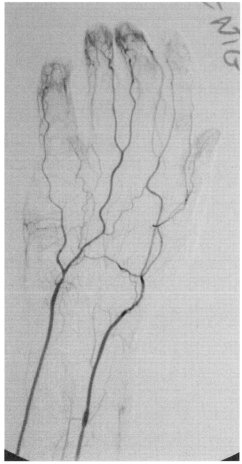

A   B

FIGURE 1.3. A: Arteriogram revealing occlusion of the left dorsalis pedis artery below the ankle and a diminutive left deep peroneal artery. **B:** Arteriogram revealing aneurysmal change of the right ulnar artery and occlusion of the lateral digital vessel of the fifth finger.

including the abdominal aorta, was normal. In addition, a skin biopsy of the right-lower-extremity ulcer demonstrated nonspecific acute hemorrhagic dermal necrosis, which was not consistent with vasculitis.

Upon presentation, the immediate initial consideration for this patient should be:

A. Anticoagulation
B. Thrombolysis
C. Thrombectomy–embolectomy
D. Emergent revascularization
E. Cardiovascular assessment and stabilization
F. All of the above

The initial assessment of a patient with evidence of ischemia in different vascular territories must include a search for evidence of vascular compromise in vital organs and systems. Much of the mortality in patients with acute limb ischemia is due to cardiovascular complications, illustrating the importance of a careful initial cardiovascular assessment. After ensuring cardiovascular stability, further evaluation should determine the severity of limb ischemia. Indicators of ischemia include the presence of imminent or actual tissue loss, such as the presence of ulcers or gangrene, persistent severe rest pain, decreased capillary refill, sensory or motor deficits, and inaudible arterial Doppler signals. The seriousness of these findings should not be underestimated, as acute arterial occlusion has been associated with a 7% to 37% mortality rate and a 10% to 30% amputation rate (15).

Therapeutic options include medical, interventional, and surgical modalities. The choice of therapy is determined by individual patient factors, including operative risk, location of vascular occlusion, collateral circulation, presence of local infection, mechanism of vascular occlusion, contraindications to anticoagulation and/or thrombolysis, as well as the experience of the medical team and available resources. Initial medical management involves anticoagulation in order to prevent propagation of the thrombus and development of new arterial thrombosis or further embolism. The risks and benefits of anticoagulation must be considered before starting anticoagulation. For instance, holding anticoagulation may be appropriate in patients with suspected endocarditis, atheroembolic disease, or absolute contraindications to anticoagulation.

The status of the ischemic digit or limb also guides the approach to management. Although the need for surgical intervention should be assessed in most patients, a viable extremity at presentation is best treated nonoperatively. Arteriography helps delineate the location of the occlusion and allows for intervention in appropriate cases. Arteriography can also help to guide the proper surgical approach but should not delay an operative procedure when one is indicated.

Surgical intervention is the preferred option for revascularization in many patients with ischemic limbs. Surgical interventions include thromboembolectomy, bypass grafting, endarterectomy, lumbar sympathectomy, and amputation. Embolectomy results in limb salvage rates of 85% to 95%; however, mortality rates may approach 10% to 15%, mainly as a result of cardiovascular complications (16). A retrospective study by Nypaver et al. (17) reported an initial 63% limb salvage rate using arterial bypass reconstruction in acute limb ischemia. Of those patients with initial successful limb salvage, 77% had patent grafts and 76% had preserved limbs at 1 year.

Thrombolysis should be reserved for patients with viable extremities in centers familiar with the use and complications of thrombolytics. Intraarterial thrombolysis has replaced intravenous administration of the lytic agent in arterial occlusion of the limbs. Intraarterial thrombolysis has been reported to result in 93% limb salvage rate at 30 days (18). Some studies have shown similar benefit from thrombolysis and surgical intervention in occlusion of native vessels (19). Recent trials have also suggested that lysis may be superior for acute occlusion of synthetic bypass grafts (i.e., occlusion occurring within 14 days of graft insertion) in patients with limb-threatening ischemia (20). Combining thrombolytics and other agents may also be beneficial. One study using reteplase and the glycoprotein IIb/IIIa inhibitor abciximab demonstrated 93% patency after 30 days (21). However, before performing thrombolysis, the risk of bleeding needs to be carefully considered. The optimal pharmacologic approach and dosing regimen remains under investigation.

Other potentially beneficial therapeutic options include calcium channel blockers, sympatholytic agents, antiplatelet agents, topical nitroglycerin, corticosteroids, plasmapheresis, pentoxifylline, and local warming (Rooke boots). One case series reported benefit with cilostazol in three patients with digital ischemia and ulcers (22). However, there is a paucity of evidence supporting the use of these agents in acute ischemia.

Hospital Course Continued. The patient initially was treated with intravenous unfractionated heparin, analgesics, amlodipine, and clonidine. Catheter-guided intraarterial thrombolysis of the left lower extremity with reteplase was unsuccessful. The patient was transferred to our institution for further evaluation and management because of persistent symptoms and ischemia.

Upon transfer to our institution, anticoagulation was continued. The ischemic changes in the left toes progressed, and on the third day following transfer, the patient developed chest pain. Elevation of cardiac enzymes, with a troponin T of 0.42 ng/mL, and ECG findings were consistent with a non-ST segment elevation acute myocardial infarction. The patient received metoprolol, aspirin, nitrates, and tirofiban, which controlled her symptoms and led to resolution of the acute coronary syndrome (ACS). The patient was also noted to have new-onset thrombocytopenia.

Which of the following is a potential cause of this patient's persistent ischemia and concomitant acute coronary syndrome?

A. **Heparin-induced thrombocytopenia (HIT)**
B. **Malignancy-associated hypercoagulability**
C. **Catastrophic antiphospholipid antibody syndrome**
D. **All of the above**

Progression or the occurrence of new thrombotic events may occur in all of the preceding clinical situations. Heparin-induced thrombocytopenia (HIT) is an immune-mediated complication of heparin administration. IgG antibodies, and less commonly, IgA or IgM antibodies, are formed against the heparin–platelet factor 4 (PF4) complex. These antibodies bind the platelet-bound heparin–PF4 complex and induce activation and aggregation of platelets. These antibodies may also cause immune-mediated endothelial injury, which leads to thrombotic events. This syndrome is known as heparin-induced thrombocytopenia with thrombosis [HIT (T)] (23). Thrombotic events may develop in venous and arterial structures.

HIT usually develops 5 to 14 days after initial exposure to heparin, although it may occur earlier in individuals with prior exposure to heparin. The diagnosis is based on clinical presentation and should be suspected in individuals who develop thrombocytopenia while receiving heparin. A 50% decrease in platelet count, a 30% decrease in platelet count associated with thrombosis, development or progression of thrombosis while receiving heparin, and heparin-associated skin necrosis also favor the diagnosis of HIT. Similarly, HIT (T) is a clinical diagnosis.

Diagnostic assays such as the heparin-induced platelet aggregation, heparin-PF4 enzyme-linked immunosorbent assay (ELISA), and C^{14} serotonin release assay (C^{14}-SRA) are supportive but not required for the diagnosis of HIT or HIT (T). Treatment of HIT includes immediate discontinuation of all heparin products, including heparin-coated catheters and heparin flushes, and the use of a direct thrombin inhibitor, such as lepirudin or Argatroban, for anticoagulation (24).

Malignancies are associated with thrombosis. Detectable changes in hemostasis have been reported in 50% of all patients with cancer and 90% of patients with metastatic disease (25). Adenocarcinoma is the predominant histologic type of cancer associated with digital ischemia, which occurs most frequently in older women. The malignancies most frequently associated with limb ischemia are gastrointestinal, hematologic, pulmonary, gynecologic, urologic, and unknown primary. Nearly two-thirds of these patients have metastatic disease. The most common sites of ischemia are fingers alone (50.1%), followed by fingers and toes (31%), and toes alone (8.6%) (26). The etiology of digital ischemia associated with malignancy is typically multifactorial. Although most cases of ischemia progress to gangrene, complete cure of the malignancy can result in resolution of the digital ischemia. A modest response to treatment has been observed with sympatholytics, vasodilators, and anticoagulation (26).

Antiphospholipid antibody (APA) syndrome is associated with thrombosis in venous and arterial beds, involving vessels of all sizes. Embolic events may also occur. Any organ may be involved, although the most common finding is venous thrombosis, with pulmonary embolism associated in up to 50% of cases. Arterial thrombosis is less common but can involve the brain, coronary vessels, kidneys, retina, or extremities (27). Other manifestations of APA syndrome include thrombocytopenia, hemolytic anemia, livedo reticularis, and recurrent pregnancy loss (27). The three antibody groups most frequently identified with APA syndrome are circulating lupus anticoagulant, anticardiolipin antibodies, and β 2-glycoprotein I antibodies. Potential mechanisms of hypercoagulability include endothelial cell activation due to binding of the antibodies, oxidant-mediated endothelial injury, and interference with phospholipid binding proteins involved in the regulation of coagulation (28–30).

APA syndrome is typically diagnosed based on a combination of clinical and laboratory criteria. Clinical features consistent with the syndrome include the presence of one or more episodes of vascular thrombosis and/or a complication of pregnancy associated with the presence of high levels of anticardiolipin antibodies or lupus anticoagulant confirmed on two separate occasions at least 6 weeks apart (31). Complications of pregnancy associated with APA syndrome include three or more consecutive unexplained abortions, one or more premature births of a normal fetus, or at least one unexplained death of a normal fetus after the tenth week of gestation. APA syndrome may be primary or secondary, with secondary forms occurring in association with autoimmune disorders, infections, malignancy, medications, or hemodialysis.

Catastrophic APA syndrome is associated with vascular occlusion in at least three different organ systems. This may occur over the course of weeks or months. In decreasing order of frequency, the kidneys, lungs, central nervous system, heart, and skin are involved. Catastrophic APA syndrome carries a 50% mortality rate, with death usually due to multiorgan failure. Precipitants of catastrophic APA syndrome include infection, surgery, and medications such as oral contraceptives. Treatment of this condition includes long-term anticoagulation, typically life-long, because of the nearly 70% risk of recurrent thrombosis. Other treatment modalities that have been utilized in conjunction with anticoagulation include corticosteroids, plasmapheresis, and intravenous immunoglobulin. These treatments have only been variably successful and have never been validated in randomized trials (27).

Case Conclusion: A hypercoagulable panel revealed strongly positive IgG and IgM anticardiolipin antibodies

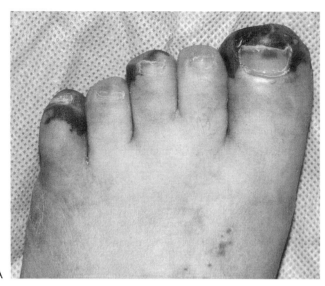
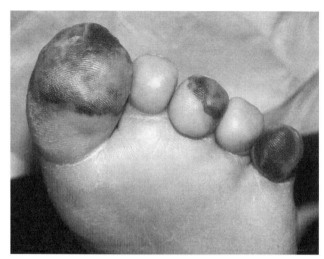

FIGURE 1.4. A,B: Photographs of the left foot demonstrating demarcation of necrosis in the first, third, and fifth toes following therapeutic anticoagulation.

and a positive lupus anticoagulant. Antiplatelet factor 4 antibody ELISA was also positive.

This patient presented with a combination of disorders, resulting in limb ischemia and an acute coronary syndrome, demonstrating the complexities potentially involved in these types of cases. The clinical diagnosis of APA was suspected and supported by the presence of anticardiolipin antibodies and a positive lupus anticoagulant. Heparin-induced thrombocytopenia with thrombosis was also thought likely to be based on the combination of the clinical course (persistent limb ischemia and an acute coronary syndrome while on heparin), new-onset thrombocytopenia, and the positive heparin-PF4 antibody ELISA. In addition, the patient's underlying ovarian cancer was believed to be a contributing factor to the development of her ischemic complications.

Heparin was discontinued at the time of the ACS, and the direct thrombin inhibitor Argatroban was started. Two cycles of plasmapheresis were performed. Oral anticoagulation with warfarin was initiated. The patient was discharged on warfarin after therapeutic anticoagulation was confirmed. Upon discharge, resolution of symptoms and demarcation of ischemic changes were observed in the first, third, and fifth toes of the left foot, with resolution of the more proximal ischemic changes (Fig. 1.4).

CONCLUSION

Limb ischemia is a serious condition, with the potential for life-threatening complications. Patients who present with acute limb ischemia need to undergo a prompt evaluation to begin appropriate treatment. The differential diagnosis

of limb ischemia is broad, and the evaluation should be guided by the clinical presentation and a careful history and physical examination. The immediate therapeutic goals include cardiovascular stabilization, preservation of limb viability, and relief of symptoms. These goals can be achieved through a combination of medical and surgical options. Clinicians need to be vigilant in watching for complications associated with the treatment.

REFERENCES

1. Angle N, Quinones-Baldrich WJ. Acute arterial and graft occlusion. In: Moore WS, ed. *Vascular surgery: a comprehensive review,* 6th ed. Philadelphia: WB Saunders, 2002:697–718.
2. Halperin JL, Creager MA. Arterial obstructive diseases of the extremities. In: Loscalzo J, Creager MA, Dzau VJ, eds. *Vascular medicine: a textbook of vascular biology and diseases,* 2nd ed. Boston: Little, Brown, 1996:825–852.
3. Applebaum RM, Kronzon I. Evaluation and management of cholesterol embolization and the blue toe syndrome. *Curr Opin Cardiol* 1996;11:533–542.
4. Broussard RK, Baethge BA. Peripheral gangrene in polyarteritis nodosa. *Cutis* 1990;46:53–55.
5. Dupuy R, Mercie P, Neau D, et al. Giant cell arteritis involving the lower limbs. *Rev Rhum Engl Ed* 1997;64:500–503.
6. Pistorius MA, Jego P, Sagan C, et al. Arterial embolic manifestations in the legs revealing isolated aorto-iliac Takayasu's disease. *J Mal Vasc* 1993;18:331–335.
7. Mills JL, Friedman EI, Taylor LM Jr, et al. Upper extremity ischemia caused by small artery disease. *Ann Surg* 1987;206:521–528.
8. Le Thi Huong D, Wechsler B, Papo T, et al. Arterial lesions in Behçet disease: a study in 25 patients. *J Rheumatol* 1995;22:2103–2113.
9. Shimizu T, Kagawa M, Katsura K, et al. Polyangiitis overlap syndrome. *Intern Med* 1997;36:524–525.

10. Tomita S, Chung K, Mas M, et al. Peripheral gangrene associated with Kawasaki disease. *Clin Infect Dis* 1992;14:121–126.
11. Herrick AL, Oogarah PK, Freemont AJ, et al. Vasculitis in patients with systemic sclerosis and severe digital ischaemia requiring amputation. *Ann Rheum Dis* 1994;53:323–326.
12. Olin JW. Thromboangiitis obliterans (Buerger's disease). *N Engl J Med* 2000;343:864–869.
13. Subar M. Clinical evaluation of hypercoagulable states. *Clin Geriatr Med* 2001;17:57–70.
14. Thomas RH. Hypercoagulability syndromes. *Arch Intern Med* 2001;161:2433–2439.
15. Neuzil DF, Edwards WH Jr, Mulherin JL, et al. Limb ischemia: surgical therapy in acute arterial occlusion. *Am Surg* 1997;63:270–274.
16. Fogarty TJ, Daily PO, Shumway NE, et al. Experience with balloon catheter technic for arterial embolectomy. *Am J Surg* 1971;122:231–237.
17. Nypaver TJ, Whyte BR, Endean ED, et al. Nontraumatic lower-extremity acute arterial ischemia. *Am J Surg* 1998;176:147–152.
18. Diffin DC, Kandarpa K. Assessment of peripheral intraarterial thrombolysis versus surgical revascularization in acute lower-limb ischemia: a review of limb-salvage and mortality statistics. *J Vasc Intern Radiol* 1996;7:57–63.
19. Ouriel K. Thrombolysis or operation for peripheral arterial occlusion. *Vasc Med* 1996;1:159–161.
20. Working Party on Thrombolysis in the Management of Limb Ischemia. Thrombolysis in the management of lower limb peripheral arterial occlusion: a consensus document. *Am J Cardiol* 1998;81:207–218.
21. Drescher P, Crain MR, Rilling WS. Initial experience with the combination of reteplase and abciximab for thrombolytic therapy in peripheral arterial occlusive disease: a pilot study. *J Vasc Interv Radiol* 2002;13:37–43.
22. Dean SM, Satiani B. Three cases of digital ischemia successfully treated with cilostazol. *Vasc Med* 2001;6:245–248.
23. Kwaan HC, Sakurai S. Endothelial cell hyperplasia contributes to thrombosis in heparin-induced thrombocytopenia. *Semin Thromb Hemost* 1999;25(Suppl 1):23–27.
24. Deitcher SR, Carman TL. Heparin-induced thrombocytopenia: natural history, diagnosis, and management. *Vasc Med* 2001;6:113–119.
25. Edwards RL, Rickles FR, Moritz TE, et al. Abnormalities of blood coagulation tests in patients with cancer. *Am J Clin Pathol* 1987;88:596–602.
26. Chow SF, McKenna CH. Ovarian cancer and gangrene of the digits: case report and review of the literature. *Mayo Clin Proc* 1996;71:253–258.
27. Levine JS, Branch DW, Rauch J. The antiphospholipid syndrome. *N Engl J Med* 2002;346:752–763.
28. Meroni PL, Raschi E, Camera M, et al. Endothelial activation by aPL: a potential pathogenetic mechanism for the clinical manifestations of the syndrome. *J Autoimmun* 2000;15:237–240.
29. Ames PR. Antiphospholipid antibodies, thrombosis and atherosclerosis in systemic lupus erythematosus: a unifying "membrane stress syndrome" hypothesis. *Lupus* 1994;3:371–377.
30. Kandiah DA, Krilis SA. Beta 2-glycoprotein I. *Lupus* 1994;3:207–212.
31. Brandt JT, Triplett DA, Alving B, et al. Criteria for the diagnosis of lupus anticoagulants: an update. *Thromb Haemost* 1995;74:1185–1190.

2

AN 86-YEAR-OLD WOMAN WITH CHEST PAIN

YASSER M. BHAT
ALLEN JEREMIAS
SABBA MAQBOOL
AMIR K. JAFFER

CASE PRESENTATION

Four hours after the onset of retrosternal, "pressing," non-radiating chest pain, an 86-year-old woman presented to the emergency room. Her pain increased with activity but was not associated with shortness of breath, diaphoresis, back pain, nausea, or vomiting. Before her arrival in the emergency department, she took aspirin and nitroglycerin, which improved her symptoms somewhat. She reported a similar episode of pain that lasted 1 hour 2 days earlier that was precipitated by eating and was relieved on its own.

The patient's past medical history included diabetes mellitus, hypertension, congestive heart failure, peripheral vascular disease, and diverticulosis. She had abdominal aortic and iliac aneurysms, for which stents had been inserted 2 years earlier. The patient had been admitted 3 months earlier with abdominal pain. Work-up at that time included computed tomography (CT) of the abdomen that showed a stable 4-cm infrarenal abdominal aneurysm, a normal upper gastrointestinal endoscopy, a normal colonoscopy, and a normal mesenteric vascular ultrasound. Her medications at the time of presentation included metoprolol, lisinopril, aspirin, hydrochlorothiazide, tolterodine, and mirtazapine. She was an ex-smoker (40 pack-years) and denied alcohol use.

On physical examination, she appeared anxious and chronically ill. Her temperature was 37.2°C, blood pressure was 191/99 mm Hg, and her pulse was 66 beats per minute and regular. Oxygen saturation was 100% on room air. There were bilateral basilar crackles on lung examination. Cardiac examination revealed regular heart sounds with a grade II/VI systolic murmur over the right sternal border. Abdominal examination revealed a soft abdomen with normal bowel sounds, a palpable aortic pulsation, and mild left lower quadrant tenderness. Examination of the extremities revealed equal pulses in all four limbs. The rest of the examination was normal.

An initial portable chest radiograph (Fig. 2.1) showed a slightly enlarged cardiac silhouette, a tortuous aorta, and clear lung fields. An electrocardiogram (ECG) revealed normal sinus rhythm, right bundle branch block, and T-wave inversions in leads V4 to V6. All these findings were unchanged when compared with a prior ECG. Serum electrolytes and liver function tests were normal. The white cell count was 7.8 K/μL with a normal differential, hematocrit was 35%, and the platelet count was 141 K/μL. The first set of cardiac enzymes was normal.

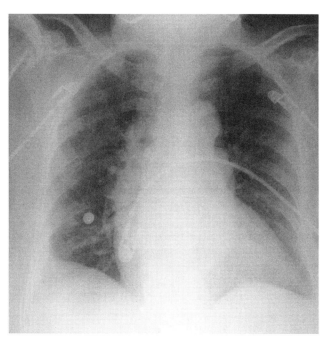

FIGURE 2.1. Portable chest radiograph on admission demonstrating a slightly enlarged cardiac silhouette, a tortuous aorta, and clear lung fields.

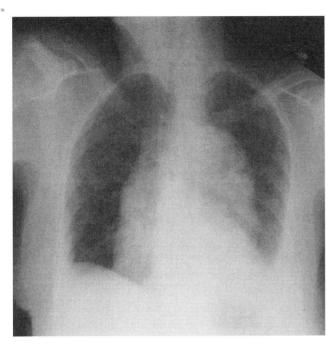

FIGURE 2.2. Posteroanterior view of a chest radiograph obtained 1 day after presentation demonstrating a dilated thoracic aorta with calcifications within the intima.

The patient was monitored overnight in the observation unit to exclude myocardial infarction. Serial cardiac enzymes, including creatinine kinase and troponin T, were negative. A dipyridamole–thallium stress test done the next day did not reveal ischemia or scar. However, the patient developed nausea, vomiting, low-grade fever to 38.2°C, and periumbilical cramping pain. She continued to have intermittent chest pain, which was similar to the pain she experienced upon presentation. At this point, the patient was transferred to a regular medical floor.

Her physical examination at that time was unchanged from her initial examination. Vital signs were significant for a pulse of 62 beats per minute and a blood pressure of 161/87 mm Hg. A repeat posteroanterior and lateral chest radiograph (Fig. 2.2) did not show any infiltrates but was concerning for a widened mediastinum. Given the patient's continued chest pain and hypertension, the possibility of a thoracic aortic dissection was raised.

QUESTIONS/DISCUSSION

Which of the following tests would be least useful in the diagnosis of thoracic aortic dissection?

A. Cardiac magnetic resonance imaging (MRI)
B. CT scan of the chest with contrast
C. Transthoracic echocardiogram
D. Transesophageal echocardiogram
E. Aortogram

Acute aortic dissection can be diagnosed using several different modalities. Chest radiograph may demonstrate findings that are suggestive of aortic dissection, but it is not sensitive enough to be used as a primary diagnostic test. Mediastinal widening may be seen as the aorta expands. However, widening may not be seen early in the course of dissection. A pleural effusion may be seen, which may be indicative of the development of a hemothorax due to a ruptured or leaking aorta.

In the past, retrograde aortography was the most definitive test, with a sensitivity of 88% and specificity of 94% (1). However, with the proliferation of more noninvasive modalities, aortography is typically reserved for patients in whom the suspicion is high but noninvasive methods are not available or nondiagnostic.

MRI is considered the best noninvasive tool, with 98% diagnostic sensitivity and specificity (2). The disadvantages of MRI are its limited availability, especially in emergencies; its inconvenience (patients have to remain motionless for about 30 minutes); and its difficulty in patients with hemodynamic instability.

CT scan with intravenous contrast is 94% sensitive and 87% specific. However, the intimal flap is seen in less than 75% of cases, and site of entry is rarely identified (3,4). The advantages of CT are that it is readily available at most institutions and it is noninvasive.

Transthoracic echocardiography (TTE) has limited utility in diagnosing aortic dissection primarily because of its inability to visualize the ascending, transverse, and descending aorta (5). Therefore, TTE would not be an appropriate initial test in a patient with a high suspicion for aortic dissection. In contrast, transesophageal echocardiography (TEE) is an excellent modality for diagnosing dissection. TEE can easily visualize the proximal aorta, which allows for detection of the intimal flap and the true and false lumens. Although the procedure is invasive, it is portable and can yield a diagnosis promptly. The sensitivity and specificity for diagnosing aortic dissection by TEE can vary, depending on monoplane or multiplane imaging. One study using multiplane imaging demonstrated 98% sensitivity and 95% specificity (6). In general, the selection of testing depends on the availability of the different diagnostic modalities and the hemodynamic stability of the patient.

An emergent CT of the chest was performed, which revealed a type A aortic dissection (Figs. 2.3 and 2.4).

Which of the following treatment choices would not be indicated in the initial management of thoracic aortic dissection?

A. Parenteral β-blockers
B. Sodium nitroprusside
C. Oral clonidine
D. Cardiothoracic surgery consultation

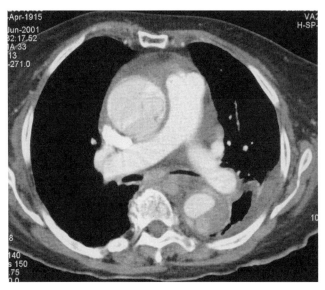

FIGURE 2.3. Computed tomography of the chest. The ascending aorta has an intimal flap with true and false lumina. The descending aorta shows a large false lumen and a true lumen with thrombus.

Emergent surgery is the treatment of choice for acute ascending aortic dissections (type A). Prompt cardiothoracic surgery consultation is imperative in these cases. Patients with type A dissections are at high risk for aortic valve dysfunction, myocardial infarction, cardiac tamponade, and extension of dissection to the great vessels. In type A dissection, there is a greater than 70% mortality rate in patients who do not undergo surgery (7). Operative mortality is high, ranging between 7% and 36% at experienced medical centers. However, outcomes after successful surgery are good, with some centers reporting 10-year survival rates of up to 56% (8). Patients with dissections not involving the ascending aorta (type B) are best treated medically.

The goal of preoperative medical therapy is to reduce aortic shear stresses to prevent further dissection. Heart rate

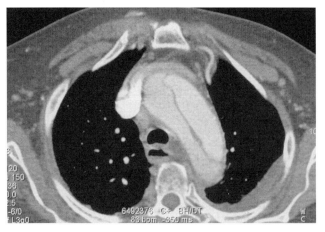

FIGURE 2.4. Computed tomographic scan of the chest demonstrating the intimal flap within the arch of the aorta.

and blood pressure control is essential. Parenteral agents should be used, as they have a faster onset of action and can be titrated more easily than oral agents. Heart rate should be controlled first, as it is a large determinant of wall shear stress in the aorta. β-blockers are suitable first-line agents. Sodium nitroprusside can provide potent and rapid blood pressure control; it is an appropriate agent to use in this setting after heart rate has been controlled. The use of sodium nitroprusside warrants admission to an intensive care unit, as patients need continuous arterial blood pressure monitoring while receiving this medication. Oral clonidine is not indicated, as it has a slower onset of action and can result in rebound tachycardia, which could increase shear forces and worsen the dissection.

This patient was transferred to the cardiac intensive care unit. Intravenous labetalol and sodium nitroprusside were started, and an urgent cardiothoracic surgery consult was obtained. Because of the patient's numerous comorbidities and poor baseline functional status, her perioperative mortality was deemed to be unacceptably high. After discussion with the patient's family, it was decided to treat her conservatively. Her chest pain resolved after her heart rate and blood pressure were controlled. She was started on oral labetolol and eventually discharged to hospice care.

CONCLUSION

Aortic dissection is a relatively common and potentially catastrophic disease. There are more than 2,000 cases per year in the United States. Aortic dissection occurs most frequently in men between the ages of 60 and 80 years with a long history of hypertension. However, in younger patients, disorders of collagen (Marfan syndrome, Ehler–Danlos syndrome), coarctation of the aorta, and a bicuspid aortic valve may be predisposing factors (9).

Patients with aortic dissection present with sudden-onset, severe, "tearing" retrosternal chest pain that is maximal at its inception (10). Severe back pain correlates more with a descending aortic dissection and may migrate as the dissection advances (10). Elevated blood pressure is commonly seen, often as a manifestation of underlying hypertension or due to abnormal baroreceptor responses. Fifty percent of proximal dissections will present with unequal pulses, and the blood pressure difference between the arms can be considerable (greater than 30 mm Hg). Acute aortic insufficiency is present in two-thirds of patients, and a new diastolic rumbling murmur should alert the clinician to this possibility. Myocardial infarction can occur due to coronary occlusion, as can cardiac tamponade with sudden death due to rupture into the pericardial space. Patients may also present with neurologic signs such as a stroke or Horner syndrome. The lack of specific signs makes the detection of an acute aortic dissection a challenge. About half of all patients with type A dissections are misdiagnosed at presentation, usually as myocardial infarction, pulmonary embolism, or pericarditis (11,12).

The patient in this case presented with chest pain and hypertension but had no signs of back pain, aortic valve insufficiency, or unequal pulses. The picture was further confounded by the development of fever and nausea, which led to a delay in her diagnosis. Clinicians must maintain a very high index of suspicion for aortic dissection in the presence of advanced age, elevated blood pressure, and peripheral vascular disease.

REFERENCES

1. Cigarroa JE, Isselbacher EM, DeSanctis RW, et al. Diagnostic imaging in the evaluation of suspected aortic dissection: old standards and new directions. *N Engl J Med* 1993;328:35–43.
2. Nienaber CA, Spielmann RP, von Kodolitsch Y, et al. Diagnosis of thoracic aortic dissection: magnetic resonance imaging versus transesophageal echocardiography. *Circulation* 1992;85:434–447.
3. Shuford WH, Sybers RG, Weens HS. Problems in the aortographic diagnosis of dissecting aneurysms of the aorta. *N Engl J Med* 1969;280:225–231.
4. Vasile N, Mathieu D, Keita K, et al. Computed tomography of thoracic aortic dissection: accuracy and pitfalls. *J Comput Assist Tomogr* 1986;10:211–215.
5. Khandheria BK, Tajik AJ, Taylor CL, et al. Aortic dissection: review of value and limitations of two-dimensional echocardiography in a six-year experience. *J Am Soc Echocardiogr* 1989;2:17–24.
6. Keren A, Kim CB, Eyngorina I, et al. Accuracy of biplane and multiplane transesophageal echocardiography in diagnosis of typical acute aortic dissection and intramural hematoma. *J Am Coll Cardiol* 1996;28:627–636.
7. Scholl FG, Coady MA, Davies R, et al. Interval or permanent nonoperative management of acute type A aortic dissection. *Arch Surg* 1999;134:402–406.
8. Bachet J, Goudot B, Dreyfus GD, et al. Surgery for acute type A aortic dissection: the Hopital Foch experience (1977–1998). *Ann Thorac Surg* 1999;67:2006–2009.
9. Larson EW, Edwards WD. Risk factors for aortic dissection: a necropsy study of 161 cases. *Am J Cardiol* 1984;53:849–855.
10. Spittell PC, Spittell JA Jr, Joyce JW, et al. Clinical features and differential diagnosis of aortic dissection: experience with 236 cases (1980 through 1990). *Mayo Clin Proc* 1993;68:642–651.
11. Butler J, Ormerod OJ, Giannopoulos N, et al. Diagnostic delay and outcome in surgery for type A aortic dissection. *Q J Med* 1991;79:391–396.
12. Jamieson WR, Munro AI, Miyagishima RT, et al. Aortic dissection: early diagnosis and surgical management are the keys to survival. *Can J Surg* 1982;25:145–149.

3

A 75-YEAR-OLD WOMAN WITH BILATERAL LOWER-EXTREMITY EDEMA

ANNE KANDERIAN
SASAN GHAFFARI

CASE PRESENTATION

A 75-year-old white woman presented with a 2-week history of bilateral ankle edema. She noticed dyspnea on exertion for 3 months, which had worsened over the preceding 3 weeks. Her exertional dyspnea had progressed such that she became short of breath with minimal activity. In the previous 3 months, she had gained 10 pounds but denied any increase in abdominal girth. She had worsening orthopnea, requiring two pillows instead of her customary one pillow, but denied any paroxysmal nocturnal dyspnea. Her symptoms raised suspicion for congestive heart failure (CHF).

QUESTIONS/DISCUSSION

Which of the following can cause heart failure in the elderly?

A. **Ischemic heart disease**
B. **Valvular heart disease**
C. **Hypertension**
D. **Hypertrophic cardiomyopathy**
E. **All of the above**

CHF is one of the leading causes of hospitalization in the United States, and more than 75% of patients with CHF are more than 65 years of age (1). Because of the aging population, both the incidence and prevalence of CHF are increasing (2).

Ischemic heart disease is the most common cause of left ventricular systolic dysfunction in the United States (2). Ischemic heart disease may manifest as angina, an arrhythmia, or heart failure, or it may be clinically silent. Myocardial ischemia produces an imbalance between myocardial oxygen demand and supply, as a result of either decreased coronary blood flow or increased oxygen requirements. Myocardial contractility can be affected, leading to diminished stroke volume and cardiac output.

In valvular heart disease, mitral valve insufficiency allows blood to leak from the left ventricle (LV) into the left atrium during systole, which increases left atrial volume and pressure. Once the capacity of the left ventricle to adapt to chronic volume overload is exceeded, systemic congestion and heart failure ensue (3). Mitral stenosis causes an obstruction between the left atrium and left ventricle. To maintain cardiac output, the left atrium enlarges, and left atrial pressure must increase to provide the greater pressure gradient necessary to fill the LV adequately. This adaptation leads to the development of pulmonary vasoconstriction, pulmonary hypertension, and ultimately, symptomatic pulmonary congestion (3).

Aortic regurgitation causes chronic volume overload, which leads to eccentric left ventricular hypertrophy and dilatation. As dilatation progresses, impaired emptying of the left ventricle develops, which produces left ventricular systolic dysfunction (2). In aortic stenosis, a pressure gradient exists across the aortic valve. The left ventricle responds to this gradient by developing concentric hypertrophy in an attempt to maintain cardiac output. As a result, diastolic and systolic left ventricular dysfunction occurs (3–5).

Hypertension is also a leading cause of heart failure. Uncontrolled hypertension leads to pressure overload and increased afterload, which can produce concentric hypertrophy. Left ventricular hypertrophy causes increased ventricular stiffness and impaired ventricular relaxation, leading to diastolic dysfunction. Systolic dysfunction occurs due to impaired myocardial contractility (2).

Hypertrophic cardiomyopathy occurs in 0.2% of the adult population (6). It is the most common genetic cardiovascular disease and is an autosomal dominant condition (6). The disease is primarily a disorder of sarcomeres that causes left ventricular hypertrophy. The hypertrophy is asymmetric, with the most prominent hypertrophy typically in the anterior septum. Outflow obstruction is more common in the elderly. Diastolic dysfunction is caused by increased left ventricular stiffness and impaired relaxation. Patients often develop congestive symptoms and exertional limitation (7).

Any of the preceding etiologies may result in CHF in the elderly.

Case Continued

The patient did not have any known history of hypertension, coronary artery disease, hyperlipidemia, or diabetes mellitus. She denied any angina, nausea, diaphoresis, light-headedness, or syncope. She denied any tobacco or alcohol use. Her daily medications were a baby aspirin and calcium supplements.

Physical examination revealed a temperature of 37.2°C, heart rate 108 beats per minute, blood pressure pf 130/78 mm Hg, and respirations of 20 per minute. Her jugular venous pressure was 6 cm above the sternal notch when measured at a 45-degree angle; her carotid pulses were decreased and delayed. Her left ventricular impulse was sustained and diffuse. The heart rhythm was regular, with a single second heart sound. There was a mid-to-late-peaking grade III/VI systolic ejection murmur at the right upper sternal border that radiated to the neck. There was also a grade II/VI holosystolic murmur at the left lower sternal border that increased with respiration. Her lungs were clear bilaterally. She did not have hepatosplenomegaly or ascites. She had 2+ pitting ankle edema bilaterally and intact distal pulses.

Which of the following cardiac disorders is not associated with a systolic murmur?

A. **Aortic stenosis**
B. **Pulmonic stenosis**
C. **Mitral regurgitation**
D. **Ventricular septal defect**
E. **Mitral stenosis**

Systolic murmurs may be midsystolic (systolic ejection), holosystolic, early systolic, or mid-to-late systolic. Midsystolic murmurs often have a crescendo–decrescendo pattern and occur when blood is ejected across the aortic and pulmonic valves (3,5). In aortic stenosis, blood flow across the valve is impaired, and the resulting turbulence increases the afterload on the left ventricle. Similarly, pulmonic stenosis increases afterload on the right ventricle. Obstruction to ventricular outflow, as is seen with hypertrophic cardiomyopathy, can also cause a midsystolic murmur.

Mitral regurgitation results when the mitral valve fails to close fully during systole and blood regurgitates from the left ventricle into the left atrium. This process produces a holosystolic murmur (3). A ventricular septal defect (VSD) is usually a congenital abnormality. The murmur of a VSD is a holosystolic murmur caused by blood flowing through the defect from the high-pressure left ventricle into the lower-pressure right ventricle.

Mitral stenosis generates a diastolic murmur, not a systolic murmur. The murmur of mitral stenosis has a mid-diastolic component, because of rapid ventricular filling, and a late diastolic component, because of atrial contraction (3). This murmur is heard best during exhalation.

Diagnostic Testing

Laboratory evaluation showed a normal complete blood count, serum electrolytes, and renal function. Troponin T was less than 0.01 ng/mL. An electrocardiogram displayed a sinus rhythm with a rate of 102, left axis deviation, left ventricular hypertrophy, and ST- and T-wave abnormalities. A chest x-ray showed small bilateral pleural effusions and cardiomegaly.

Based on the patient's history and physical examination, valvular heart disease was suspected. A transthoracic echocardiogram revealed severely decreased left ventricular systolic function, with an ejection fraction of 20%. There was moderate left ventricular hypertrophy, as well as biatrial enlargement. The aortic valve appeared thickened and calcified, and the aortic valve orifice measured 0.4 cm^2 (Fig. 3.1). The peak and mean gradients across the aortic valve were 76 mm Hg and 51 mm Hg, respectively. Moderate tricuspid regurgitation was also noted.

Because of her severe systolic dysfunction, a cardiac catheterization was performed to assess for coronary artery disease. The catheterization confirmed severe aortic stenosis (AS) and demonstrated only mild atherosclerotic heart disease.

All of the following are causes of aortic stenosis except:

A. **Degenerative calcific aortic valve**
B. **Rheumatic aortic valve**
C. **Fibromuscular obstruction**
D. **Bicuspid aortic valve**
E. **Marfan syndrome**

Age-related degenerative calcific aortic stenosis is the most common cause of aortic stenosis in adults (5). Degeneration and calcification of the aortic valve lead to immobilization of the valve and stenosis, which is more prevalent in the seventh and eighth decades of life. Abnormal calcium metabolism, as seen in Paget disease of the bone and end-stage renal disease, may lead to progression of AS. Other risk factors that may contribute to the progression of aortic stenosis are diabetes, smoking, and hypercholesterolemia (3,4,8–10). Recent evidence has shown that treatment with HMG–CoA reductase inhibitors reduced the progression of aortic stenosis by 45% (9).

It is uncommon to acquire rheumatic aortic stenosis without involvement of the mitral valve. Patients with

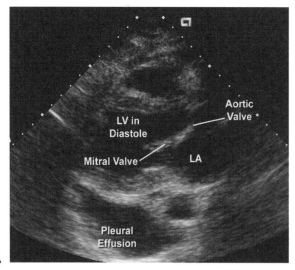 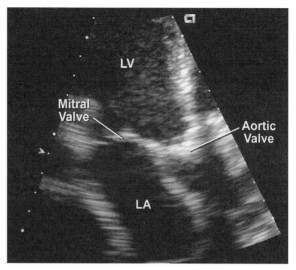

FIGURE 3.1. Transthoracic echocardiogram revealing moderate left ventricular hypertrophy and a thickened and calcified aortic valve. The aortic valve orifice measured 0.4 cm². Ejection fraction was estimated at 20%, and the peak and mean gradients across the aortic valve were 76 mm Hg and 55 mm Hg, respectively.

rheumatic aortic stenosis commonly become symptomatic in the fourth decade of life. Calcification occurs on both surfaces of the valve, and there is often concomitant regurgitation (3,5). In developed countries, the frequency of rheumatic fever and subsequent rheumatic aortic stenosis has decreased with the widespread use of antibiotics.

Congenital lesions can produce several forms of left ventricular outflow tract obstruction. The obstruction may be above the valve (supravalvular) or below it (subvalvular). Supravalvular aortic stenosis can occur as part of Williams syndrome (10). Examples of causes of subvalvular stenosis include hypertrophic cardiomyopathy and congenital fibromuscular obstruction (4).

Congenital malformation of the aortic valve can cause unicuspid, bicuspid, or tricuspid valves. Unicuspid valves can produce severe obstruction and are the most common aortic valve malformation in children under 1 year of age. Bicuspid aortic valves are the most frequent congenital abnormality in adults. Turbulence due to abnormal flow across the valve causes progressive degeneration and fibrosis, leading to stenosis and/or regurgitation (3,5). Symptoms develop in the fifth and sixth decades of life.

Marfan syndrome is not associated with aortic stenosis. Cystic medial necrosis of the aorta often leads to aortic regurgitation.

All of the following are indications for aortic valve replacement (AVR) except

A. An asymptomatic patient with an aortic orifice area of 0.7 cm² undergoing coronary artery bypass surgery
B. A patient with an aortic orifice area of 0.5 cm² and heart failure
C. A patient with an aortic orifice area of 0.8 cm² and syncope
D. A patient with an aortic orifice area of 0.9 cm² and no symptoms
E. A patient with an aortic orifice area of 0.7 cm² and angina

In normal adults, the aortic orifice area is 3.0 to 4.0 cm². The ACC/AHA Task Force grades the severity of aortic stenosis according to the aortic orifice area. Mild aortic stenosis is defined as an area greater than 1.5 cm², moderate stenosis is an area of 1.0 to 1.5 cm², and severe stenosis is defined as an area of less than or equal to 1.0 cm² (5).

Symptoms Related to Aortic Stenosis

The most common symptoms of aortic stenosis are angina pectoris, syncope, and dyspnea. Angina pectoris occurs in 35% of patients with aortic stenosis. Without valve replacement, approximately 50% of these patients will die within 5 years (4,5,8,11). Syncope occurs in 15% of patients, and 50% will die within 3 years without valve replacement (4,5,8,11). Fifty percent of those patients presenting with dyspnea related to heart failure will die within 2 years without valve replacement (4,5,8,11). Symptoms are less likely to be related to aortic stenosis when the aortic orifice is greater than 1.0 cm².

Angina may occur in the presence or absence of coronary artery disease. Angina results from an imbalance between myocardial oxygen demand and supply (5,8, 11,12). Syncope occurs due to reduced cerebral perfusion; it is often related to exertion, as cardiac output is fixed in the face of systemic vasodilation (3,5,11). Dyspnea may occur with the development of progressive heart failure (5,11).

Indications for Aortic Valve Replacement

In patients with aortic stenosis, AVR is indicated in all patients with syncope, angina, or CHF that is felt to be due to aortic stenosis (class I recommendation). Sudden death can occur in patients with severe aortic stenosis but does not usually precede the onset of symptoms (4,5,8,13). Both symptoms and survival improve following AVR.

The management of asymptomatic patients with severe AS is controversial. The risk of sudden death in asymptomatic patients is less than 1%. However, surgical mortality is about 2% to 5%, and the prevalence of postoperative valve-related complications is approximately 2% to 3% (3,5,13). In asymptomatic patients with severe aortic stenosis, class II recommendations for AVR include the presence of LV dysfunction, an abnormal response to exercise (hypotension), and the presence of ventricular tachycardia. Debate persists as to whether AVR is indicated in asymptomatic patients with marked left ventricular hypertrophy (>15 mm) or a valve area of less than 0.6 cm^2.

In patients with asymptomatic severe aortic stenosis, AVR is indicated if the patient will be undergoing another cardiovascular surgery, such as coronary artery bypass surgery or surgery on the aorta or other heart valves (5). Based on the preceding information, the patient with a valve area of 0.9 cm^2 and no symptoms would not have an indication for AVR.

The ACC/AHA Task Force recommends that transthoracic echocardiography be performed every 5 years in patients with mild aortic stenosis, every 2 years in patients with moderate aortic stenosis, and yearly in patients with severe aortic stenosis (5). The rate of progression of stenosis is about 0.12 cm^2 per year (8). Controversy exists regarding the use of exercise testing in aortic stenosis, especially in symptomatic patients. However, in asymptomatic patients, exercise testing may unmask diminished functional capacity that may reveal the need for AVR (3–5,13).

Hospital Course

The only effective treatment for severe aortic stenosis is aortic valve replacement; there is no medical therapy (3,5). Patients with aortic stenosis are usually elderly, but in the absence of coexisting illnesses, prognosis is very good with surgery, and age should not be considered a contraindication to surgery (3). Since this patient had CHF symptoms and severe aortic stenosis, AVR was recommended.

CONCLUSION

The patient was diuresed with intravenous furosemide, which improved her dyspnea and ankle edema. She underwent AVR with a bioprosthetic valve and had an uncomplicated postoperative course. A transthoracic echocardiogram performed after surgery demonstrated an intact valve, with improved peak and mean gradients of 22 mm Hg and 11 mm Hg, respectively. Ejection fraction was 30%. Her symptoms improved considerably before discharge, and she was doing well at 6-month follow-up.

REFERENCES

1. Ghali JK, Cooper R, Ford E. Trends in hospitalization rates for heart failure in the United States, 1973–1986: evidence for increasing population prevalence. *Arch Intern Med* 1990;150:769–773.
2. Rich MW. Epidemiology, pathophysiology, and etiology of congestive heart failure in older adults. *J Am Geriatr Soc* 1997;45:968–974.
3. Carabello BA, Crawford FA Jr. Valvular heart disease. *N Engl J Med* 1997;337:32–41.
4. Carabello BA. Clinical practice. Aortic stenosis. *N Engl J Med* 2002;346:677–682.
5. ACC/AHA guidelines for the management of patients with valvular heart disease. A report of the American College of Cardiology/American Heart Association Task Force on Practice Guidelines (Committee on Management of Patients with Valvular Heart Disease). *J Am Coll Cardiol* 1998;32:1486–1588.
6. Towbin JA, Bowles NE. The failing heart. *Nature* 2002;415:227–233.
7. Maron BJ. Hypertrophic cardiomyopathy: a systematic review. *JAMA* 2002;287:1308–1320.
8. Faggiano P, Aurigemma GP, Rusconi C, et al. Progression of valvular aortic stenosis in adults: literature review and clinical implications. *Am Heart J* 1996;132:408–417.
9. Novaro GM, Tiong IY, Pearce GL, et al. Effect of hydroxymethylglutaryl coenzyme A reductase inhibitors on the progression of calcific aortic stenosis. *Circulation* 2001;104:2205–2209.
10. Morris CA. Genetic aspects of supravalvular aortic stenosis. *Curr Opin Cardiol* 1998;13:214–219.
11. Ross J Jr, Braunwald E. Aortic stenosis. *Circulation* 1968;38 (1 Suppl):61–67.
12. Gould KL. Why angina pectoris in aortic stenosis. *Circulation* 1997;95:790–792.
13. Pellikka PA, Nishimura RA, Bailey KR, et al. The natural history of adults with asymptomatic, hemodynamically significant aortic stenosis. *J Am Coll Cardiol* 1990;15:1012–1017.

4

A 47-YEAR-OLD MAN WITH A PAINFUL, BLUE FINGER

AHMED A. ABSI
SUSAN M. BEGELMAN

CASE PRESENTATION

A previously healthy 47-year-old right-handed man presented to the outpatient department with a 1-month history of sensory and color changes involving the third digit of his right hand. He first noticed pain and numbness while hitting golf balls on a cold day. Initially, he noted intermittent pain, which he described as an ache, as well as numbness and tingling. Gradually, the pain became constant, and after 2 weeks, he developed bluish discoloration of the digit.

The patient denied any history of injury to his hand or other limbs, frostbite, previous cold intolerance, chemical or heavy metal exposure, or venous thromboembolic disease. His medical history was significant for right knee surgery to repair a torn anterior cruciate ligament. He denied any family history of hypercoagulable states, Raynaud disease, or autoimmune disorders. The patient worked as a pipe fitter and was an avid golfer. Upon presentation, he had smoked one pack of cigarettes a day for 15 years.

On physical examination, the patient was a healthy-appearing man with a blood pressure of 120/75 mm Hg and pulse of 78 beats per minute. Examination of the right upper extremity demonstrated normal range of motion of his shoulder, elbow, hand, and wrist. The radial pulse was normal, but the ulnar pulse was not palpable. The third digit of the right hand was circumferentially cyanotic and cool to the level of the proximal interphalangeal joint. An area of discoloration extended from the medial aspect of the finger to the palmar surface of the hand. There was delayed capillary refill in all of his fingers, with a more prominent delay in the third digit. Decreased sensation to light touch involving the third and medial fourth digits was noted. An Allen test of the right ulnar artery was positive, with an absence of normal color in the hand upon release of the ulnar artery. There was delayed filling of the radial artery. Normal color in the hand did return upon release of the radial artery, but it did not occur immediately. The left hand appeared normal and was warm to the touch. An Allen test of the left ulnar and radial arteries was negative,

but there was delayed filling in both vessels. The physical examination was otherwise unremarkable.

QUESTIONS/DISCUSSION

Based on the history and physical examination, what is the most likely explanation of this patient's findings?

A. **Acute arterial ischemia**
B. **Chronic arterial ischemia**
C. **Venous hemorrhage**
D. **Vasospasm**

Any decision regarding treatment of a blue, painful digit or limb requires identification of the vascular structures involved and the time course of the process. Although this patient presents with symptoms limited to his hand, the possibility that the disease extends more proximally needs to be considered.

Acute arterial ischemia occurs as a result of the abrupt cessation of arterial blood flow. Features that commonly characterize an acute arterial occlusion include pain, pallor, pulselessness, poikilothermia (decreased skin temperature), paresthesias (which can lead to anesthesia), and paralysis distal to the occlusion. The latter two symptoms portend a poorer prognosis and may not completely resolve with emergent intervention. Individuals can often recall the exact moment when their symptoms began. In addition, these symptoms typically persist due to the presence of a fixed defect. However, not all of the classic signs and symptoms are always present in cases with limited digital involvement (1). This patient's symptoms started abruptly and progressed over a 1-month period. His presentation is consistent with acute arterial ischemia.

Acute arterial ischemia needs to be differentiated from chronic arterial ischemia. Patients with chronic arterial ischemia present with slowly progressive symptoms. These patients are frequently asymptomatic initially due to the development of extensive collateral blood vessels. Like acute arterial disease, the obstructions are fixed in chronic arterial ischemia. With severe chronic arterial disease, signs and symptoms of ischemia may be present. Necrosis most often develops after a traumatic event with associated ulceration and failure of the wound to heal. Chronic arterial insufficiency of the upper extremity is much less common than chronic lower-extremity arterial insufficiency (2,3).

Venous hemorrhage results from capillary rupture, which can occur either spontaneously or in association with trauma. Venous hemorrhage is a painless, benign condition in which the finger is blue but warm. These patients are usually asymptomatic, but the presence of a discolored digit can cause the patient considerable concern. The discoloration usually resolves within days (1). Venous hemorrhage is unlikely in this patient, who had both pain and evidence of a sensory deficit.

Vasospasm, more commonly known as Raynaud phenomenon, is a reversible event that usually occurs in response to a cold stimulant. It is characterized by well-demarcated color changes and paresthesias that are limited to the fingers and, less frequently, the toes. Classically, the digits of these patients first turn white from cessation of blood flow, then blue due to blood desaturation, and finally red from reactive hyperemia. However, not all individuals experience all three phases. Raynaud phenomenon is characterized by its episodic nature; signs and symptoms are usually absent between episodes. This vasospastic disorder can occur as a primary disease or in association with an underlying condition (1–4). The fixed nature of this patient's symptoms makes Raynaud phenomenon less likely in this case.

Which of the following is/are possible causes of this patient's acute hand ischemia?

A. **Embolism**
B. **Thrombosis *in situ***
C. **Vasculitis**
D. **Occupational injury**
E. **Thromboangiitis obliterans (Buerger disease)**
F. **All of the above**

Embolism of either an atherosclerotic plaque or a thrombus is a common cause of acute hand ischemia. Embolic disease is characterized by the sudden onset of localized symptoms, which persist due to an absence of perfusion distally. Cardiac conditions, including atrial fibrillation, diminished left ventricular function, endocarditis, atrial myxomas, and a patent foramen ovale, are the source of emboli in most cases. Subclavian aneurysms, arterial injury due to thoracic outlet syndrome, and fibromuscular dysplasia are the most common noncardiac sources of embolic disease. Significant atherosclerosis in the aortic arch or proximal limb arteries can also result in atheroembolism. Sudden onset of symptoms, identification of an embolic source, and the absence of significant peripheral atherosclerotic disease characterize thromboembolic disease (1,2).

Thrombosis *in situ* is a less common cause of acute arterial ischemia. A history significant for venous and/or arterial thrombosis should be elicited. Causes of thrombotic occlusions include atherosclerotic plaques, aneurysms, arteritis, connective-tissue disorders, hypercoagulable disorders, and thrombosis associated with malignancy. Factors that may predispose to acute thrombosis include dehydration, hypotension, malignancy, and unusual posture or activity. Thrombosis is more likely to be the cause of acute ischemia in cases with more proximal lesions (1,2). Differentiating embolic disease from thrombosis *in situ* is difficult solely on the basis of history and physical examination. Therefore, an extensive work-up is often required in order to distinguish these two entities, which are managed differently.

Vasculitis describes a group of immune-mediated disorders that are characterized by the presence of vascular inflammation and necrosis. Scleroderma, its variant CREST syndrome (characterized by *c*alcinosis, *R*aynaud phenomenon, *e*sophageal motility disorders, *s*clerodactyly, and *t*elangiectasia), and systemic lupus erythematosus are the most common connective-tissue diseases causing small-vessel arterial disease. However, vasculitides that affect large and medium-sized vessels cause stenosis and thromboembolic disease, which can ultimately produce hand ischemia. A thorough history and physical examination are required to look for stigmata of autoimmune disease. In addition, inflammatory markers and disease markers may be abnormal (1,5). Although the absence of other symptoms and physical examination findings in this patient make vasculitis less likely, further investigations to evaluate for autoimmune disease and vasculitis are appropriate.

Occupational causes of hand ischemia include toxic and chemical exposures, vibration injury, and repetitive injury. Traumatic vasospastic disease, sometimes called Raynaud phenomenon of occupational origin, is an example of an occupational cause of hand ischemia. Use of vibrating tools, such as pneumatic hammers, chainsaws, riveting machines, and brush saws, can cause arterial narrowing, vasospasm, and palmar artery occlusive disease over time. Some improvement in symptoms may occur after cessation of use of the tool, but the arterial damage is often permanent (4). Hypothenar hammer syndrome develops in individuals who repetitively use their hands to pound or grip objects. This type of trauma compresses the ulnar artery against the hamate bone, resulting in vasospasm, ulnar aneurysm formation, and multiple digital artery occlusions due to distal embolization. An Allen test is usually positive with delayed filling in the ulnar distribution (4). Although working as a pipe fitter should not cause excessive trauma to this patient's hands, the degree of this trauma is still more excessive and repetitive than that which an average individual experiences. Diagnosing an occupational cause of hand ischemia typically relies on the angiographic appearance of affected arteries, as well as ruling out other disorders and studying the arterial circulation of the lower extremities, which should be normal in these cases.

Thromboangiitis obliterans (TAO, Buerger disease) is a nonatherosclerotic segmental inflammatory disease that affects the small and medium-sized arteries, veins, and nerves of the extremities. The pathogenesis of Buerger disease is unknown, but the use of tobacco, including smokeless tobacco, plays a central role in the initiation and progression of the disease (6). Buerger disease typically occurs in male smokers under 50 years of age; however, the prevalence of the disease has increased in women, mostly due to the increased number of female smokers (6). Symptomatic patients note claudication involving the arch of the foot, hands, and calves. Disease involving larger arteries is rare. If the disease progresses, ischemic rest pain and digital ulcers may develop (7–10).

This patient presented with acute occlusion of his right ulnar artery and bilateral involvement of his small digital arteries, as evidenced by delayed filling in both hands with the Allen test. All the above causes of acute arterial occlusion could present in this fashion. Therefore, further investigations are warranted.

All of the following tests are appropriate to evaluate this patient's symptoms except:

A. **Angiogram of the upper extremities**
B. **Ankle–brachial index with tracings**
C. **Transthoracic echocardiogram**
D. **C-reactive protein, antinuclear antibody, and cryoglobulins**
E. **Blood vessel biopsy**

Often, patients with evidence of acute digit ischemia need to be admitted to the hospital for further evaluation. An angiogram of the upper extremities is appropriate, since it can identify a culprit lesion that might be amenable to intervention. Furthermore, angiography may help identify the underlying disease. Patients who present with hand ischemia should undergo an angiogram of both extremities, not just the symptomatic one. Otherwise, diseases with a predilection for diffuse limb involvement may go undetected. Angiography is routinely used to confirm the diagnosis of Buerger disease and to rule out other etiologies of peripheral limb ischemia, such as proximal atheromatous plaques (8–10).

Measuring the ankle–brachial index (ABI) and obtaining tracings of peripheral vascular flow is an important tool to assess for involvement of asymptomatic limbs. This study can help rule out occupational causes of upper limb ischemia, in which the lower-extremity vasculature would be unlikely to be involved. In addition, these noninvasive vascular studies can help in diagnosing diseases with a predilection for diffuse limb involvement, especially Buerger disease. Multiple series have shown that almost all patients with Buerger disease had multivessel involvement at the time of presentation (8–10).

It is essential to rule out other causes of arterial occlusion, especially embolic disease. A transthoracic echocardio-

gram and/or a transesophageal echocardiogram can help to evaluate for potential cardiac sources of embolic disease (1).

As mentioned previously, small-vessel vasculitis can present with acute arterial ischemia. A thorough history and physical examination and appropriate laboratory investigation typically allow clinicians to determine if vasculitis is present. An appropriate laboratory evaluation typically includes acute phase reactants, such as serum C-reactive protein, erythrocyte sedimentation rate, and immunologic markers, such as complement levels, cryoglobulins, antinuclear antibodies, and Scl-70 for scleroderma (5). All of these tests should be normal in disease processes such as Buerger disease.

Blood vessel biopsy is rarely required as part of the work-up of acute limb ischemia. Patients with seemingly atypical presentations of their suspected disease may need this type of testing. In this case, blood vessel biopsy would not be appropriate, especially not until the patient undergoes further evaluation.

Case Continued. The patient was admitted to the hospital for anticoagulation and further testing. Neither transthoracic nor transesophageal echocardiography revealed any evidence of valvular disease, intracardiac thrombi, or arch atheroma. A patent foramen ovale was not identified. Laboratory testing—including C-reactive protein, erythrocyte sedimentation rate, fibrinogen, anticardiolipin antibodies, and lupus anticoagulant—was unremarkable. Screening tests for autoimmune disease (antinuclear antibodies and Scl-70) and viral hepatitis were also negative. A fasting lipid panel revealed total cholesterol of 169 mg/dL, low-density lipoprotein of 112 mg/dL, high-density lipoprotein of 34 mg/dL, and triglycerides of 116 mg/dL.

Noninvasive physiologic vascular testing revealed an ankle–brachial index of 1.0 bilaterally. However, there was evidence of mild small-vessel disease in the left foot. An angiogram of his upper extremities was performed upon admission. His aortic arch was free of disease, as were his subclavian, axillary, brachial, and radial arteries. The left ulnar artery was also normal, but the right ulnar artery was occluded. The right second, third, and fourth proper digital arteries were also occluded. All of the digital arteries in both hands were diminutive and abnormal in appearance (Figs. 4.1 and 4.2).

The negative laboratory tests, angiographic appearance of disease limited to the small vessels in the hand and distal forearm, and evidence of disease in multiple extremities favored thromboangiitis obliterans, or Buerger disease, as the most likely diagnosis.

Which of the following signs or symptoms is not consistent with Buerger disease?

A. **Superficial thrombophlebitis**
B. **Raynaud phenomenon**
C. **Ischemic ulcers**

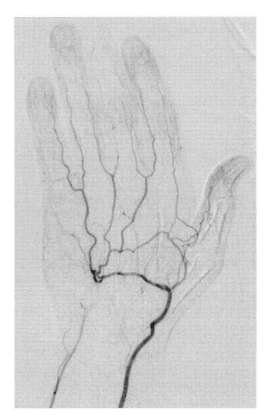

FIGURE 4.1. Right hand angiogram demonstrating an occluded distal right ulnar artery, consistent with an occlusive thrombus. There is a paucity of perfusion into the third digit, with occlusion of several proper digital arteries. There is also diffuse irregular narrowing of the second, third, and fourth digital arteries.

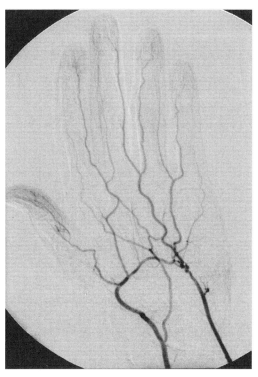

FIGURE 4.2. Left hand angiogram demonstrating diffuse irregular narrowing of the second, third, and fourth digital arteries. These findings were also consistent with underlying disease of the small arteries.

D. "Corkscrew" collaterals on angiogram
E. Subclavian artery aneurysm

In addition to typical features of ischemia, such as gangrene, nonhealing ulcers, and rest pain, features commonly seen in Buerger disease include a history of claudication, Raynaud phenomenon, and superficial thrombophlebitis. Raynaud phenomenon may occur in up to one-third of patients with Buerger disease. The superficial thrombophlebitis typically occurs early in the disease in a migratory, recurrent fashion; it may be present for 1 to 2 years before arterial symptoms (6,7).

Although there are no pathognomonic angiographic findings for Buerger disease, typical findings include segmental occlusive lesions (areas of disease alternating with normal-appearing areas), more severe distal disease, and normal proximal arteries without evidence of atherosclerosis. Collateral vessels, often referred to as "corkscrew collaterals," form around areas of occlusion (7).

Subclavian artery aneurysms can be primary or secondary in nature. Secondary causes include extrinsic compression from thoracic outlet obstruction, prior fracture, and chronic trauma, such as that associated with the use of

crutches. However, Buerger disease is not associated with subclavian artery aneurysms (2).

Which of the following is the most important therapeutic intervention in patients with Buerger disease?

A. Anticoagulation
B. Thrombolysis
C. Surgical revascularization
D. Smoking cessation

Upon admission to the hospital, most individuals with hand ischemia are started on anticoagulation while undergoing evaluation. Many individuals with Buerger disease are taken off anticoagulants prior to discharge. Despite a lack of data to support its use, thrombolysis is occasionally performed. Thrombolysis may be indicated in individuals with angiographic findings consistent with acute thrombosis of the ulnar or radial artery. If thrombolysis is successful, anticoagulation is often continued. Surgical revascularization is usually not feasible because of the segmental and distal nature of vessel involvement in patients with Buerger disease (2,3). Other therapies that have been tried include infusion of iloprost and sympathectomy as a means to treat pain or prevent amputation (7).

Smoking cessation is the only intervention that prevents progression of Buerger disease. Avoidance of all forms of

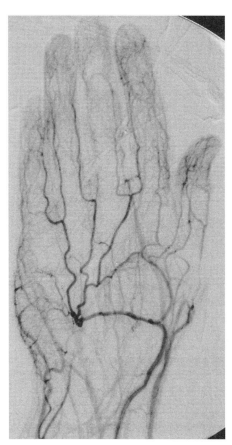

FIGURE 4.3. Right hand angiogram following attempted thrombolysis of the occluded ulnar artery. There was dissolution of the previously identified thrombus in the distal ulnar artery; however, irregular narrowing of the digital arteries persisted.

tobacco, including nicotine replacement therapy, is necessary. Urinary nicotine and cotinine levels should be measured in any patient with Buerger disease that denies tobacco use but has evidence of disease progression (11). Arterial damage in these patients is not reversible, but cessation of all tobacco products is a must to prevent disease progression.

Case Conclusion

Thrombolysis was attempted due to the acuity of his symptoms and the presence of the occluded ulnar artery. Despite some resolution of the thrombus in the ulnar artery, the patient did not have significant improvement in arterial flow (Figure 4.3). He was discharged from the hospital on oral anticoagulation. Upon outpatient follow-up, the patient had stopped smoking. Except for paresthesias in the third digit of his right hand, he was asymptomatic.

CONCLUSION

Acute ischemia of the upper extremities is uncommon compared with acute lower-extremity ischemia. However, similar to acute lower-extremity ischemia, the consequences of impaired function or an upper-extremity amputation are devastating. Therefore, acute ischemia of the upper extremity should initiate prompt action. Thromboangiitis obliterans (Buerger disease) needs to be considered in the differential diagnosis of acute limb ischemia. While certain historical features and findings on examination suggest the diagnosis of Buerger disease, other causes of limb ischemia still need to be ruled out. Although anticoagulation and thrombolysis may play a role in the treatment of Buerger disease, smoking cessation remains the only intervention that prevents disease progression.

REFERENCES

1. Edwards JM, Porter JM. Upper extremity arterial disease: etiologic considerations and differential diagnosis. *Semin Vasc Surg* 1998;11:60–66.
2. Mills JL, Fujitani RM. Acute and chronic upper extremity ischemia. II. Small vessel arterial occlusive disease. *Ann Vasc Surg* 1993;7:195–199.
3. Callum K, Bradbury A. Acute limb ischaemia. *BMJ* 2000;320: 764–767.
4. Coffman JD. Vasospastic diseases. In: Young JR, Olin JW, Bartholomew JR, et al., eds. *Peripheral vascular diseases.* 2nd ed. St. Louis: Mosby Year Book, Inc., 1996:407–424.
5. Calabrese LH, Hoffman GS, Clough JD. Systemic vasculitis. In: Young JR, Olin JW, Bartholomew JR, et al., eds. *Peripheral vascular diseases.* 2nd ed. St. Louis: Mosby Year Book, Inc., 1996:380–406.
6. Olin JW, Young JR, Graor RA, et al. The changing clinical spectrum of thromboangiitis obliterans (Buerger's disease). *Circulation* 1990;82(5 Suppl):IV3–IV8.
7. Olin JW. Thromboangiitis obliterans (Buerger's disease). *N Engl J Med* 2000;343:864–869.
8. McKusick VA, Harris WS, Ottesen OE, et al. Buerger's disease: a distinct clinical and pathologic entity. *JAMA* 1962;181:93–100.
9. Shionoya S. Diagnostic criteria of Buerger's disease. *Int J Cardiol* 1998;66(Suppl 1):S243–S245.
10. Joyce JW. Thromboangiitis obliterans (Buerger's disease). In: Young JR, Olin JW, Bartholomew JR, et al., eds. *Peripheral vascular diseases.* 2nd ed. St. Louis: Mosby Year Book, Inc., 1996:371–379.
11. Matsushita M, Shionoya S, Matsumoto T. Urinary cotinine measurements in patients with Buerger's disease—effects of active and passive smoking on the disease process. *J Vasc Surg* 1991;14:53–58.

5

A 46-YEAR-OLD MAN WITH RIGHT LEG PAIN

SIBYLL GOETZE
JOHANNES BRECHTKEN
CHRISTOPHER T. BAJZER

CASE PRESENTATION

A 46-year-old man presented to the outpatient clinic for evaluation of right leg pain. The patient described a cramping sensation in his calf that occurred with walking progressively shorter distances. Upon presentation, the patient could walk less than 100 feet before developing calf pain. If he walked through the discomfort, he would subsequently experience right foot numbness. The cramping sensation did not involve the thigh or buttocks, and the patient did not have any symptoms in the left leg. The patient experienced relief of his symptoms after resting for approximately 3 minutes. He denied any discoloration of his feet or toes, leg ulcers, or leg pain at rest.

The patient's past medical history included hypertension and hyperlipidemia. He had no history of cardiac disease, diabetes mellitus, stroke, or transient ischemic attacks. Medications upon presentation included aspirin, lisinopril, triamterene/hydrochlorothiazide, and a number of herbs and supplements. Because of erectile dysfunction, the patient had recently been switched from extended-release metoprolol to lisinopril. Upon presentation, the patient had smoked one to two packs of cigarettes per day for 30 years. Family history was notable for a father with hypertension, diabetes, and myocardial infarction at age 52.

QUESTIONS/DISCUSSION

Based on the history, which of the following is the most likely cause of the *patient's* leg pain?

A. Arthritis of the right hip and knee
B. Intermittent claudication
C. Lumbosacral spinal stenosis
D. Chronic compartment syndrome

The patient's symptoms are most compatible with intermittent claudication, which is the most common symptom of peripheral arterial disease (PAD) of the lower extremities. Intermittent claudication is defined as pain, aching, cramping, numbness, or sense of fatigue in the muscles of one or both legs during exercise or walking. Patients who develop these symptoms with walking typically describe the onset of symptoms with walking a predictable distance. The pain does not cease with continued walking but is relieved by rest, including standing, within a few minutes (1–3).

The site of claudication is distal to the location of occlusive disease. Aortoiliac disease leads to pain in the area of the buttocks, hips, thighs, and calves. Femoral and popliteal disease leads to calf pain. Progression of peripheral arterial disease can lead to rest pain, cool limbs, and numbness. Further progression of PAD leads to ulceration and gangrene. Although atherosclerotic disease is the most common cause of vascular compromise of the lower extremities, clinicians also need to consider etiologies such as fibromuscular dysplasia, vasculitis, and arteriovenous fistula formation.

Arthritis of the hips and knees can mimic thigh and buttock claudication. Osteoarthritic pain is usually associated with variable amounts of exercise. It is typically relieved after prolonged, rather than short, periods of rest, and the intensity of pain varies on a daily basis. This patient's pain was in the calf, rather than in a joint. Furthermore, his pain was reproducible after walking a certain distance, and he consistently experienced prompt relief with rest.

Osteophytic narrowing of the neural canal causes leg pain due to spinal stenosis of the lumbosacral area (neurogenic claudication). The pain associated with spinal stenosis can be chronic, intermittent, or progressive and is commonly exacerbated by standing, walking, or carrying. Lying down or bending forward often relieves the symptoms. Many patients also experience back pain, as nearly 50% of affected individuals have radicular pain. The leg pain is frequently associated with symptoms such as burning, tingling, and numbness. Spinal stenosis is less likely in this patient, whose progressive symptoms were clearly reproducible with walking and were quickly relieved with rest.

Chronic compartment syndrome usually afflicts younger people, especially athletes. Vigorous exercise typically precedes the onset of pain. Unlike this patient's symptoms, pain associated with chronic compartment syndrome does not resolve quickly with rest.

Which of the following statements about peripheral arterial disease is false?

A. **Its incidence increases with age.**
B. **In 80% to 90% of symptomatic patients, the femoropopliteal segment is affected.**
C. **It affects greater than 10% of the adult population.**
D. **Increased homocysteine level is not a risk factor.**
E. **Routine screening for asymptomatic patients without risk factors is not recommended.**
F. **Up to one-half of patients with PAD are asymptomatic.**

Peripheral arterial disease represents chronic obstruction of the arteries supplying the extremities. Atherosclerosis (arteriolosclerosis obliterans) is the leading cause of occlusive arterial disease of the extremities in patients greater than 40 years of age, with the greatest incidence in the sixth and seventh decades (4,5). Large to medium-sized arteries are most commonly affected. Sites of PAD include the abdominal aorta and iliac arteries (30% of symptomatic patients), femoral and popliteal arteries (80% to 90% of symptomatic patients), and distal tibial and peroneal arteries (40% to 50% of symptomatic patients) (4).

Although the exact prevalence of atherosclerotic PAD depends in part on the specific population studied and the diagnostic tools used, the prevalence approaches 12% in the adult population (6,7). The prevalence increases with age, ranging from 2.5% in patients 40 to 59 years of age up to 18.8% in patients 70 to 79 years of age (2,3). Patients over age 65 have an annual incidence of 2% (7).

Risk factors for PAD include smoking, systemic hypertension, diabetes mellitus, hyperlipidemia, and hyperhomocysteinemia (2–3,5–6). Elevated homocysteine levels are thought to represent a more substantial risk for PAD compared with its risk in association with coronary artery disease (2,5). Until about age 70, men are at increased risk for PAD compared with women (2,3). Other potentially significant risk factors include elevations in C-reactive protein, lipoprotein (a), fibrinogen, and hematocrit (2,3,5,6).

While routine screening for asymptomatic patients without risks for PAD is neither recommended nor cost-effective, evaluation for PAD should be pursued in at-risk patients and in patients with symptoms such as leg pain on exertion or distal limb ulceration without an obvious alternative explanation (3). Furthermore, clinicians need to have a healthy suspicion for PAD, since 20% to 50% of patients

with PAD based on ankle–brachial indices are asymptomatic (3,6). Nearly 90% of patients with intermittent claudication do not report their symptoms to their physicians, thinking that their diminished walking distance is an effect of aging (8).

The physical examination of patients with leg pain and suspected PAD should include measurement of the blood pressure in both arms while sitting and standing, funduscopic examination, cardiac examination, and palpation of pulses in the upper and lower extremities (Fig. 5.1). The intensity of pulses is usually graded from 0 to 2, with 0 representing absent pulses; 1, diminished pulses; and 2, normal pulses. The presence of decreased or absent pulses on physical examination is suggestive of PAD. Clinicians should also auscultate for the presence of carotid, subclavian, axil-

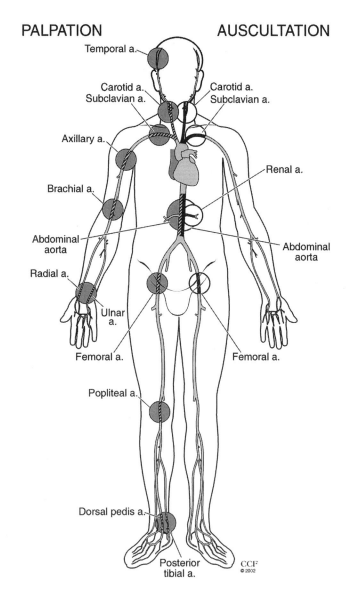

FIGURE 5.1. Schematic demonstrating appropriate palpation and auscultation of peripheral pulses.

lary, abdominal, and femoral bruits. Other findings suggestive of PAD include trophic changes, such as muscle atrophy, hair loss, thickened nails, and smooth, shiny skin. Decreased temperature, pallor, cyanosis, ulcers, and gangrene are signs of potential arterial occlusion. A thorough neurologic examination can help to distinguish true claudication from neurogenic claudication.

This patient's physical examination revealed a blood pressure of 150/80 mm Hg in both arms, pulse of 80 beats per minute, respiratory rate of 14 per minute, and temperature of 36.9°C. There were no carotid bruits or jugular venous distension. Pulmonary and cardiac examinations were normal. The abdomen was slightly protuberant, nontender, with normal bowel sounds. There was no palpable enlargement of the abdominal aorta. A systolic bruit was heard over the right lower quadrant extending from the umbilicus into the right groin. There was no cyanosis, clubbing, or edema. Peripheral pulses were intact and symmetric throughout except for the right lower extremity, in which the popliteal and dorsalis pedis pulses were absent. The right posterior tibial pulse was 1+.

Which of the following is the most appropriate next step in evaluating this patient?

A. Arterial duplex ultrasound of the lower extremities
B. Pulse volume recordings with measurement of ankle–brachial index
C. Contrast angiography of the aorta and lower extremities
D. Magnetic resonance angiography (MRA) of the lower extremities
E. No further testing is indicated.

This patient's history and physical examination were highly suspicious for peripheral arterial disease. Goals of subsequent evaluation include quantification of the degree of limb ischemia and localization of the obstructing lesion. Noninvasive investigations are appropriate as the initial evaluation for PAD. Noninvasive modalities to assess the peripheral arterial system include pulse volume recordings (PVRs), segmental pressure measurements, stress testing, Doppler flow velocity waveform analysis, arterial duplex ultrasound, reactive hyperemia testing, and transcutaneous oximetry.

Arterial pressures in the extremities can be measured noninvasively with pulse volume recordings, which involve the placement of blood pressure cuffs and the use of a Doppler device to auscultate blood flow. In this patient, PVRs with measurement of the ankle–brachial index (ABI) are the most appropriate next test. The ankle–brachial index is the ratio of the ankle systolic blood pressure to the brachial artery systolic blood pressure. The systolic blood pressure is measured in each arm and in the dorsalis pedis (DP) and tibialis posterior (TP) arteries in each ankle. The greater of the two arm pressures is selected, as is the greater

of the ankle pressures (6). Ankle–brachial indices of 1 or slightly higher are normal. In hemodynamically significant stenoses of the lower extremities, the ABIs will be decreased. Ankle–brachial indices are 95% sensitive and 99% specific for diagnosing PAD (1). Table 5.1 summarizes the interpretation of ABI measurements.

Doppler segmental pressures involve the use of PVRs and the measurement of systolic blood pressure at several levels in the lower extremity (proximal thigh, distal thigh, proximal calf, and ankle/foot) (9). These measurements are useful in determining the level of obstructive PAD. A drop in pressure of at least 20 mm Hg between two segments in the lower extremities predicts arterial occlusion between the two levels (2,5,8,9). Doppler segmental pressures are 97% accurate for detecting the level of stenosis (5).

When noninvasive testing is equivocal at rest, stress testing can help clarify the diagnosis of PAD. A decreased ABI with exercise can support the diagnosis of PAD (8). Using standard treadmill exercise testing protocols, the patient walks at a rate of 2 miles per hour on a 12% grade for 5 minutes or until claudication symptoms prohibit exercise (5). The decrease in ABI and the time required for the ABI to return to resting values are proportional to the severity of stenosis (9). In addition, these noninvasive tests are useful in assessing progression of disease or response to therapy (9). A change in ABI of greater than or equal to 0.15 in consecutive studies is considered significant (5).

Duplex ultrasound may be used in special circumstances to assess the patency of a single arterial segment, such as a bypass graft (2). It is not useful to assess the patency of the entire arterial system of an extremity.

Contrast angiography is not routinely used in the initial evaluation of a patient with suspected peripheral arterial disease. It is typically used before potential revascularization (percutaneous transluminal angioplasty or surgery) in order to define anatomy and plan for surgery (2,8). Although contrast angiography remains the gold standard for defining the arterial system, MRA has comparable diagnostic accuracy and is being used more frequently in place of contrast

TABLE 5.1. CLASSIFICATION OF ANKLE–BRACHIAL INDEX MEASUREMENTS

Ankle–Brachial Index	Clinical Significance
>1.3	Noncompressible, calcified vessel
1.0–1.3	Normal
0.9–1	Borderline (variability)
0.7–0.89	Mild disease (intermittent claudication often associated)
0.5–0.69	Moderate disease (intermittent claudication)
<0.5	Severe peripheral arterial disease (rest pain, critical limb ischemia)
<0.2	Tissue loss

Data from refs. 2–3 and 5–7.

angiography. However, similar to contrast angiography, MRA is not an appropriate initial test to diagnose peripheral arterial disease (2).

In addition to an assessment of the peripheral vascular system, a basic laboratory evaluation focusing on the risk factors and sequelae of atherosclerotic disease is warranted. Appropriate tests include a complete blood count, glucose, renal function, fasting lipid panel, and electrocardiogram (2,5). A hypercoagulable work-up may be indicated in patients with repeated failures of revascularization procedures or in young individuals with accelerated atherosclerosis (2).

Case Continued. The patient underwent PVRs of the lower extremities, which revealed ABIs of 0.79 on the right and 1.17 on the left (Fig. 5.2). Segmental pressures were consistent with a high-grade single-level occlusion, thought to be located in the iliac system. The right ABI markedly decreased with exercise, and the patient began to experience right calf claudication after about 90 seconds of exercise. His blood work was unremarkable.

Following the PVRs, the patient underwent an MRA of the pelvis and lower extremities, which revealed a high-grade focal stenosis of the right external iliac artery (Fig. 5.3). This lesion was thought to be amenable to angioplasty and stent placement. There was also mild left external iliac artery stenosis. Otherwise, the visualized arteries in the lower extremity appeared normal.

Which of the following statements regarding the prognosis of patients with peripheral arterial disease is true?

A. Infection is the most common cause of mortality.
B. Complications associated with revascularization are the most common cause of mortality.
C. The 10-year survival rate of patients with intermittent claudication is approximately 50%.
D. The 5-year risk of amputation is approximately 20%.
E. Approximately 50% of nondiabetic patients with claudication remain stable or improve.

The prognosis of peripheral arterial disease is influenced by several factors, most notably the extent of coexisting coronary artery disease (CAD) and cerebrovascular disease (CVD). Up to 50% of patients with symptomatic PAD have significant CAD, as compared with 11% of the general population (1,3,5). Patients with intermittent claudica-

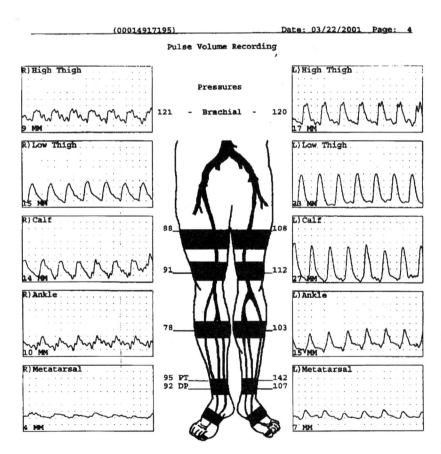

FIGURE 5.2. Resting and stress noninvasive arterial testing of the lower extremities. The study illustrates a segmental pressure gradient between the right brachial artery and the right thigh (121 to 88 mm Hg). The right ankle–brachial index is 0.79, and the left ankle–brachial index is 1.17, without a significant segmental pressure gradient in the left lower extremity. No significant segmental pressure gradients are identified below the low right thigh. These findings are consistent with a high-grade focal stenosis, likely involving the iliac system.

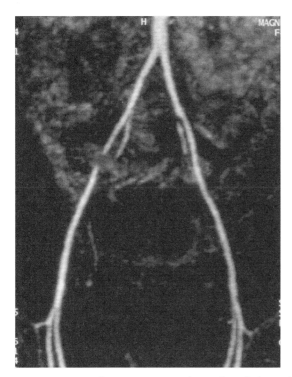

FIGURE 5.3. Magnetic resonance angiography of the pelvis and lower extremities revealing a high-grade focal stenosis of the right external iliac artery and mild left external iliac artery stenosis.

tion have 70% 5-year, 50% 10-year, and 30% 15-year survival rates (3–5). Cardiovascular events represent the most common cause of mortality in association with PAD, with up to 80% of mortality due to cardiovascular events (2,3,7). Patients with PAD carry a relative risk of mortality from cardiovascular causes similar to that of patients with known CAD or CVD (6). Patients with critical limb ischemia have an annual mortality approaching 20% to 25% (2,6). Since patients with PAD often have impaired functional status, clinicians need to recognize that these patients may not develop symptoms of angina pectoris.

Approximately 75% of nondiabetic patients with mild to moderate claudication remain symptomatically stable or improve (1,4,5). Up to 20% of patients develop worsening claudication, and 5% to 10% of patients progress to ischemic pain at rest, ulcers, or gangrene. Five percent of this group will need amputation within 5 years (1,5,6,8). The risk of amputation is much higher in smokers and diabetics (1,4,5).

All of the following are treatment options for peripheral vascular disease except:

A. Control of diabetes mellitus and other risk factors
B. Aspirin
C. Warfarin
D. Surgical revascularization
E. Walking programs

The goals of therapy for peripheral vascular disease include preventing or treating cardiovascular complications, maintaining or improving functional status and quality of life, preventing disease progression, and reducing or eliminating symptoms.

These goals are achieved by a variety of methods:

Supportive measures: These include meticulous foot care, smoking cessation, and exercise programs. An exercise program of 30 to 45 minutes per day will help to increase maximum and pain-free walking distances, improve cardiovascular risk factors, and enhance functional capacity. Optimal results with an exercise program are achieved in a supervised setting (1,3,6,8).

Risk factor modification: Despite a lack of prospective data on cardiovascular risk in patients with peripheral arterial disease, these patients should be treated based on the current recommendations for other manifestations of atherosclerosis. Patients with PAD are not typically treated as aggressively as those with CAD in terms of risk factor modification and antiplatelet therapy (7).

Though specific data on the effects of treatment of hypertension on the natural history of PAD have not been fully evaluated, current recommendations include following established hypertension guidelines (JNC VI) and maintaining blood pressure below 130/85 mm Hg (5,7,8). Traditionally, β-blockers have been thought to have negative effects on symptoms of PAD. However, recent data evaluating their use concluded that these agents are safe in PAD, except in the most severely affected patients, in whom the drugs should be administered with caution (6).

Consensus supports the treatment of hyperlipidemia according to National Cholesterol Education Program III guidelines, which recommend maintaining low-density lipoprotein (LDL) cholesterol below 100 mg/dL and triglycerides below 150 mg/dL (3,5–8). The current guidelines for treating patients with diabetes mellitus recommend a target hemoglobin A1c under 7% and fasting blood sugar between 80 and 120 mg/dL (5–8). Elevated homocysteine levels are emerging as a prevalent and strong risk factor for atherosclerotic vascular disease. However, because of the paucity of data regarding the treatment of hyperhomocysteinemia, no specific recommendations are available (6,7).

Medications: Pharmacologic therapy for PAD has not proven to be as successful as pharmacologic treatment for CAD. Antiplatelet therapy with aspirin or clopidogrel is the most crucial pharmacologic intervention and the only therapy shown to improve long-term survival in patients with PAD. The benefits of antiplatelet therapy are likely secondary to its ability to prevent adverse cardiovascular events. Although the specific benefits of antiplatelet therapy on the course of PAD itself are less clearly defined, it is an important part of the management of patients who undergo vascular intervention or graft surgery (3,5–8).

Cilostazol, a phosphodiesterase inhibitor with vasodilatory and antiplatelet properties, is the only agent specifically recommended for PAD. Studies have shown that cilostazol increases the distance patients can walk before developing claudication (1–3,6–7). It is contraindicated in congestive heart failure, and its major side effect is headache.

Recent data suggest that angiotensin converting enzyme (ACE) inhibitors such as ramipril are likely to be effective in the treatment of PAD and in decreasing cardiovascular morbidity and mortality in patients with PAD (6,7). However, prospective randomized trials about the role of ACE inhibitors in patients with PAD are needed before making definite treatment recommendations.

Pentoxifylline, a methylxanthine derivative, has been reported to increase blood flow by decreasing blood viscosity and increasing cell flexibility. However, its efficacy is questionable, as existing clinical trials and data have failed to provide sufficient evidence to support its widespread use (1–3,6–8). Among the agents shown not to be beneficial for PAD are vasodilators (papaverine), α-adrenergic blockers, heparin, and warfarin (1,5,6). Agents under investigation for a role in PAD include angiogenic growth factor, carnitine, propionyl-L-carnitine, prostaglandins (PGE1 and PGI2), and L-arginine (2,3,6).

Revascularization: Revascularization is particularly successful for aortoiliac disease and is reserved for patients with disabling symptoms, ischemia at rest, critical limb ischemia, and/or failure of medical therapy (1,3,4,6,8). Most available data suggest that surgical revascularization has greater long-term durability than does endovascular therapy; however, periprocedural complications are lower with percutaneous modalities (2).

Percutaneous transluminal angioplasty (PTA), especially when combined with stent placement, is most successful in the proximal vessels and in focal, short stenoses. The initial patency associated with PTA/stent placement is 90% to 95% for the aortoiliac vessels and 80% for femoropopliteal vessels. Patency at 3 years is 75% for the aortoiliac vessels and 60% for femoral and popliteal vessels (4).

Surgical intervention for aortoiliac disease typically involves aortobifemoral bypass, with 99% immediate patency, 90% patency at 5 years, and 80% patency at 10 years (4,8). Surgical options for femoropopliteal disease include *in situ* and reverse autologous saphenous vein bypass grafting, thromboendarterectomy, and polytetrafluoroethylene (PTFE) grafts. Patency with saphenous vein grafts is 90% at 1 year and 70% to 80% at 5 years; patency rates associated with PTFE grafts are significantly lower (4). The overall perioperative mortality typically ranges from 1% to 3% (4).

CONCLUSION

PTA of the isolated high-grade stenosis of the right iliac artery was recommended. The patient opted for medical management with aggressive risk factor modification. He has remained adherent to a walking program but has struggled to quit smoking completely. He underwent a dobutamine echocardiogram, which was negative for ischemia and showed normal ventricular function. Following the results of the dobutamine echocardiogram, the patient was started on cilostazol.

REFERENCES

1. Beebe HG. Intermittent claudication: effective medical management of a common circulatory problem. *Am J Cardiol* 2001;87:14D–18D.
2. Ouriel K. Peripheral arterial disease. *Lancet* 2001;358:1257–1264.
3. Schainfeld RM. Management of peripheral arterial disease and intermittent claudication. *J Am Board Fam Pract* 2001;14:443–450.
4. Creager MA, Dzau VJ. Vascular diseases of the extremities. In: Braunwald E, Fauci AS, Kasper DL, et al., eds. *Harrison's principles of internal medicine,* 15th ed. New York: McGraw-Hill, 2001:1434–1442.
5. Schmieder FA, Comerota AJ. Intermittent claudication: magnitude of the problem, patient evaluation, and therapeutic strategies. *Am J Cardiol* 2001;87:3D–13D.
6. Hiatt WR. Medical treatment of peripheral arterial disease and claudication. *N Engl J Med* 2001;344:1608–1621.
7. Regensteiner JG, Hiatt WR. Current medical therapies for patients with peripheral arterial disease: a critical review. *Am J Med* 2002;112:49–57.
8. Santilli JD, Rodnick JE, Santilli SM. Claudication: diagnosis and treatment. *Am Fam Physician* 1996;53:1245–1253.
9. Creager MA. Clinical assessment of the patient with claudication: the role of the vascular laboratory. *Vasc Med* 1997;2:231–237.

6

A 66-YEAR-OLD MAN WITH CHEST PAIN AND COCAINE ABUSE

BENJAMIN J. FREDA
AMJAD ALMAHAMEED
RITESH GUPTA
W. FRANK PEACOCK IV

CASE PRESENTATION

A 66-year-old man presented to the emergency department (ED) with several hours of chest pain and dyspnea, which developed several hours after smoking cocaine. The patient described the chest pain as substernal, and it did not radiate. His past medical history included hepatitis B and C, hypertension, and chronic renal insufficiency with a baseline serum creatinine of 5.8 mg/dL. He had a known history of cocaine, tobacco, and alcohol abuse, as well as a remote history of intravenous heroin use. He denied fevers, chills, cough, or any use of intravenous drugs over the last 10 years.

On examination, the patient was afebrile and mildly dyspneic. His blood pressure was 240/140 mm Hg; heart rate, 87 beats per minute; respiratory rate, 20 per minute; and pulse oximetry 96% on 2 L of oxygen. A 6-day-old clonidine patch was present on his arm. Lung examination revealed scattered bibasilar crackles. Cardiac examination revealed third and fourth heart sounds and a grade I/VI early systolic murmur at the left sternal border. There was no jugular venous distension. His peripheral pulses were equal, and his abdominal and neurologic examinations were normal.

QUESTIONS/DISCUSSION

His 12-lead electrocardiogram (ECG) is shown in Fig. 6.1A along with a previous tracing (Fig. 6.1B). All the following electrocardiographic diagnoses apply to his current ECG except:

A. Left ventricular hypertrophy
B. Normal sinus rhythm
C. Left bundle branch block
D. Pseudonormalization of T waves

The ECG recorded while the patient was experiencing chest pain shows normal sinus rhythm. Voltage criteria for left ventricular hypertrophy are fulfilled. A left bundle branch block is not present, as the QRS interval is less than 0.12 second. The ECG performed 1 month earlier (Fig. 6.1B) shows inverted T waves throughout the precordial leads. The current ECG shows "pseudonormalization" of previously inverted T waves. In patients with baseline T-wave inversion, T waves may return to an upright position during myocardial ischemia. This may occur in the setting of spontaneous or provoked (e.g., stress test-induced) ischemia (1).

Cocaine acts as a potent sympathomimetic agent by blocking presynaptic reuptake of biogenic amines (norepinephrine) in the peripheral and central nervous system (2). Cocaine is a commonly used drug of abuse. A 1998 national survey estimated that nearly 11% of the population had used cocaine at least once (3). Patients present to emergency departments with a variety of complaints attributed to cocaine intoxication. The most common complaints include chest pain, syncope, dyspnea, palpitations, and dizziness. As many of the complaints are related to the cardiovascular system, the main clinical concern is often acute myocardial ischemia. Other potential cardiovascular complications associated with cocaine include myocardial infarction, arrhythmia, cardiomyopathy, myocarditis, and aortic dissection. Neurologic complications include intracerebral hemorrhage and cerebral infarction. The pathophysiologic effects of cocaine on the cardiovascular system are numerous, as shown in Table 6.1. Identification of cocaine use in patients with cardiovascular complaints is important, as the diagnosis and treatment of patients with cocaine-associated myocardial ischemia are unique.

Chest pain is the most common complaint of patients presenting to the ED after cocaine use. In one study at an urban hospital, the urine of 14% to 25% of patients presenting with nontraumatic chest pain was positive for cocaine (4). However, only 6% of patients with cocaine-associated chest pain will have cardiac marker elevations consistent with myocardial infarction (5). There are no clin-

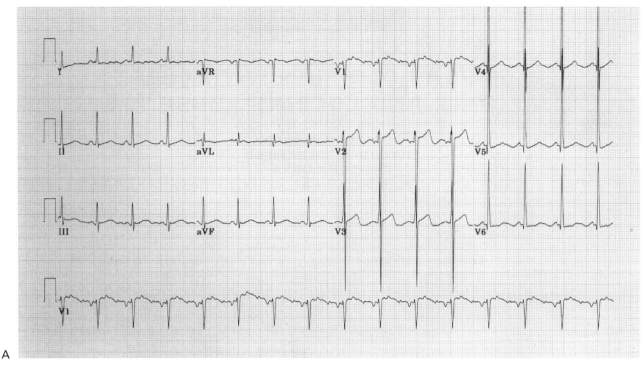

A

FIGURE 6.1. Electrocardiogram (ECG) on admission **(A)** and from one month prior **(B)**.

ical predictors capable of identifying ischemic chest pain in this setting. Furthermore, roughly half of patients with cocaine-induced myocardial infarction have coronary angiograms without evidence of atherosclerotic disease (6). There is a high prevalence of false-negative and false-positive ECG changes in patients with cocaine-associated chest pain (5,7). Cocaine can produce ECG changes mimicking ischemia with ST-segment and J-point elevation due to early repolarization.

Troponin T or troponin I is the biomarker of choice to identify myocardial necrosis. Cocaine use can lead to elevations of serum creatine kinase (CK) and the MB fraction of creatine kinase (CK-MB) in the absence of myocardial infarction, presumably due to skeletal muscle damage (8,9).

Most patients with cocaine-associated chest pain do well, with a low incidence of cardiovascular complications. When complications occur, such as a malignant arrhythmia, they almost always occur within the first 12 hours of presentation (10).

Initial management of this patient should include all the following diagnostic and/or therapeutic strategies except:

A. Chest radiograph
B. Aspirin
C. Oral nonselective β-blocker, such as propranolol
D. Parenteral antihypertensive medication
E. Benzodiazepines

TABLE 6.1. CARDIOVASCULAR EFFECTS OF COCAINE

Immediate	Intermediate	Delayed
↑Myocardial oxygen demand	Thrombosis due to *de novo* endothelial injury	Hypertension
↑Heart rate, afterload		Myocarditis
↓Coronary flow	Thrombosis on preexisting plaque	Cardiomegaly
↓Coronary diameter (especially in diseased arteries)	Platelet aggregation	Left ventricular hypertrophy
	↑Plasminogen-activator inhibitor	Accelerated atherosclerosis
Arrhythmias		
Coronary dissection		

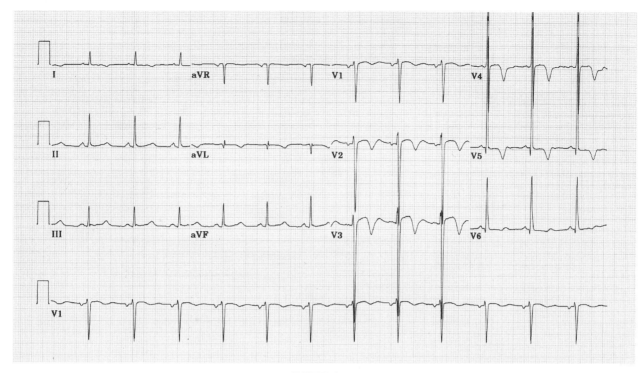

B

FIGURE 6.1B.

Chest radiograph: A chest radiography (CXR) is a useful tool to look for nonischemic causes of chest pain. Table 6.2 lists the differential diagnosis of cocaine-associated chest pain. Excessive Valsalva-type maneuvers can sometimes lead to pneumothorax or pneumomediastinum in cocaine smokers (11). Although CXR is an insensitive tool to screen for aortic dissection, the clinician should carefully inspect the mediastinal silhouette for widening or asymmetry. Careful inspection for pulmonary hemorrhage, infiltrates, and abnormal vascular distribution may help the clinician to focus on a particular diagnosis. In this patient, the chest x-ray showed mild pulmonary venous congestion, an enlarged cardiac silhouette, and an unremarkable mediastinum.

Aspirin: This patient had chest pain, hypertensive emergency, and ECG changes suggestive of ischemia. The most likely diagnosis at this point is an acute coronary syndrome

(ACS). Aspirin (ASA) is a first-line agent for the treatment of ACS. This is also true for cocaine-associated myocardial ischemia (12). In humans, cocaine is a potent stimulator of platelet activation and aggregation; therefore, ASA needs to be considered in this setting. However, cocaine use has also been associated with the development of subarachnoid hemorrhage (SAH), which, before the administration of ASA, must be ruled out if clinically suspected (13).

Oral nonselective β-blockers: This clinical scenario clearly meets the definition of a hypertensive emergency, in which case a slow-acting oral medication is not indicated. Additionally, nonselective β-blockers may augment the myocardial toxicity of cocaine. In one study, intracoronary administration of propranolol was shown to increase coronary vascular resistance and decrease coronary sinus blood flow when given to volunteers after administration of intranasal cocaine (14). Cocaine use results in high catecholamine levels that stimulate α-receptors and enhance coronary vasoconstriction. Blockade of β-receptors could theoretically produce unopposed α-receptor stimulation in the setting of cocaine intoxication. These theoretical concerns have not been tested in clinical trials. However, some small animal studies suggest that these concerns may be warranted (14).

Parenteral antihypertensives: Intravenous medications are preferred in the management of hypertensive emergencies, as they have a faster onset of action and can be easily titrated. Rapid diminishment of the blood pressure is required to prevent permanent end-organ damage, but care

TABLE 6.2. DIFFERENTIAL DIAGNOSIS OF COCAINE-ASSOCIATED CHEST PAIN

Myocardial ischemia/infarction
Pneumothorax
Pulmonary hemorrhage
Aortic dissection
Endocarditis (intravenous drug abuse)
Musculoskeletal
Asthma exacerbation
Pulmonary embolism

must be taken not to induce too great a drop in pressure over a short period of time, because this may put the patient at risk for cerebral ischemia.

Benzodiazepines: Experts recommend benzodiazepines as first-line agents in the treatment of cocaine-associated myocardial ischemia (2,12). Cocaine toxicity is associated with psychomotor agitation, hypertension, tachycardia, and hyperthermia. Sedation is required in most cases, especially when concerns of limiting myocardial oxygen demand exist. Animal studies have shown that benzodiazepines are beneficial in cocaine toxicity (15,16). In humans, benzodiazepines can decrease myocardial oxygen demand by lowering heart rate and blood pressure (17).

Case Continued. In the ED, the patient was given ASA 325 mg, intravenous furosemide 80 mg, morphine 4 mg intravenously, and two doses of sublingual nitroglycerin. His blood pressure remained elevated, with the systolic pressure between 200 and 240 mm Hg and the diastolic pressure between 100 and 130 mm Hg. His heart rate was between 60 and 70 beats per minute. His respirations were less labored, and he remained stable on 2 L of oxygen. His chest pain resolved. There was no evidence of arrhythmia on telemetry.

Initial laboratory studies revealed a white blood cell count of 11 K/μL, hemoglobin of 12.6 g/dL, platelets of 128 K/μL, blood urea nitrogen of 78 mg/dL, and creatinine of 6.1 mg/dL. Amylase, lipase, calcium, alkaline phosphatase, and bilirubin were normal. Urinalysis showed 11 to 25 white blood cells, six to ten red blood cells, 2+ hemoglobin, and no casts. Urine toxicology was negative for alcohol and positive for cocaine. CK-MB was 6.6 ng/mL, and troponin T was 0.17 ng/mL. One month earlier, during a similar hospitalization, troponin T had been 0.05 ng/mL. The patient's serum creatinine was 5.9 mg/dL at that time. He was asymptomatic but remained hypertensive and was transferred to a monitored cardiology bed.

On arrival to the medical floor, he denied chest pain but noted some mild nausea. His vital signs included a blood pressure of 228/115 mm Hg, heart rate of 60 beats per minute, and respiratory rate of 19 breaths per minute. He appeared comfortable and in no acute distress. He urinated about 500 mL following the administration of furosemide in the ED.

Which of the following therapies would be contraindicated in this patient?

A. **Intravenous nitroglycerin**
B. **Intravenous phentolamine**
C. **Intravenous calcium-channel blockers**
D. **Intravenous labetalol**
E. **Intravenous thrombolytic therapy**

Nitroglycerin: Minimal data are available from randomized clinical trials to suggest evidence-based approaches to the management of cocaine-associated myocardial ischemia or hypertensive emergency. In cases of myocardial ischemia or infarction not associated with cocaine, the beneficial effects of intravenous nitroglycerin are well known. Nitroglycerin is effective after cocaine ingestion, by reversing cocaine-induced coronary vasoconstriction, decreasing chest pain, and reducing the development of heart failure (18,19). Nitroglycerin can produce favorable hemodynamic effects by lowering afterload and preload, while protecting coronary circulation.

Phentolamine: Phentolamine is a reversible α-adrenergic antagonist, used most commonly in the short-term management of pheochromocytoma-induced hypertension. Phentolamine has a rapid onset and short duration of action. It has been recommended as a second-line agent for cocaine-induced myocardial ischemia, if signs or symptoms persist despite use of nitrates, benzodiazepines, and ASA (2,12). Phentolamine offers the theoretical advantage of reversing cocaine-induced coronary vasoconstriction by its blockade of α-receptors (20). Although there is a paucity of data on the clinical benefit of phentolamine in this setting, some small reports suggest its efficacy (20,21). Low doses should be used to avoid hypotension. An intravenous dose of 1 to 5 mg is a reasonable starting dose. The duration of action is short, and multiple doses may be necessary.

Calcium-channel blockers: Calcium-channel blockers (CCBs) do not have a proven benefit in the setting of myocardial ischemia in the absence of cocaine ingestion. The results of small animal studies do not provide a clear consensus regarding the safety and efficacy of CCBs in the treatment of cocaine-associated myocardial ischemia (22). However, one small study of human volunteers showed that intravenous *verapamil* relieved cocaine-induced coronary vasospasm (23). These agents should probably be avoided in clinical settings such as volume overload and bradycardia, in which negative inotropic action could be harmful.

Labetalol: In the setting of cocaine-associated myocardial ischemia, the use of labetalol is controversial (2). Although labetalol produces both nonselective β-blockade and α-blockade, most of its effect is a result of β-receptor antagonism (24). In one study, labetalol lowered mean arterial pressure but failed to reverse cocaine-induced coronary vasoconstriction in humans undergoing cardiac catheterization (25). As discussed previously, cocaine causes catecholamine-mediated α- and β-receptor activation. Nonselective β-blockers are thought to result in unopposed α-activity, which can worsen hypertension. Although the α-blocking effect of labetalol may counteract some of the vasoconstrictions produced by cocaine, there are no good data to support this. Labetalol is not necessarily contraindicated, but its use as a first-line agent is controversial.

Thrombolytics: The presence of contiguous ST-segment elevation or new left bundle branch block are the classic criteria for urgent revascularization in patients with an acute chest pain syndrome. Many patients with cocaine-associated chest pain meet these criteria even though a small minority has elevated cardiac enzymes. Prior ECGs should be reviewed carefully to ensure that any ST-segment elevation seen is not "old" and possibly an effect of early repolarization. Patients with cocaine intoxication and elevated blood pressure are also at risk for aortic dissection and intracerebral hemorrhage, two conditions with potentially fatal outcomes if intravenous thrombolytics are administered. Additionally, many patients with cocaine-induced myocardial infarction do not have significant coronary atherosclerosis by angiography. Therefore it is recommended that patients with cocaine intoxication and ECG findings suggestive of acute myocardial infarction have urgent coronary angiography with catheter-based revascularization rather than peripherally administered thrombolytics (12). Since this patient did not have ST-elevation or a new left bundle branch block, he would not have been a candidate for intravenous thrombolysis, even in the absence of cocaine use. Furthermore, his elevated blood pressure is a contraindication to the use of intravenous thrombolytics.

Case Concluded

Shortly after arrival on the medical floor, the patient developed recurrent substernal chest pain with a blood pressure of 220/100 mm Hg and a heart rate of 55 beats per minute. He was given a total of 20 mg of phentolamine intravenously over four divided doses. His blood pressure decreased to 165/78 mm Hg; his heart rate remained in the range of 50 to 60 beats per minute. His chest pain resolved. A repeat ECG showed T-wave inversions similar to his ECG from 1 month earlier. He remained free of chest pain, but his blood pressure increased 1 hour later, and he required an intravenous nitroglycerin drip to keep his systolic blood pressure around 150 to 160 mm Hg. Since the patient was not tachycardic and showed no evidence of hyperthermia or anxiety, benzodiazepines were not given. Subsequent troponin T levels did not change. Total CK and CK-MB remained within normal limits. An echocardiogram revealed moderate left ventricular hypertrophy, diastolic dysfunction, and a normal ejection fraction. A dipyridamole (Persantine)-nuclear stress test was negative for ischemia. He was discharged on ASA, isosorbide mononitrate 30 mg daily, clonidine patch, labetalol 200 mg twice a day, and amlodipine 10 mg daily. The patient refused to participate in a detoxification program, and plans for cardiac catheterization were deferred secondary to his tenuous renal status.

CONCLUSION

Cocaine-associated myocardial ischemia and hypertensive emergency require special attention regarding diagnosis and treatment. In this setting, there are no clinical predictors that accurately differentiate ischemic and nonischemic

chest pain. Patients should be monitored while troponin T or I is followed to rule out myocardial infarction. The incidence of myocardial infarction is low, and most patients with cocaine-associated chest pain have a benign course, especially after the first 12 hours of presentation. The goals of medical therapy include decreasing thrombogenesis with ASA, limiting possible myocardial ischemia with oxygen and benzodiazepines, and reversing hypertension and coronary vasoconstriction with nitrates, phentolamine, and calcium channel blockers. In the acute setting, monotherapy with β-blockers alone is not recommended, and the use of combination α/β-blocking agents is controversial. In the setting of acute ST-elevation or new left bundle branch block, thrombolytics can be dangerous and treatment should be guided by coronary angiography.

REFERENCES

1. Noble RJ, Rothbaum DA, Knoebel SB, et al. Normalization of abnormal T waves in ischemia. *Arch Intern Med* 1976;136:391–395.
2. Lange RA, Hillis LD. Cardiovascular complications of cocaine use. *N Engl J Med* 2001;345:351–358.
3. National Household Survey on Drug Abuse: Main Findings. Department of Health and Human Services, Substance Abuse and Mental Health Services Administration, Rockville, MD 2000.
4. Hollander JE, Todd KH, Green G, et al. Chest pain associated with cocaine: an assessment of prevalence in suburban and urban emergency departments. *Ann Emerg Med* 1995;26:671–676.
5. Hollander JE, Hoffman RS, Gennis P, et al. Prospective multicenter evaluation of cocaine-associated chest pain. *Acad Emerg Med* 1994;1:330–339.
6. Minor RL Jr, Scott BD, Brown DD, et al. Cocaine-induced myocardial infarction in patients with normal coronary arteries. *Ann Intern Med* 1991;115:797–806.
7. Gitter MJ, Goldsmith SR, Dunbar DN, et al. Cocaine and chest pain: clinical features and outcomes of patients hospitalized to rule out myocardial infarction. *Ann Intern Med* 1991;115:277–282.
8. Tokarski GF, Paganussi P, Urbanski R, et al. An evaluation of cocaine-induced chest pain. *Ann Emerg Med* 1990;19:1088–1092.
9. McLaurin MD, Henry TD, Apple FS, et al. Cardiac troponin I, T and CK-MB in patients with cocaine related chest pain. *Circulation* 1994;90:I-278 [abstract].
10. Hollander JE, Hoffman RS, Burstein JL, et al. Cocaine-associated myocardial infarction: mortality and complications. *Arch Intern Med* 1995;155:1081–1086.
11. Salzman GA, Khan F, Emory C. Pneumomediastinum after cocaine smoking. *South Med J* 1987;80:1427–1429.
12. Hollander JE. The management of cocaine-associated myocardial ischemia. *N Engl J Med* 1995;333:1267–1272.
13. Fessler RD, Esshaki CM, Stankewitz RC, et al. The neurovascular complications of cocaine. *Surg Neurol* 1997;47:339–345.
14. Lange RA, Cigarroa RG, Flores ED, et al. Potentiation of cocaine-induced coronary vasoconstriction by beta-adrenergic blockade. *Ann Intern Med* 1990;112:897–903.
15. Derlet RW, Albertson TE. Diazepam in the prevention of seizures and death in cocaine-intoxicated rats. *Ann Emerg Med* 1989;18:542–546.
16. Guinn MM, Bedford JA, Wilson MC. Antagonism of intravenous cocaine lethality in nonhuman primates. *Clin Toxicol* 1980;16:499–508.

17. Baumann BM, Perrone J, Hornig SE, et al. Randomized, double-blind, placebo-controlled trial of diazepam, nitroglycerin, or both for treatment of patients with potential cocaine-associated acute coronary syndromes. *Acad Emerg Med* 2000;7:878–885.

18. Brogan WC 3rd, Lange RA, Kim AS, et al. Alleviation of cocaine-induced coronary vasoconstriction by nitroglycerin. *J Am Coll Cardiol* 1991;18:581–586.

19. Hollander JE, Hoffman RS, Gennis P, et al. Nitroglycerin in the treatment of cocaine associated chest pain—clinical safety and efficacy. *J Toxicol Clin Toxicol* 1994;32:243–256.

20. Lange RA, Cigarroa RG, Yancy CW Jr, et al. Cocaine-induced coronary-artery vasoconstriction. *N Engl J Med* 1989;321:1557–1562.

21. Hollander JE, Carter WA, Hoffman RS. Use of phentolamine for cocaine-induced myocardial ischemia. *N Engl J Med* 1992;327:361.

22. Hoffman RS, Hollander JE. Evaluation of patients with chest pain after cocaine use. *Crit Care Clin* 1997;13:809–828.

23. Negus BH, Willard JE, Hillis LD, et al. Alleviation of cocaine-induced coronary vasoconstriction with intravenous verapamil. *Am J Cardiol* 1994;73:510–513.

24. Kaplan NM. Treatment of hypertension: drug therapy. In: *Kaplan's clinical hypertension,* 8th ed. Philadelphia: Lippincott Williams & Wilkins, 2002:237–338.

25. Boehrer JD, Moliterno DJ, Willard JE, et al. Influence of labetalol on cocaine-induced coronary vasoconstriction in humans. *Am J Med* 1993;94:608–610.

7

A YOUNG MAN WITH AORTIC DISSECTION

RITA SHI-MING LEE
MARK E. MAYER

CASE PRESENTATION

A 37-year-old man presented to his primary care physician for routine health maintenance. He was in good health until several months before, when he presented to the emergency department with numbness and a "dead feeling" in his right leg. On physical examination at that time, he was found to have a pulseless right lower extremity. During the evaluation he became hemodynamically unstable, developing hypotension and requiring intubation. Transthoracic echocardiography revealed a type A aortic dissection arising from the noncoronary sinus. He underwent emergent repair of the dissection.

Intraoperative transesophageal echocardiography showed a normal mitral valve and a tricuspid aortic valve with a flap over the noncoronary cusp. There was 1+ aortic regurgitation and a type A dissection involving the ascending aorta, arch, and proximal descending aorta with a complex spiral flap. Intraoperative examination revealed dissection into the right coronary artery without evidence of luminal compromise.

The patient underwent aortic valve replacement with a St. Jude's valve conduit using the Bentall procedure. Pathologic evaluation of the resected aorta revealed cystic medial necrosis. He did well postoperatively and was discharged home with instructions to establish a primary care physician for ongoing medical care.

He had no other past medical or surgical history prior to these events. There was no family history of coronary artery disease or any other medical illnesses.

Upon presentation to his primary care physician, his blood pressure was 121/76 mm Hg and his pulse was 90 beats per minute. In general, he was a tall, thin male with mild retrognathia. His skin appeared loose on his body. He had long, thin fingers and mildly increased flexibility. Examination of the chest revealed pectus excavatum and clear lung sounds. On cardiac examination, there was a mechanical valve click and a harsh systolic murmur at the right upper sternal border. Peripheral pulses were 4+ and symmetric.

QUESTIONS/DISCUSSION

What is the most likely diagnosis?

A. Homocystinuria
B. Ehlers–Danlos, type IV
C. Marfan syndrome
D. Beals syndrome
E. MASS phenotype

Homocystinuria is an autosomal recessive disease caused by a deficiency of cystathionine β-synthase. Physical features include tall, dolichostenomelic habitus (excessively long limbs), scoliosis, ectopia lentis, mental retardation, and anterior chest deformity. Although they physically resemble the patient described earlier, patients with homocystinuria do not classically have aortic dilation or dissection. However, vascular complications can occur in the form of thrombosis and tissue infarction (1).

Ehlers–Danlos, type IV is a rare, autosomal dominant connective-tissue disease leading to an increased risk of uterine, gastrointestinal, and arterial rupture. Physical examination reveals thin, translucent skin; easy bruising; thin lips; and a prematurely aged appearance of the hands and feet (2). Although patients with Ehlers–Danlos, type IV are at risk for aortic dissection and rupture, there is less joint hypermobility and skin hyperextensibility than seen in this patient.

Beals syndrome, or congenital contractural arachnodactyly, is an autosomal dominant disorder characterized by a tall, thin appearance; "crumpled" external ears; and contractures of major joints. There has been no definite linkage to aortic root dilatation and dissection (3).

The MASS phenotype describes a set of patients with mitral valve prolapse, myopia, minimal or no aortic dilatation, subtle skeletal changes, and striae atrophicae. Inheritance appears to be autosomal dominant (4).

Marfan syndrome is the correct diagnosis.

MARFAN SYNDROME

Antonine-Bernard Marfan first described this phenotype in 1896 in a 5-year-old girl with disproportionately long, thin limbs and digits; contractures of the fingers and knees; anterior chest deformity; and scoliosis. Aortic involvement in Marfan syndrome was described in 1943.

Marfan syndrome is inherited in an autosomal dominant manner, although 15% to 25% of cases occur via spontaneous mutation. It is estimated to affect one in 10,000 people. Organ systems classically involved include the skeleton, eye, heart, and aorta (4). The diagnostic criteria are presented in Table 7.1. Cardiovascular abnormalities are present in more than 80% of patients with Marfan syndrome. The predominant pathologic finding in aortic involvement is cystic medial necrosis (5).

The differential diagnosis of Marfan syndrome can be broad due to phenotypic variation. For the skeletal manifestations, the differential diagnosis includes homocystinuria, Stickler syndrome, classic Ehlers–Danlos syndrome, Klinefelter syndrome, Beals syndrome, and familial tall stature. Causes of aortic root dilatation and dissection include familial aortic aneurysm/dissection, Ehlers–Danlos type IV, tertiary syphilis, ankylosing spondylitis, relapsing polychondritis, and Reiter syndrome. However, these diseases are not associated with the skeletal and ocular manifestations of Marfan syndrome (4,5).

Before the development of advanced surgical techniques for aortic repair, the estimated life expectancy was 32 ± 16 years. Most deaths were due to cardiovascular causes (6). Advances in surgical repair have resulted in an increase in life expectancy by nearly 10 years, to 41 ± 18 years (7).

Where is the genetic/molecular defect in Marfan syndrome?

A. Fibrillin 1
B. Fibrillin 2
C. Type III collagen
D. Type I collagen

Fibrillin 2 (FBN2) mutations have been linked to Beals syndrome at chromosome 5q23–31. Mutations that cause congenital contractural arachnodactyly tend to cluster in exons that encode the epidermal growth factor (EGF)-like motifs (3).

Type III collagen defects have been associated with Ehlers–Danlos syndrome, type IV. Decreased secretion or unstable type III collagen has been implicated as the etiology for the tissue fragility seen in these patients (2).

Mutations in one of two genes (COLIA1 and COLIA2) that encode type I collagen have been involved in the pathogenesis of osteogenesis imperfecta (8). Type I collagen defects have also been found in Ehlers–Danlos, types VII and VIII (2).

Mutations in the fibrillin 1 (FBN1) gene have been associated with Marfan syndrome, but also have been found in individuals with familial aortic aneurysm and familial ectopia lentis. The detection rate of FBN1 mutations in patients with Marfan syndrome is 66% (9). Marked heterogeneity of mutations exists, without any correlation between the type of mutation and phenotypic presentation. However, no FBN1 defect was found in 35% of cases, which is due to either a failure to detect the mutation or to the presence of another locus causing the Marfan phenotype. Because of low sensitivity, genetic analysis is currently not recommended as a tool for diagnosing Marfan syndrome. However, it can help identify susceptible individuals within family cohorts in which the mutation has been identified.

Routine management of patients with Marfan syndrome includes all of the following except:

A. Chronic β-blocker therapy
B. Advise vigorous exercise
C. Routine transthoracic echocardiography
D. Endocarditis prophylaxis

Because of the increased risk of aortic rupture or dissection, routine vigorous exercise and high-impact sports are not advised for patients with Marfan syndrome. Regular low-impact exercise in the form of walking or swimming is safe. Generally, the maximum heart rate achieved should be 100 beats per minute (10).

Chronic β-blocker therapy has been shown to slow the rate of increase in aortic root size and to reduce the risk for aortic dissection (11). Therefore β-blocker therapy is recommended as a prophylactic agent once the diagnosis of Marfan syndrome is made. While there are no data on patients who have undergone operative repair of aortic aneurysms and dissections, the consensus is to place these patients on chronic β-blocker therapy as well. This helps prevent postgraft dilatation and extension of any dissection in the remaining aorta.

All patients with Marfan syndrome should have routine transthoracic echocardiography to monitor aortic root dimensions and valvular abnormalities. Current recommendations include annual monitoring for those with aortic root diameters less than 40 mm and additional evaluation every 6 months once the aortic root diameter is greater than 40 mm. If transthoracic echocardiography is not technically feasible due to pectus deformities, then transesophageal echocardiography or magnetic resonance imaging is recommended. Patients should be evaluated for elective surgical repair once the aortic root reaches 50 to 55 mm in diameter (10). If a family history of dissection at a smaller aortic root diameter exists, then surgical repair should be performed earlier (12). In addition, routine monitoring with computed tomography or magnetic res-

TABLE 7.1. DIAGNOSTIC CRITERIA FOR MARFAN SYNDROME

Skeletal System

Major criteria:
Presence of at least four of the following manifestations:
Pectus carinatum or pectus excavatum requiring surgery
Reduced upper- to lower-body segment ratio or arm-span-to-height ratio >1.05
Positive wrist and thumb signs
Scoliosis of >20° or spondylolithesis
Reduced extension of elbows (<170°)
Medial displacement of the medial malleolus causing pes planus
Protrusio acetabulae

Minor criteria:
Pectus excavatum of moderate severity
Joint hypermobility
Highly arched palate with dental crowding
Facial appearance (malar hypoplasia, retrognathia, down-slanting palpebral fissures)
Osteoporosis

Cardiovascular System

Major criteria:
Presence of at least one of the following:
Dilatation of the ascending aorta with or without aortic regurgitation and involving at least the sinuses of Valsalva
Dissection of the ascending aorta

Minor criteria:
Mitral valve prolapse
Dilatation of main pulmonary artery, in absence of valvular or peripheral pulmonic stenosis or any other obvious cause, age <40 years
Calcification of the mitral annulus, age <40 years
Dilatation or dissection of the descending thoracic or abdominal aorta, age <50 years

Ocular System

Major criteria:
Ectopia lentis

Minor criteria:
Abnormally flat cornea (measured by keratometry)
Increased axial globe length
Hypoplastic iris or hypoplastic ciliary muscle

Pulmonary System

Major criteria:
None

Minor criteria:
Spontaneous pneumothorax
Apical blebs

Skin and Integument

Major criteria:
Lumbosacral dural ectasia by CT or MRI

Minor criteria:
Striae atrophicae not associated with marked weight changes, pregnancy, or repetitive stress
Recurrent or incisional herniae

Family History

Major criteria:
History of a parent, child, or sibling who meets the diagnostic criteria independently
Presence of a mutation in FBN1 known to cause the Marfan syndrome
Presence of a haplotype around FBN1, inherited by descent, known to be associated with unequivocally diagnosed Marfan syndrome in the family

Minor criteria:
None

Note: For the index case, the patient must have major criteria in at least two different organ systems and involvement of a third organ system. For a family member, there must be a presence of a major criterion in the family history and one major criterion in an organ system and involvement of a second organ system.
CT, computed tomogram; FBN1, mutations in fibrillin 1; MRI, magnetic resonance imaging.
Adapted from Pyeritz RE. The Marfan syndrome. *Annu Rev Med* 2000;51:481–510.

onance imaging has been recommended to evaluate the remainder of the aorta.

Patients with Marfan syndrome are at high risk for endocarditis both before and after cardiac surgery, given their valvular abnormalities. Broad-spectrum intravenous antibiotics are recommended for dental and surgical procedures (10).

CONCLUSION

The patient had β-blocker therapy titrated to achieve a goal resting heart rate of 60 beats per minute. He started a walking program and returned to work on a part-time basis. Routine follow-up transthoracic echocardiogram and CT scan have revealed excellent valve function and a persistent but stable aortic dissection in the remaining native aorta.

REFERENCES

1. Longo N. Inherited disorders of amino acid metabolism and storage. In: Braunwald E, Fauci AS, Kasper DL, et al., ed. *Harrison's principles of internal medicine,* 15th ed. New York: McGraw-Hill, 2001:2301–2309.
2. Yeowell HN, Pinnell SR. The Ehlers-Danlos syndromes. *Semin Dermatol* 1993;12:229–240.
3. Viljoen D. Congenital contractural arachnodactyly (Beals syndrome). *J Med Genet* 1994;31:640–643.
4. Pyeritz RE. The Marfan syndrome. *Annu Rev Med* 2000;51: 481–510.
5. Tsipouras P, Silverman DI. The genetic basis of aortic disease. Marfan syndrome and beyond. *Cardiol Clin* 1999;17:683–696.
6. Murdoch JL, Walker BA, Halpern BL, et al. Life expectancy and causes of death in the Marfan syndrome. *N Engl J Med* 1972; 286:804–808.
7. Silverman DI, Burton KJ, Gray J, et al. Life expectancy in the Marfan syndrome. *Am J Cardiol* 1995;75:157–160.
8. Grahame R. Heritable disorders of connective tissue. *Baillieres Best Pract Res Clin Rheumatol* 2000;14:345–361.
9. Loeys B, Nuytinck L, Delvaux I, et al. Genotype and phenotype analysis of 171 patients referred for molecular study of the fibrillin-1 gene FBN1 because of suspected Marfan syndrome. *Arch Intern Med* 2001;161:2447–2454.
10. Nienaber CA, Von Kodolitsch Y. Therapeutic management of patients with Marfan syndrome: focus on cardiovascular involvement. *Cardiol Rev* 1999;7:332–341.
11. Shores J, Berger KR, Murphy EA, et al. Progression of aortic dilatation and the benefit of long-term beta-adrenergic blockade in Marfan's syndrome. *N Engl J Med* 1994;330:1335–1341.
12. Child AH. Marfan syndrome-current medical and genetic knowledge: how to treat and when. *J Card Surg* 1997;12(2 Suppl):131–136.

8

A 55-YEAR-OLD MAN WITH CHEST PAIN FOLLOWING VALVE REPAIR SURGERY

KHALDOUN G. TARAKJI
CURTIS M. RIMMERMAN

CASE PRESENTATION

A 55-year-old man underwent mitral valve repair for mitral regurgitation secondary to myxomatous valve disease. There were no perioperative complications. One month later, he presented to the emergency department complaining of chest pain. The pain started suddenly when he woke up, was substernal without radiation, was worse with deep inspiration, and was relieved upon sitting up and leaning forward. On presentation, he was afebrile (temperature 37.1°C), had a blood pressure of 115/85 mm Hg, and had a heart rate of 85 beats per minute without orthostatic changes. Oxygen saturation on room air was 100% by pulse oximetry. His physical examination was normal except for a grade II/VI holosystolic murmur heard best at the left sternal border. Chest x-ray showed clear lungs. A 12-lead electrocardiogram (ECG) was done (Fig. 8.1).

QUESTIONS/DISCUSSION

The ECG most likely suggests:

A. Pulmonary embolism
B. Pneumonia
C. Acute pericarditis
D. Acute myocardial infarction

Pulmonary embolism is the most common cause of an acute rise in pulmonary artery and right-sided heart pressures. Sinus tachycardia is commonly seen with pulmonary embolism. Other ECG changes that may be seen with an acute pulmonary embolism are:

- *Lead III:* Increase in Q-wave amplitude with slight ST-segment elevation and T-wave inversion. In contrast with inferior infarction, there are minimal changes in leads II and aVF.

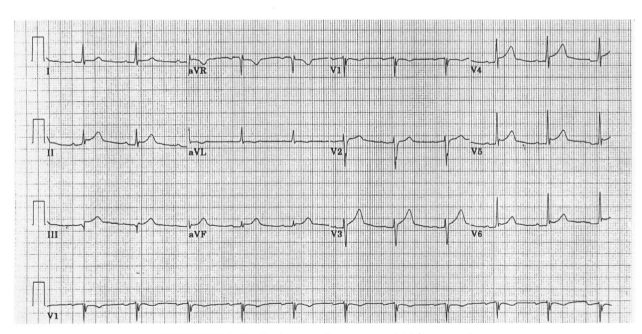

FIGURE 8.1. Patient's electrocardiogram upon initial presentation.

TABLE 8.1. ELECTROCARDIOGRAM IN ACUTE PERICARDITIS VS. ACUTE ISCHEMIA

	Acute Pericarditis	Acute Ischemia
J-ST	Diffuse concave elevation, without reciprocal depression	Localized deviation, usually convex, with reciprocal changes
PR segment depression	Yes	No
Abnormal Q waves	None unless with infarction	Common with infarction
T waves	Inverted after J points return to baseline	Inverted while ST segment still elevated
Arrhythmia	Often find atrial arrhythmias, premature beats	Frequent
Conduction abnormalities	None	Frequent

From Spodick DH. Acute, clincally noneffusive ("dry") pericarditis. In: Spodick DH, ed. *The pericardium: a comprehensive textbook.* New York: Marcel Dekker, 1997:108, with permission.

- *Lead I:* Increase in S-wave amplitude.
- *Precordial leads (V1–V3):* Right ventricular conduction delay and T-wave inversion reflecting slowed conduction and right ventricular strain.
- *QRS complex:* Right axis deviation.

Pneumonia has no specific ECG changes. Findings may include sinus tachycardia, atrial dysrhythmias, and nonspecific ST-T changes.

Typically, the ECG changes in acute pericarditis evolve through four stages, regardless of the etiology. These changes occur in most patients, although their absence does not exclude acute pericarditis (1).

- *Stage I:* This stage is the most important in the diagnosis of pericarditis. It represents epicardial injury (ST elevation) that develops when pericardial inflammation is contiguous to the epicardial surface. Stage I ECG changes are most useful in confirming the diagnosis of acute pericarditis when they involve all leads. PR segments are frequently depressed except in leads aVR and V1, in which depressed J points and elevated PR segments are seen. T waves in stage I generally remain normal (2,3). Clinically, it is important to differentiate acute pericarditis, acute myocardial injury, and early repolarization (3a) (Table 8.1).
- *Stage II:* ST segments return to baseline with progressive T-wave flattening and subsequent T-wave inversion.
- *Stage III:* Generalized T-wave inversion is present in most or all leads.
- *Stage IV:* T waves become upright, and the ECG returns to its baseline.

The ECG in this patient is most consistent with acute pericarditis.

Postcardiac Injury Syndrome

Pericarditis following myocardial infarction is referred to as postmyocardial infarction syndrome (PMIS), whereas peri-carditis following cardiac surgery or trauma is referred to as postpericardiotomy syndrome (PCS) (4). The term *postcardiac injury syndrome* (PCIS) is used to encompass both of these entities. Soloff (5) first described this syndrome in 1953 in patients undergoing mitral valve commissurotomy. He referred to it as the postcommissurotomy syndrome and attributed the etiology to the reactivation of rheumatic fever. In 1958, Itoh (6) noted the same syndrome following various types of cardiac surgery and labeled the condition *postpericardiotomy syndrome.* Dressler (7) first described pericarditis following a myocardial infarction in 1956, when he described similar findings among 44 patients who had suffered a recent myocardial infarction.

The prevalence of postpericardiotomy syndrome is estimated to be between 10% and 40% (4,8,9). The prevalence of postmyocardial infarction syndrome is estimated to be less than 5% (7,10,11). It is substantially reduced when thrombolytic therapy is administered to manage an acute myocardial infarction (12). The term *postpericardiotomy syndrome* was substituted for *postcardiotomy syndrome* since it was observed after pericardiotomy without cardiac muscle surgery (4). The syndrome has also been reported after pulmonary embolism (13,14). It may also occur after minor cardiac insults, such as cardiac catheterization, implantation of epicardial and transvenous pacemakers (13–16), and chest traumas (17,18).

Pathogenesis

Although the exact etiology of the postcardiac injury syndrome remains uncertain, an autoimmune explanation appears to be the most plausible. The initial cardiac insult is thought to release cardiac antigens and stimulate an immune response (4). The generated immune complexes deposit onto the lung parenchyma, pericardial, and pleural surfaces, eliciting an inflammatory response (4). This hypothesis is supported by multiple observations and studies. The latent period from cardiac injury to the clinical onset of PCIS and the resolution of the syndrome spontaneously or following therapy with nonsteroidal antiinflammatory drugs (NSAIDs) or corticosteroids both support an immunopathogenic etiology (19–21).

Clinical Features and Diagnosis

The presentation and clinical course of PCIS are independent of the etiology. The most frequent complaint is chest pain occurring a few days to several weeks after the cardiac insult (4,6,9). The syndrome manifests as fever, leukocytosis, high erythrocyte sedimentation rate, pericardial and sometimes pleural effusion, with or without an associated pulmonary infiltrate. Infection and other causes of postoperative fever should be ruled out.

The physical examination may disclose a pericardial friction rub. Rubs are common after cardiac surgery, but their continued presence coupled with other features consistent with pericarditis should alert the clinician to consider PCIS. The chest x-ray may show an enlarged cardiac silhouette in a patient with a pericardial effusion, which should be confirmed or excluded by echocardiography. The chest x-ray may also reveal a pleural effusion, which is usually unilateral.

Which one of the following statements regarding the management of postcardiac injury syndrome is/are true?

A. **Aspirin (ASA) or NSAIDs are usually sufficient to treat postpericardiotomy pericarditis.**

B. **Corticosteroids should be used only in refractory cases.**

C. **ASA is usually the first-line agent in postmyocardial infarction pericarditis.**

D. **NSAIDs and corticosteroids should be avoided early after an acute myocardial infarction.**

E. **All the above are true.**

Patients with postpericardiotomy syndrome are treated conservatively with ASA or NSAIDs, such as indomethacin or ibuprofen. Corticosteroids should be reserved for patients who do not respond to standard nonsteroidal agents. ASA is usually the first choice in patients with the postmyocardial infarction syndrome. NSAIDs and corticosteroids should be avoided early in the course after an acute MI. NSAIDs may cause coronary vasoconstriction and may affect the healing process following infarction (22,23). Some studies have linked the use of corticosteroids after acute MI with the development of ventricular aneurysms and myocardial rupture (24,25).

Case Continued. The patient was started on ibuprofen and his chest pain resolved over the following few days. One week later, he presented to the emergency department complaining of palpitations. Upon presentation, his heart rate was 105 beats per minute, and his blood pressure was 110/73 mm Hg. A 12-lead electrocardiogram was performed (Fig. 8.2).

Which rhythm is demonstrated in the ECG?

A. **Sinus tachycardia**
B. **Atrial flutter**
C. **Atrial fibrillation**
D. **Atrial tachycardia with 2:1 AV block**

At first glance, the ECG may be interpreted as sinus tachycardia with a heart rate of approximately 100 beats per minute. With careful inspection, two P waves are identified

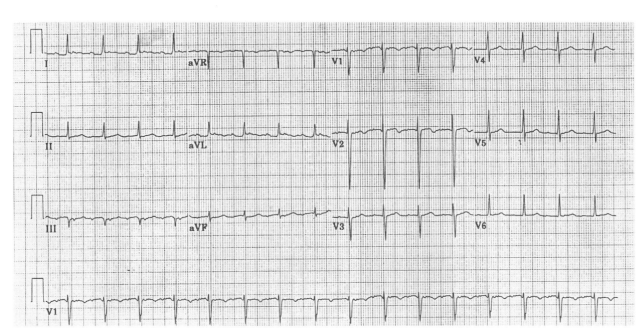

FIGURE 8.2. Patient's electrocardiogram upon his return to the emergency department.

for each QRS complex. The ECG represents atrial tachycardia with 2:1 A-V conduction. A higher rate of A-V conduction ratio, perhaps 1:1, likely explains the symptomatic palpitations.

The following morning, the patient complained of mild dyspnea. He remained afebrile but his blood pressure dropped to 85/55 mm Hg with a heart rate of 90 beats per minute. His lungs were clear, and cardiac auscultation revealed muffled heart sounds. A chest x-ray showed an enlarged cardiac silhouette with clear lung fields. An emergent echocardiogram was performed and revealed a large posterolateral pericardial effusion with mild right atrial diastolic collapse.

All of the following are true regarding cardiac tamponade except:

A. **Tamponade is a clinical diagnosis supported by echocardiographic findings.**
B. **Tamponade affects the right side of the heart before the left side.**
C. **The finding of a small pericardial effusion rules out tamponade.**
D. **Drainage is the ultimate treatment in acute tamponade.**

The prevalence of cardiac tamponade in PCIS is estimated to range from 0.1% to 6% (4). Cardiac tamponade develops when an increased volume of pericardial fluid causes an increase in the intrapericardial pressure, impairing diastolic heart filling. Tamponade occurs when pericardial contents increase at a rate exceeding the rate of stretch of the parietal pericardium.

Tamponade represents a physiologic continuum ranging from mild cases, which can be managed conservatively, to serious, life-threatening cases, which require immediate intervention. The interaction between the rate of fluid accumulation and parietal pericardial stretch determines the shape of the pericardial pressure–volume curve. With a rapid accumulation of fluid, the limit of stretch is quickly reached, and even a small increase in pericardial fluid will shift the hemodynamics to the steep portion of the pressure–volume curves. Beyond a critical volume, small fluid increases provoke large pressure increments. With slow fluid accumulation, the initial portion of the pressure–volume curve remains flat, and relatively large fluid volume increases cause relatively little pressure rise.

The rising intrapericardial pressure first affects the right side of the heart, causing an equilibration of right atrial and ventricular diastolic pressures. Compensatory mechanisms maintain cardiac filling by a rise in the systemic and pulmonary venous pressures (26,27). The rate of the venous expansion plays a key compensatory role. Since it requires time, this mechanism is ineffective in rapidly developing tamponade. As the compensatory mechanisms are overcome, cardiac filling decreases, and

pericardial pressure equilibrates with left ventricular diastolic pressure. Cardiac output decreases significantly and the characteristic hemodynamics of tamponade develop (26,27), with equilibration of the diastolic pressures in both ventricles, the pulmonary artery, and the mean right and left atrial pressures.

Clinical Findings

Tamponade is almost always associated with tachycardia. Heart sounds may be distant, and a pericardial rub may or may not be heard. With significant tamponade, hypotension may develop. However, hypotension may be initially absent due to the compensatory adrenergic response. Fever related to the underlying etiology may be present; this may be misdiagnosed as septic shock. If the patient is not hypovolemic, the jugular venous pressure is elevated. Pulsus paradoxus is defined as an exaggeration of the normal inspiratory fall in arterial flow and systolic pressure (28). To demonstrate pulsus paradoxus, a cuff is inflated to 15 mm Hg above the apparent highest systolic level while the patient breathes normally. The cuff is slowly deflated until Korotkoff sounds are first heard. At this point, the Korotkoff sounds are expiratory because of the lower systolic pressure during inspiration. Deflation is continued until beats are heard throughout the respiratory cycle. The difference between the pressures when systolic sounds are first heard and when they are continuously heard is the size of the pulsus paradoxus.

There are a number of conditions in which pulsus paradoxus may be absent despite cardiac tamponade. Examples include patients with rapid heart rates, an irregular rhythm, left ventricular diastolic pressures and stiffness in excess of right ventricular pressures, extreme hypotension in shock, severe aortic regurgitation, atrial septal defect, and some cases of acute left ventricular infarction. There are also non-pericardial causes for pulsus paradoxus. These include chronic obstructive lung disease and acute asthma, right ventricular infarction, tension pneumothorax, hemorrhagic shock, restrictive cardiomyopathy, and cardiac compression by a mass lesion.

Electrocardiogram

The ECG may be normal or may show sinus tachycardia. Low voltage is due to the interposed pericardial effusion. Electrical alternans also may be seen. This refers to alternating high and low voltages of all ECG waveforms between cardiac cycles within a given lead, resulting from the free swinging of the heart suspended within the pericardial effusion.

Transthoracic Echocardiography

Although tamponade is a clinical diagnosis, echocardiography plays a major role in the identification of a pericardial effusion and in assessing its hemodynamic significance. Signs of cardiac tamponade include diastolic collapse of the right atrium, right ventricle, and left atrium; congestion of the inferior vena cava (IVC), with loss of inspiratory collapse of the IVC; increased respiratory variation of Doppler inflow and outflow velocities; and shift of the interventricular septum to the left upon inspiration.

Diagnosis

Tamponade should be suspected in every patient with hypotension, especially in patients with active pericarditis or predisposing factors for pericarditis who have elevated systemic venous pressure, pulsus paradoxus, tachycardia, dyspnea, and tachypnea with clear lungs. Tamponade should be distinguished from an acute myocardial infarction, especially when it involves the right ventricle, and from a dissecting aneurysm without tamponade.

Treatment

Drainage is the definitive treatment for cardiac tamponade. Optimal medical management, including volume expansion and inotropic support may be used as temporizing and adjunctive measures (29). Pericardial drainage may be accomplished using catheter-based pericardiocentesis or surgical pericardiectomy. Catheter pericardiocentesis, with echocardiographic guidance, permits selection of the best location for puncture. It is also less expensive, is faster, and requires minimal preparation. Surgical drainage allows for more complete drainage, and permits biopsies to be taken and pericardiectomy to be performed if necessary. However, it requires general anesthesia and is time-consuming.

The patient underwent pericardiocentesis under echocardiographic guidance. Four hundred milliliters of serosanguinous fluid were drained. The blood pressure immediately rose to 110/80 mm Hg. A repeat echocardiogram showed a trivial amount of pericardial fluid. The patient was discharged in good condition.

CONCLUSION

Postpericardiotomy syndrome develops days to months after cardiac and pericardial injury. The presentation is similar to that of pericarditis and may mimic atelectasis, infection, or myocardial infarction. Treatment consists of ASA, or in severe cases, corticosteroids. Pericardial effusion and tamponade may complicate this syndrome. Early recognition of cardiac tamponade is crucial, and rapid management with pericardial drainage may be lifesaving.

REFERENCES

1. Spodick DH. Mechanisms of acute epicardial and myocardial injury in pericardial disease. *Chest* 1998;113:855–856.
2. Spodick DH. Electrocardiographic abnormalities in pericardial disease. In: Spodick DH, ed. *The pericardium: a comprehensive textbook.* New York: Marcel Dekker, 1997:40–64.
3. Spodick DH. Pericardial dieases. In: Braunwald E, Zipes DP, Libby P, eds. *Heart disease: a textbook of cardiovascular medicine,* 6th ed. Philadelphia: WB Saunders, 2001:1823–1876.
3a. Spodick DH. Acute, clinically noneffusive ("dry") pericarditis. Spodick DH, ed. *The pericardium: a comprehensive textbook.* New York: Marcel Dekker,1997:108.
4. Khan AH. The postcardiac injury syndromes. *Clin Cardiol* 1992;15:67–72.
5. Soloff LA. Pericardial cellular response during the post-myocardial infarction syndrome. *Am Heart J* 1971;82:812–816.
6. Ito T, Engle MA, Goldberg HP. Postpericardiotomy syndrome following surgery for nonrheumatic heart disease. *Circulation* 1958;17:549–556.
7. Dressler W. The post-myocardial infarction syndrome: a report on 44 cases. *Arch Intern Med* 1959;103:28.
8. McGuiness JB, Taussig HB. The postpericardiotomy syndrome: its relation to ambulation in the presence of "benign" pericardial and pleural reaction. *Circulation* 1962;26:500–507.
9. Miller RH, Horneffer PJ, Gardner TJ, et al. The epidemiology of the post-pericardiotomy syndrome: a common complication of cardiac surgery. *Am Heart J* 1988;116:1323–1329.
10. Thadani U, Chopra MP, Aber CP, et al. Pericarditis after acute myocardial infarction. *Br Med J* 1971;2:135–137.
11. Lichstein E, Arsura E, Hollander G, et al. Current incidence of postmyocardial infarction (Dressler's) syndrome. *Am J Cardiol* 1982;50:1269–1271.
12. Oliva PB, Hammill SC, Talano JV. Effect of definition on incidence of postinfarction pericarditis: Is it time to redefine postinfarction pericarditis? *Circulation* 1994;90:1537–1541.
13. Sklaroff HJ. The post-pulmonary infarction syndrome. *Am Heart J* 1979;98:772–776.
14. Jerjes-Sanchez C, Ibarra-Perez C, Ramirez-Rivera A, et al. Dressler-like syndrome after pulmonary embolism and infarction. *Chest* 1987;92:115–117.
15. Peters RW, Scheinman MM, Raskin S, et al. Unusual complications of pericardial pacemakers: recurrent pericarditis, cardiac tamponade and pericardial constriction. *Am J Cardiol* 1980;45:1088–1094.
16. Snow ME, Agatston AS, Kramer HC, et al. The postcardiotomy syndrome following transvenous pacemaker insertion. *Pacing Clin Electrophysiol* 1987;10:934–936.
17. Tabatznik B, Isaac JP. Postpericardiotomy syndrome following traumatic hemopericardium. *Am J Cardiol* 1961;7:83–96.
18. Loughlin V, Murphy A, Russell C. The post-pericardiotomy syndrome and penetrating injury of the chest. *Injury* 1987;18:412–414.
19. Dressler W. A post-myocardial infarction syndrome: preliminary report of a complication resembling idiopathic, recurrent, benign pericarditis. *JAMA* 1956;160:1379–1383.
20. Lichstein E, Liu HM, Gupta P. Pericarditis complicating acute myocardial infarction: incidence of complications and significance of electrocardiogram on admission. *Am Heart J* 1974;87:246–252.
21. Dressler W. Flare-up of pericarditis complicating myocardial infarction after two years of steroid therapy. *Am Heart J* 1959;57:501–506.
22. Lessof MH. Postcardiotomy syndrome: pathogenesis and management. *Hosp Prac* 1976;11:81–86.

23. Hammerman H, Kloner RA, Schoen FJ, et al. Indomethacin-induced scar thinning after experimental myocardial infarction. *Circulation* 1983;67:1290–1295.

24. Jugdutt BI, Basualdo CA. Myocardial infarct expansion during indomethacin or ibuprofen therapy for symptomatic postinfarction pericarditis: influence of other pharmacologic agents during early remodelling. *Can J Cardiol* 1989;5:211–221.

25. Roberts R, DeMello V, Sobel BE. Deleterious effect of methylprednisolone in patients with myocardial infarction. *Circulation* 1976;53(3 Suppl):I204–206.

26. Ofori-Krakye SK, Tyberg TI, Geha AS, et al. Late cardiac tamponade after open heart surgery: incidence, role of anticoagulants in its pathogenesis and its relation to the postpericardiotomy syndrome. *Circulation* 1981;63:1323–1328.

27. Spodick DH. Pathophysiology of cardiac tamponade. *Chest* 1998;113:1372–1378.

28. Reddy PS, Curtiss EI, Uretsky BF. Spectrum of hemodynamic changes in cardiac tamponade. *Am J Cardiol* 1990;66:1487–1491.

29. Spodick DH. Pulsus paradoxus. In: Spodick DH, ed. *The pericardium: a comprehensive textbook.* New York: Marcel Dekker, 1997:191–199.

9

A 26-YEAR-OLD POSTPARTUM WOMAN WITH DYSPNEA

TYLER STEVENS
MARK A. ROTH

CASE PRESENTATION

A 26-year-old $G_3 P_2 Ab_1$ black woman with known asthma presented to the emergency room with acute onset of shortness of breath and chest tightness. She denied fever, productive cough, wheezing, orthopnea, paroxysmal nocturnal dyspnea, pleurisy, sick contacts, recent upper respiratory infection, or other complaints. She noted no previous similar episodes, and her dyspnea felt different from her usual asthma.

Of note, she had delivered a healthy, full-term infant 5 days before presentation. She denied any complications or significant shortness of breath during her pregnancy. Review of her prenatal record revealed normal blood pressures, blood sugars, and blood tests, including thyroid function tests.

Her past medical history was significant for moderate obesity, seasonal allergies, and mild intermittent asthma. Her only medications included twice-weekly use of β-agonist inhalers and occasional use of ibuprofen. Social history was negative for smoking or significant alcohol use. Family history and the rest of her review of systems were noncontributory.

QUESTIONS/DISCUSSION

Which of the following are differential considerations in this postpartum patient with dyspnea?

A. **Asthma exacerbation**
B. **Pulmonary embolism**
C. **Cardiomyopathy**
D. **Amniotic fluid embolism**
E. **Physiologic dyspnea of peripartum state**

Pregnancy has a variable effect on asthma, with approximately one-third of asthmatics experiencing fewer symptoms while pregnant, another one-third experiencing more severe symptoms, and the remaining third with unchanged asthma. Some studies have shown improvement in asthma symptoms, reflecting an improvement in bronchial hyperresponsiveness, which gradually returns to baseline in the months postpartum (1). Patients may cease taking their asthma medications because of fear of birth defects, leading to worsening of asthma control during pregnancy.

Pregnancy, as well as the peripartum state, is a well-known risk factor for the development of venous thromboembolism (2). The pathogenesis includes venous stasis secondary to compression of large veins by the gravid uterus as well as increased venous capacitance secondary to physiologic changes. Furthermore, pregnancy is itself a hypercoagulable state, associated with an increase in several procoagulant factors and a decrease in anticoagulant factors.

Acute onset of dyspnea due to congestive heart failure in a 26-year-old would be rare, but the relationship to recent pregnancy makes postpartum cardiomyopathy a consideration.

Amniotic fluid embolism is a catastrophic complication that usually presents with abrupt onset of hypoxia, cardiogenic shock, and disseminated intravascular coagulation (DIC) during delivery or in the early peripartum period (3). Amniotic fluid embolism rarely occurs later than 48 hours after delivery and thus is highly unlikely in this patient.

Several physiologic changes in the cardiopulmonary systems occur during pregnancy, including an increase in circulating blood volume with secondary anemia, increase in the cardiac output, decrease in systemic vascular resistance, minor changes in lung volumes, and increased respiratory drive. Previously healthy women may experience "physiologic" dyspnea during pregnancy, often related to progesterone-induced hyperventilation and decreased partial pressure of carbon dioxide (4). The acute onset of dyspnea 5 days postpartum makes this etiology unlikely.

Physical examination revealed an obese woman in moderate respiratory distress, sitting upright in bed, alert and oriented. Vital signs included blood pressure 124/87 mm Hg, pulse 97 beats per minute, temperature 37.0°C, respi-

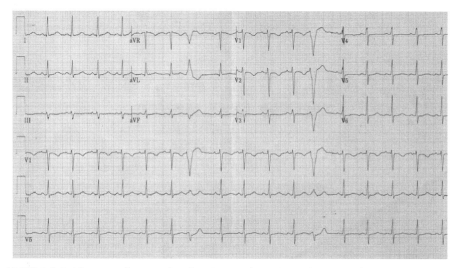

FIGURE 9.1. Electrocardiogram showing sinus tachycardia and nonspecific T-wave changes.

ratory rate 24 per minute, and pulse oximetry 89% on room air. Neck examination did not reveal jugular venous distension. Examination of the lungs was significant for fine rales at the bases. No wheezes were noted on forced expiration. Cardiac examination revealed a regular rhythm without murmurs or gallops. Trace edema was noted in the lower extremities without significant calf or leg tenderness. Pulses were normal throughout.

Laboratory studies revealed normal electrolytes, complete blood count, and serum creatinine. An electrocardiogram showed sinus tachycardia (Fig. 9.1). A chest x-ray was remarkable for an enlarged cardiac silhouette, bilateral lower lung infiltrates, increased vascularity, and a small left

pleural effusion (Fig. 9.2). The patient received diuretics while in the emergency room with mild improvement in her dyspnea. An elevated D-dimer and suspicion for pulmonary embolism led to her being anticoagulated with heparin. She was then admitted to the hospital for further diagnosis and management.

Duplex ultrasound of her legs and spiral computed tomography (CT) of her chest were negative for thromboembolism and heparin was discontinued. Repeated episodes of dyspnea and physical examination findings of congestive heart failure prompted echocardiography, which showed severe global systolic dysfunction, moderate mitral regurgitation, and an apical thrombus (Fig. 9.3).

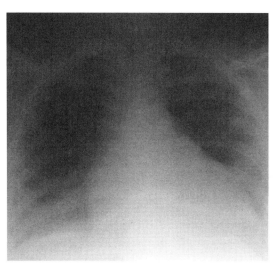

FIGURE 9.2. Chest radiograph (anterior–posterior view) showing cardiomegaly, increased pulmonary vascularity, and a small left pleural effusion.

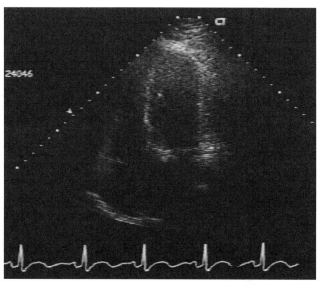

FIGURE 9.3. Echocardiogram showing left ventricular (LV) dilatation and decreased LV function (ejection fraction = 25%). The apical thrombus is not visualized well in this view.

Which of the following is not a criterion for the diagnosis of peripartum cardiomyopathy?

A. Absence of heart disease before pregnancy
B. Absence of another identifiable cause for heart failure
C. Echocardiographic evidence of left ventricular dysfunction
D. Congestive failure within the last month of pregnancy or within 6 months of delivery
E. Cardiac catheterization showing absence of coronary artery disease

Peripartum cardiomyopathy (PPCM) is rarely seen before 36 weeks' gestation. Clinical criteria for its diagnosis include the onset of congestive failure from 1 month before delivery up to 6 months postpartum, the absence of heart disease before pregnancy, and a lack of other potential etiologies of heart failure (5).

This patient had no significant coronary risk factors to suggest an ischemic cause. Her moderate mitral regurgitation was more likely a result of her cardiomyopathy rather than an etiology. The absence of alcohol, prior drug use, or chemotherapy eliminated potential toxin-induced systolic dysfunction. Her clinically euthyroid state, as well as a normal TSH, helped to rule out hypothyroidism as a factor in her heart disease. Myocarditis is difficult to diagnose without an endocardial biopsy, and some patients with presumed PPCM have been found to have an inflammatory histology similar to that seen in infectious myocarditis. A negative travel history helped rule out the most common worldwide cause of myocarditis—*Trypanosoma cruzi* (Chagas disease). Viral etiologies are possible; however, the close temporal relationship with pregnancy and the absence of prodromal symptoms make postpartum cardiomyopathy the most likely diagnosis in this patient.

Echocardiography aids in the diagnosis and the presence of left ventricular enlargement, and global systolic dysfunction has been added to the list of clinical criteria. Cardiac catheterization is not required if no obvious coronary risk factors exist.

Which of the following is not a potential risk factor for development of peripartum cardiomyopathy?

A. Multiparity
B. African-American race
C. Gestational diabetes
D. Cocaine use
E. Preeclampsia

Risk factors for development of PPCM include age greater than 30 years, multiparity, multiple gestation, African-American race, hypertension during or after pregnancy, preeclampsia, poor nutrition, cocaine, selenium deficiency, and long-term tocolytic therapy with β-agonists. Gestational diabetes is not considered a risk factor.

Which of the following treatments is absolutely contraindicated during pregnancy?

A. Digoxin
B. Diuretics
C. Hydralazine
D. Angiotensin-converting enzyme (ACE) inhibitors
E. β-Blockers

As in other forms of cardiomyopathy, afterload reduction forms the cornerstone of medical management in PPCM by improving cardiac output and slowing the rate of myocardial deterioration. Because of the potential for fetal renal teratogenicity, especially during the second and third trimesters, ACE inhibitors are absolutely contraindicated during pregnancy. Long-term experience has shown hydralazine to be a safe alternative vasodilator in the prepartum and postpartum states.

Digoxin improves myocardial contractility and contributes to rate control in patients with secondary atrial fibrillation. Though digoxin crosses the placenta to some extent, newborns generally are resistant to toxicity, and this drug is considered relatively safe. β-Blockers have been shown to have benefit in preserving myocardial function in patients with heart failure. They are usually safe in pregnancy but may gain access to the fetal circulation and cause fetal bradycardia, growth retardation, and hypoglycemia. Diuretics may cause problems by decreasing maternal blood volumes, compromising fetal oxygenation and nutrition, but should be used as needed in conjunction with salt restriction to maintain euvolemia.

Which of the following is not effective in the treatment of peripartum cardiomyopathy?

A. "Conventional" heart failure therapy (afterload reduction, diuretics, digoxin, β-blockers)
B. Immunosuppressive agents
C. Intravenous immunoglobulin
D. Cardiac transplantation
E. Anticoagulation

As in other forms of cardiomyopathy, "conventional treatment" with afterload reduction, diuretics, salt restriction, digoxin, and β-blockers form the foundation of therapy for PPCM. Because of the hypercoagulable state of pregnancy, intracardiac thrombi secondary to stasis within the cardiac chambers are particularly common in PPCM. If there is significant left ventricular dilatation and dysfunction, anticoagulation should be considered, even if thrombus is not seen on echocardiography. Warfarin is not thought to be teratogenic in the third trimester of pregnancy and may be used, but heparin is generally preferable prepartum to allow for delivery or Caesarean section as necessary. Warfarin is not secreted in breast milk and may be used postpartum.

Therapies found helpful in cases of myocarditis also have been tried in PPCM, as the pathology on cardiac biopsy is sometimes similar to that seen in myocarditis (6). Limited retrospective data have shown a benefit of intravenous immunoglobin in postpartum cardiomyopathy, but further prospective studies are needed to confirm this benefit (7). Studies have not shown immunosuppressive therapy to be helpful; moreover, immunosuppressive therapy may be harmful to mother and fetus. In cases refractory to conventional therapy, cardiac transplantation has been shown to be successful in improving long-term survival (8). Mothers who survive PPCM should be cautioned about undergoing future pregnancies, as the risk for recurrence of cardiomyopathy is significantly increased in these patients.

CONCLUSION

An ACE inhibitor was initiated and titrated to adequate blood pressure control, and the patient was diuresed until euvolemic. Given the presence of intracardiac thrombus, she was started on warfarin. Before discharge, she was seen by a cardiologist, who has followed her as an outpatient. Within months, her ejection fraction gradually improved to a low normal range (45%).

REFERENCES

1. Juniper EF, Daniel EE, Roberts RS, et al. Improvement in airway responsiveness and asthma severity during pregnancy: a prospective study. *Am Rev Respir Dis* 1989;140:924–931.
2. Toglia MR, Weg JG. Venous thromboembolism during pregnancy. *N Engl J Med* 1996;335:108–114.
3. Clark S. New concepts of amniotic fluid embolism: a review. *Obstet Gynecol Surv* 1990;45:360–368.
4. Elkus R, Popovich J Jr. Respiratory physiology in pregnancy. *Clin Chest Med* 1992;13:555–565.
5. Homans DC. Peripartum cardiomyopathy. *N Engl J Med* 1985; 312:1432–1437.
6. Midei MG, DeMent SH, Feldman AM, et al. Peripartum myocarditis and cardiomyopathy. *Circulation* 1990;81:922–928.
7. Bozkurt B, Villaneuva FS, Holubkov R, et al. Intravenous immune globulin in the therapy of peripartum cardiomyopathy. *J Am Coll Cardiol* 1999;34:177–180.
8. Rickenbacher PR, Rizeq MN, Hunt SA, et al. Long-term outcome after heart transplantation for peripartum cardiomyopathy. *Am Heart J* 1994;127:1318–1323.

10

A 62-YEAR-OLD MAN WITH POLYMORPHIC VENTRICULAR TACHYCARDIA

JOHN P. GIROD
DANIEL J. BROTMAN

CASE PRESENTATION

A 62-year-old man was admitted to the hospital with worsening shortness of breath. His past medical history was remarkable for a dilated cardiomyopathy and ventricular arrhythmias, which had been treated with amiodarone and an automated implantable cardiac defibrillator (AICD). For several weeks before presentation, his heart failure had worsened, requiring escalating doses of loop diuretics. Several days before admission, the patient was diagnosed with community-acquired pneumonia, for which he received azithromycin. His medications on admission included amiodarone, digoxin, lisinopril, metoprolol, and azithromycin, all of which were continued in the hospital. On admission, an electrocardiogram (ECG) revealed normal sinus rhythm with an interventricular conduction delay. The PR interval was normal, and the corrected QT interval (QT$_c$) was 422 msec (Fig. 10.1).

A few days later, the patient experienced recurrent firing of his AICD. Interrogation of the AICD revealed three appropriate shock therapies for ventricular tachycardia (VT). His last episode of VT for which the AICD fired was more than 2 years before this episode; he had been free of shocks before this episode. ECG on the day the AICD fired revealed a QT$_c$ of 572 msec (Fig. 10.2). Serum potassium level was 2.9 mg/dL, and serum magnesium was 2.0 mg/dL. Two days later, following correction of his potassium to 4.0 mg/dL, the QT$_c$ remained prolonged, and he had an episode of torsades de pointes with syncope (Fig. 10.3).

Torsades de pointes is a rapid polymorphic ventricular tachycardia characterized by continuous alteration of the morphology of the QRS complex and a long QT interval on baseline ECG. The prolonged QT can be congenital or acquired. Common causes of acquired long QT syndrome are medications, electrolyte disturbances (such as hypokalemia, hypomagnesemia, and hypocalcemia), severe bradycardia, and structural heart disease (Table 10.1).

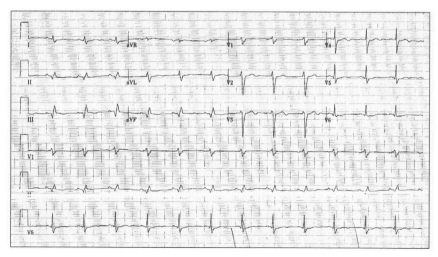

FIGURE 10.1. Electrocardiogram obtained on admission to hospital revealed normal sinus rhythm with nonspecific interventricular conduction delay and normal QT$_c$.

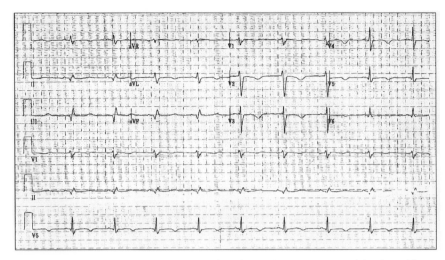

FIGURE 10.2. Electrocardiogram obtained after the patient's automated implantable cardiac defibrillator fired revealed normal sinus rhythm with QT$_c$ of 572 msec.

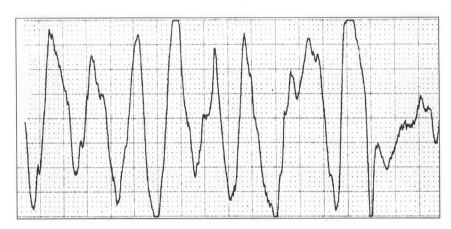

FIGURE 10.3. A rhythm strip recorded at time of the patient's syncopal episode revealed torsades de pointes.

TABLE 10.1. CAUSES OF TORSADES DE POINTES

Congenital long QT syndrome
  Romano–Ward syndrome
  Jervell and Lange–Nielsen syndrome
  Idiopathic
Acquired disorders
  Electrolyte disorders
    Hypokalemia
    Hypomagnesemia
    Hypocalcemia
  Bradyarrhythmias
  Structural heart disease
    Ischemic cardiomyopathy
    Idiopathic dilated cardiomyopathy
  Neurologic events
    Subarachnoid hemorrhage
    Cerebrovascular accident
  Medications

TABLE 10.2. MEDICATIONS CAPABLE OF INDUCING TORSADES DE POINTES

Antiarrhythmics
  Quinidine, procainamide, disopyramide
  Sotalol, amiodarone, dofetilide, ibutilide
Psychotropic medications
  Tricyclic antidepressants
  Phenothiazines
  Haloperidol
  Risperidone
Antimicrobials
  Macrolides
  Trimethoprim-sulfamethoxazole
  Ketoconazole
  Sparfloxacin
  Chloroquine
Antihistamines
  Terfenadine
  Astemizole
Cisapride

QUESTIONS/DISCUSSION

Which of the following is the most likely etiology of the patient's prolonged QTc and torsades de pointes?

A. Hypokalemia
B. Bradyarrhythmia
C. Structural heart disease
D. Medications

Electrolyte disorders are common causes of QT prolongation. Hypokalemia prolongs repolarization by interfering with the third phase of the action potential, during which the outward flow of potassium creates a current that repolarizes the membrane to near resting potential. Low extracellular potassium also results in early after-depolarizations, which likely serve to initiate torsades. Generally, torsades does not occur unless the serum potassium level is less than 3.6 mg/dL (1,2). Although this patient had hypokalemia 2 days before developing torsades, his potassium had been appropriately replaced when the torsades occurred. Hypomagnesemia and hypocalcemia are also associated with torsades, but the mechanism of initiation of polymorphic ventricular tachycardia is not well established with these electrolyte abnormalities.

Severe bradycardia can prolong the QT interval because repolarization represents most of the increase in cycle length. As in hypokalemia, slow heart rates are associated with decreased outward potassium current, which facilitates early after-depolarizations and triggered activity. However, this patient did not have significant bradycardia.

Myocardial fibrosis and the loss of cellular cohesion in ischemic and dilated cardiomyopathies prolong repolarization by down-regulation of outward potassium current. Electrical heterogeneity occurs as a result of a lack of cell-to-cell coupling, which leads to dispersion of refractoriness and early after-depolarizations. A scarred myocardium provides the substrate for maintenance of an arrhythmia by reentrant mechanisms (3,4). The patient's dilated cardiomyopathy may have contributed to the development of torsades but does not explain the appearance and resolution of the long QT interval.

Many medications have been shown to prolong the QT interval (Table 10.2). QT prolongation and torsades de pointes usually occur within a few days of initiation of a medication. In this patient, a medication is the most likely cause of his torsades.

Which of the patient's medications are known to prolong the QTc and increase the risk of torsades de pointes?

A. Amiodarone
B. Metoprolol
C. Azithromycin
D. A and C
E. All of the above

Review of this patient's medications revealed both amiodarone and azithromycin as potential culprits of the QT prolongation. Amiodarone has some class III antiarrhythmic effects and is used extensively to treat both atrial and ventricular tachycardias. Amiodarone is known to increase the QT, but rarely induces torsades de pointes. Amiodarone increases the QT interval through its potassium channel blockade, which prolongs the third phase of the action potential. The low incidence of torsades with amiodarone relative to other class Ia and class III agents may be due to its blockade of sodium and calcium channels, which are thought to be involved in the genesis of early after-depolarizations. Amiodarone also has some β-blocking properties, which can suppress myocardial automaticity and counteract some of the pro-arrhythmic effects (1).

Azithromycin is a macrolide antibiotic that has been associated with QT prolongation. Unlike erythromycin, it rarely induces torsades. The combined pro-arrhythmic effects of amiodarone and azithromycin have not been evaluated. A recent report revealed that a patient who received oral azithromycin while on long-term oral amiodarone experienced prolongation of the QT interval (5). Both amiodarone and azithromycin are frequently prescribed medications. This case illustrates the need for clinicians to recognize the effects that additional medications may have on electrophysiologic parameters and the risks of arrhythmia in patients treated with amiodarone.

Metoprolol is not known to cause QT_c prolongation.

Which of the following is/are considered appropriate management strategies for torsades?

A. Discontinuation of any offending drugs
B. Intravenous magnesium
C. Intravenous lidocaine
D. Overdrive pacing
E. All of the above

All of these are appropriate measures in the treatment of torsades. Initial management of torsades de pointes includes the withdrawal of any agent known to prolong the QT and correction of serum potassium levels. Infusion of 2 g of magnesium over 2 minutes is reported to be beneficial, although the efficacy of this strategy has not been proven (6). Lidocaine infusion designed to shorten the QT interval has shown to be beneficial (7). Atrial or ventricular pacing can shorten the QT as well as decrease the dispersion of refractoriness. Pacing may be necessary in refractory cases, especially those that are bradycardic in origin.

This patient's amiodarone and azithromycin were discontinued. He was given 2 g of magnesium sulfate and was placed on a continuous infusion of lidocaine. Two days later his QT_c interval had returned to baseline.

CONCLUSION

Clinicians should be aware that many medications predispose patients to torsades de pointes. Potentially dangerous drug interactions must be avoided, especially in patients prone to torsades due to underlying heart disease or electrolyte disturbances. Identification and discontinuation of offending drugs is essential, and proper treatment should be instituted early to prevent serious sequelae.

REFERENCES

1. Passman R, Kadish A. Polymorphic ventricular tachycardia, long Q-T syndrome, and torsades de pointes. *Med Clin North Am* 2001;85:321–341.
2. Yang T, Roden DM. Extracellular potassium modulation of drug block of Ikr. Implications for torsade de pointes and reverse use-dependence. *Circulation* 1996;93:407–411.
3. Beuckelmann DJ, Nabauer M, Erdmann E. Alterations of K+ currents in isolated human ventricular myocytes from patients with terminal heart failure. *Circ Res* 1993;73:379–385.
4. Grimm W, Steder U, Menz V, et al. QT dispersion and arrhythmic events in idiopathic dilated cardiomyopathy. *Am J Cardiol* 1996;78:458–461.
5. Samarendra P, Kumari S, Evans SJ, et al. QT prolongation associated with azithromycin/amiodarone combination. *Pacing Clin Electrophysiol* 2001;24:1572–1574.
6. Tzivoni D, Banai S, Schuger C, et al. Treatment of torsade de pointes with magnesium sulfate. *Circulation* 1988;77:392–397.
7. Schwartz PJ, Priori SG, Locati EH, et al. Long QT syndrome patients with mutations of the SCN5A and HERG genes have differential responses to Na+ channel blockade and to increases in heart rate: implications for gene-specific therapy. *Circulation* 1995;92:3381–3386.

11

A 35-YEAR-OLD WOMAN WITH HEART PALPITATIONS

TODD SCHWEDT
BRUCE WILKOFF

CASE PRESENTATION

A 35-year-old woman presented to the emergency department following a 2-minute episode of heart palpitations, chest tightness, mild shortness of breath, and lightheadedness. She reported that such episodes have occurred on an almost monthly basis since the age of 17. This episode started suddenly while watching television. The patient experienced the sudden onset of rapid heartbeat followed by diffuse chest tightness, mild shortness of breath, and the sensation that she was going to faint. These symptoms were quite similar to her past episodes. Over many years, the patient learned to hold her breath and "bear down" in order to stop these episodes. This maneuver worked for her the great majority of the time. She had never experienced a syncopal event. She had been diagnosed with panic attacks during previous evaluations of her palpitations.

The patient's past medical history was significant only for the previously mentioned "panic attacks." She was not on any regular medication. The patient had a 13-pack-year history of smoking but had quit a few years earlier. The patient reported no usage of alcohol, illicit drugs, or herbal medications. Family history was significant only for congestive heart failure in her mother. There was no known family history of anxiety disorder, coronary artery disease, or sudden cardiac death.

On physical examination, the patient was afebrile, with a blood pressure of 112/72 mm Hg, a pulse of 93 beats per minute, and normal oxygenation on room air. She was in no acute distress, had clear lungs and a normal cardiovascular examination. The rest of her physical examination was unremarkable. The patient had an electrocardiogram (ECG) performed (Fig. 11.1).

QUESTIONS/DISCUSSION

The ECG in Fig. 11.1 is most consistent with:

A. Normal ECG

B. Wolff–Parkinson–White

C. Acute myocardial infarction

D. Acute ischemia

E. Remote myocardial infarction

This electrocardiogram is most consistent with the Wolff–Parkinson–White (WPW) pattern. The WPW pattern consists of a short P-R interval (less than 0.12 sec), a prolonged QRS complex (greater than 0.12 sec), and a slow-rising upslope of the QRS complex, known as a delta (δ) wave. A patient with such an ECG and symptoms of recurrent tachyarrhythmias is said to have WPW syndrome.

The findings on the electrocardiogram can be explained by the electrophysiologic properties of the accessory pathway that is part of WPW. Accessory pathways are additional bands of conductive tissue that connect the atrium to the ventricle. These bypass tracts have different electrophysiologic properties from the normal conductive pathways of the atrioventricular (AV) node and the His–Purkinje system. Accessory pathways tend to have rapid conduction velocities and are not subject to decremental conduction (1). Structures with decremental conduction, such as the AV node, slow the conduction velocity (increase the conduction time) as earlier heartbeats reach that structure. The differences in electrical properties account for the short P-R interval and delta wave seen on the electrocardiogram. The widened QRS complex is due to slowed conduction through the ventricles. During normal conduction of a sinus impulse through the His–Purkinje system, the duration of ventricular activation is short, resulting in a narrow QRS complex on the electrocardiogram. When conduction occurs via an accessory pathway, the electrical impulse travels more slowly, resulting in a widened QRS complex (Fig. 11.2).

The presence of bypass tracts is thought to be quite prevalent in the general population. The WPW pattern on electrocardiogram is reported to have a prevalence of 0.1% to 0.3% (2). The WPW pattern is found twice as frequently in males as it is in females (3). Accessory pathways may be

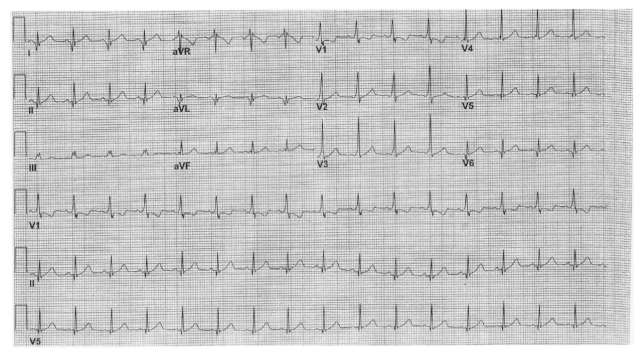

FIGURE 11.1. Patient's electrocardiogram upon presentation.

found anywhere along the AV groove but are most commonly found at the left free wall, followed by posteroseptal, right free wall, and anteroseptal locations (4). Approximately one-quarter of accessory pathways conduct only in a retrograde ventriculoatrial manner (5). These pathways are called "concealed" bypass tracts since there is no electrocardiographic evidence of them while patients are in sinus rhythm. Although the great majority of cases of WPW occur sporad-

ically, a familial tendency for accessory pathways is associated with some cases. Approximately 7% to 20% of patients with WPW syndrome have congenital cardiac defects, with Ebstein's anomaly the most common defect (1).

Case Continued. While in the emergency department, the patient again experienced palpitations and lightheadedness. Her vital signs included a pulse of 190 beats per

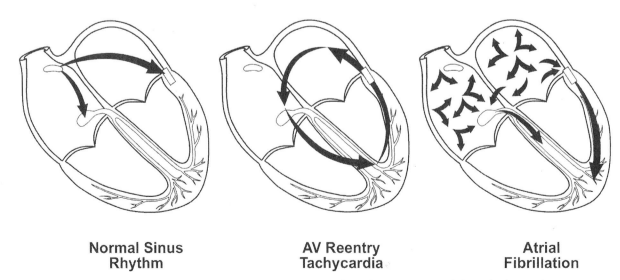

Normal Sinus Rhythm   **AV Reentry Tachycardia**   **Atrial Fibrillation**

FIGURE 11.2. Diagram demonstrating the pattern of conduction in normal sinus rhythm, atrioventricular reentry tachycardia, and atrial fibrillation.

minute and blood pressure of 115/75 mm Hg. An ECG was repeated (Fig. 11.3).

This ECG is most consistent with which type of tachy-arrhythmia?

A. **Ventricular tachycardia**
B. **Ventricular fibrillation**
C. **Atrial fibrillation with rapid ventricular response**
D. **Supraventricular tachycardia**
E. **Torsades de pointes**

The pattern on this electrocardiogram is most consistent with the diagnosis of atrial fibrillation with a rapid ventricular response (Fig. 11.2). The most common supraventricular tachycardia in patients with WPW is orthodromic atrioventricular reentrant tachycardia (6). This situation is often initiated by premature depolarization of the atrium or ventricle, which starts a reentrant circuit. The electrical impulse travels antegrade through the normal conducting system (the AV node, His bundle, and bundle branches) to the ventricles and then in a retrograde fashion back to the atrium through the accessory pathway. In a small percentage of patients with WPW syndrome, the reentry circuit travels in the opposite direction, with antegrade conduction over the accessory pathway and retrograde conduction through the normal conducting pathway. This pattern of supraventricular

tachycardia, which is more common in patients with multiple accessory pathways, is referred to as antidromic atrioventricular reentrant tachycardia (7) (Fig. 11.2).

Atrial fibrillation and flutter are also common arrhythmias in patients with WPW syndrome. These atrial arrhythmias are often initiated from an episode of atrioventricular reentrant tachycardia (8). Patients with accessory pathways are at particular risk from atrial fibrillation and flutter since they are capable of rapid ventricular responses via nondecremental conduction. This may result in ventricular fibrillation. An important measure for risk stratification of patients with atrial fibrillation is the refractory period of the accessory pathway. Patients with a refractory time of less than 250 msec are at higher risk of developing ventricular fibrillation during atrial fibrillation (9).

A markedly irregular and extremely rapid ventricular response during atrial fibrillation is suggestive of conduction over an accessory pathway. Such rapid ventricular response very rarely occurs with conduction through the AV node. An ECG alone may be insufficient to differentiate between atrial fibrillation with a rapid ventricular response and ventricular tachycardia. The patient demographics and baseline ECG may help to differentiate the rhythms. A young patient with evidence of WPW on a baseline EKG is more likely to have pre-excitation as a cause for a wide irregular tachyarrhythmia. Clinicians must keep in mind that atrial fibrillation in WPW patients may degen-

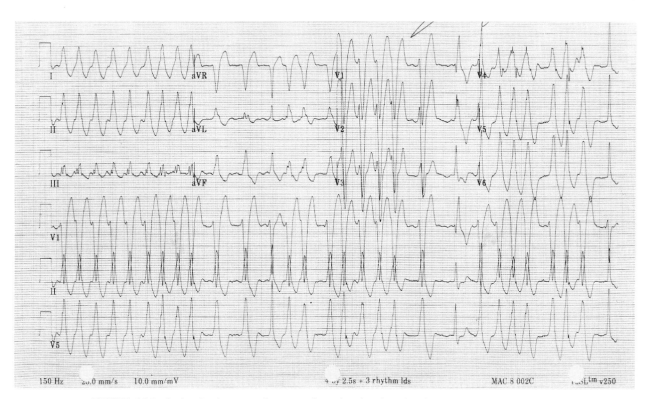

FIGURE 11.3. Patient's electrocardiogram when she developed palpitations and lightheadedness.

erate into ventricular fibrillation, likely due to the very high ventricular rates and extremely variable R-R intervals (10).

What is the initial treatment of choice for this tachyarrhythmia?

A. **Adenosine**
B. **Procainamide**
C. **Digoxin**
D. **Verapamil**
E. **Cardioversion**

WPW patients with atrial fibrillation without hemodynamic compromise may be initially treated with procainamide in an attempt to slow the rate and terminate the arrhythmia. If hemodynamic compromise is present, immediate synchronized cardioversion is the treatment of choice. Therapies that slow conduction through the AV node, such as β-blockers, digoxin, diltiazem, verapamil, and adenosine, should not be used in these patients. These agents may have detrimental effects by blocking the AV node and enhancing conduction through the accessory pathway, which may lead to ventricular fibrillation or cause hypotension (1).

WPW patients with an acute episode of supraventricular tachycardia may be treated with intravenous adenosine. Studies have shown that adenosine can successfully terminate supraventricular tachycardias in patients with reentry that involves the AV node (11). Care must be taken when using adenosine in WPW patients due to the risk of initiating atrial fibrillation or atrial flutter.

LONG-TERM TREATMENT OF WOLFF–PARKINSON–WHITE

Patients with the WPW pattern on electrocardiogram generally do not require intervention. Exceptions to this rule may include asymptomatic patients with high-risk occupations, such as police officers, bus drivers, and airplane pilots. It may be appropriate for patients in this group to undergo electrophysiologic testing to assess the risk for dangerous arrhythmias and the need for treatment.

Ablation of the accessory pathway is considered the treatment of choice for patients with WPW syndrome who have symptomatic tachyarrhythmias. Surgical ablation techniques requiring an open-chest procedure had been used, which limited the procedure to patients who did not respond to medical therapy or had life-threatening arrhythmias (12). With the advent of radiofrequency catheter ablation techniques, which are considerably less risky, ablation

may be considered first-line treatment in all WPW patients with symptomatic tachyarrhythmias. Accessory pathways are located via catheter mapping techniques, and a small radiofrequency lesion is made along the pathway. This interrupts conduction along the accessory pathway and thus prevents further episodes of tachycardia in greater than 90% of cases (6). In about 10% of patients, conduction via the accessory pathway will return within 2 months of ablation, requiring a second procedure (6).

CONCLUSION

The patient underwent an electrophysiology study the following day. An accessory conduction pathway was mapped and ablated using radiofrequency. At follow-up, the patient did not report any further episodes of palpitations, shortness of breath, or lightheadedness.

REFERENCES

1. Al-Khatib SM, Pritchett EL. Clinical features of Wolff–Parkinson–White syndrome. *Am Heart J* 1999;138:403–413.
2. Trohman RG. Supraventricular tachycardia: implications for the intensivist. *Crit Care Med* 2000;28:129–135.
3. Zardini M, Yee R, Thakur RK, et al. Risk of sudden arrhythmic death in the Wolff–Parkinson–White syndrome: current perspectives. *Pacing Clin Electrophysiol* 1994;17:966–975.
4. Reddy GV, Schamroth L. The localization of bypass tracts in the Wolff–Parkinson–White syndrome from the surface electrocardiogram. *Am Heart J* 1987;113:984–993.
5. Oren JW 4th, Beckman KJ, McClelland JH, et al. A functional approach to the preexcitation syndromes. *Cardiol Clin* 1993;11:121–149.
6. Ganz LI, Friedman PL. Supraventricular tachycardia. *N Engl J Med* 1995;332:162–173.
7. Atie J, Brugada P, Brugada J, et al. Clinical and electrophysiologic characteristics of patients with antidromic circus movement tachycardia in the Wolff–Parkinson–White syndrome. *Am J Cardiol* 1990;66:1082–1091.
8. Campbell RW, Smith RA, Gallagher JJ, et al. Atrial fibrillation in the preexcitation syndrome. *Am J Cardiol* 1977;40:514–520.
9. Klein GJ, Bashore TM, Sellers TD, et al. Ventricular fibrillation in the Wolff–Parkinson–White syndrome. *N Engl J Med* 1979;301:1080–1085.
10. Prystowsky EN, Fananapazir L, Packer DL, et al. Wolff–Parkinson–White syndrome and sudden cardiac death. *Cardiology* 1987;74(Suppl 2):67–71.
11. DiMarco JP, Sellers TD, Lerman BB, et al. Diagnostic and therapeutic use of adenosine in patients with supraventricular tachyarrhythmias. *J Am Coll Cardiol* 1985;6:417–425.
12. Stevenson WG, Ellison KE, Lefroy DC, et al. Ablation therapy for cardiac arrhythmias. *Am J Cardiol* 1997;80:56G–66G.

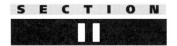

ENDOCRINOLOGY

12

A 55-YEAR-OLD WOMAN WITH POSTOPERATIVE HYPOTENSION

ANIL ASGAONKAR
AMIR H. HAMRAHIAN

CASE PRESENTATION

A 55-year-old woman with a past medical history significant for Crohn disease and hypertension presented to the emergency department with abdominal pain. Ten days prior, the patient underwent a right hemicolectomy with an ileocolic anastomosis for a cecal stricture. Following the surgery, the patient developed mild abdominal discomfort, which progressed to intense pain on the day of presentation. Her vital signs were notable for a temperature of 38.4°C and heart rate of 110 beats per minute. Abdominal examination revealed diffuse tenderness to palpation, rebound tenderness, and involuntary guarding. Computed tomography (CT scan) of the abdomen revealed an abscess at the ileocolic anastomosis site. An exploratory laparotomy with drainage of the abscess and a diverting loop ileostomy was performed the following morning, and broad-spectrum antibiotics, including ceftriaxone and gentamicin, were started.

On postoperative day 1, the patient remained febrile and was hypotensive. The patient had a temperature of 37.9°C, blood pressure of 95/60 mm Hg, heart rate of 105 beats per minute, respiratory rate of 18 per minute, and pulse oximetry of 98% on 2 L of oxygen. She was not in any distress. Her cardiovascular examination revealed normal heart sounds, with no murmurs, rubs, or gallops; pulses were strong and equal in all extremities. There were diminished breath sounds bilaterally, without focal signs of consolidation. The abdominal examination was significant for diffuse tenderness to palpation and decreased bowel sounds. The wound site was clean without significant erythema or drainage. No lower-extremity edema, rash, or skin lesion was noted.

QUESTIONS/DISCUSSION

Which of the following processes can produce postoperative hypotension?

A. Hypovolemia secondary to blood or fluid loss
B. Sepsis
C. Adrenal insufficiency
D. Perioperative myocardial infarction
E. All of the above

Intraabdominal surgery is often associated with significant perioperative fluid or blood loss. Fluid and blood losses during surgery, as well as the amount of fluid administered, should be noted in the operative notes. Clinicians also need to remember that significant insensible fluid losses can occur while the abdomen is open. Therefore the duration of surgery should be noted in order to estimate insensible fluid losses. Careful evaluation of a patient's fluid balance should help to determine whether *hypovolemia* is a potential cause for hypotension.

Surgical patients are susceptible to postoperative infections from various sources, including surgical wounds, venous catheters, bladder catheters, and pneumonia. *Sepsis* must be considered in all hypotensive surgical patients, and it should be aggressively investigated and treated when suspicion is high.

Adrenal insufficiency, either preexisting or secondary to surgical complications, can produce postoperative hypotension. This diagnosis is often overlooked, as patients can present with various nonspecific signs and symptoms. An adrenocorticotropic hormone (ACTH) analog (Cortrosyn) stimulation test can help to establish the diagnosis.

Myocardial infarction can present silently in the perioperative period, manifesting itself only with shortness of breath, hypotension, or signs of congestive heart failure. Patients with cardiac risk factors should be carefully monitored for signs of cardiac ischemia or infarction. In summary, *all of the preceding* causes of hypotension need to be considered in this patient.

The patient was treated with intravenous fluids and maintained on antibiotics. Blood and urine cultures were negative. Sputum and wound cultures grew methicillin-resistant *Staphylococcus aureus* (MRSA), and vancomycin was added to her antibiotic regimen. A chest x-ray did not demonstrate any infiltrates. An electrocardiogram revealed sinus tachycardia without any ischemic changes; cardiac enzymes were negative. Since the patient remained febrile, upper and lower extremity duplex ultrasonography was performed to exclude deep venous thrombosis (DVT). Ultrasound revealed bilateral calf DVTs, which were followed with serial ultrasounds; systemic anticoagulation was not initiated.

On postoperative day (POD) 5, the patient suffered a cardiac arrest. After she was resuscitated, she was transferred to the intensive care unit (ICU). Laboratory studies revealed a sodium of 142 mEq/L, potassium of 4.4 mEq/L, calcium of 8.7 mg/dL, hematocrit of 25% (decreased from 31% on POD 1), and white blood cell count of 14 K/µL with a normal differential. BUN was 40 mg/dL, and creatinine was 1.2 mg/dL. The patient received a transfusion of 2 units of packed red blood cells. Because of persistent hypotension despite aggressive rehydration with intravenous fluids and the use of pressor agents, intravenous hydrocortisone 100 mg every 8 hours was initiated. The patient's blood pressure improved, and her fever resolved. On postoperative day 11, hydrocortisone was discontinued, with the patient's improvement believed to be due to the antibiotics. The following day, her blood pressure again trended lower, and her fever returned. Her serum potassium was 5.3 mEq/L, with her serum creatinine unchanged. On POD 14, a CT scan of

the abdomen was done as part of the evaluation for persistent fever and revealed bilateral massive adrenal hemorrhage (BMAH) (Fig. 12.1).

Which of the following is the most appropriate method to diagnose BMAH?

A. Cortrosyn stimulation test
B. CT scan of adrenal glands
C. CT scan of adrenal glands and Cortrosyn stimulation test
D. Random plasma cortisol level

A *Cortrosyn stimulation test* is an excellent test to evaluate for primary adrenal insufficiency. The test consists of injecting 250 µg of an ACTH analog intravenously, followed by measurements of serum cortisol levels at baseline, 30 minutes after injection, and 60 minutes. Two methods for evaluating adrenal function during a Cortrosyn stimulation test have been proposed. The first is to measure the change in serum cortisol level following Cortrosyn injection (delta), and the second is a measurement of the peak serum cortisol level achieved during the test. The peak serum cortisol is more reliable than the delta to diagnose adrenal insufficiency since the rise in serum cortisol is inversely proportional to the basal cortisol level (1). The incremental rise in

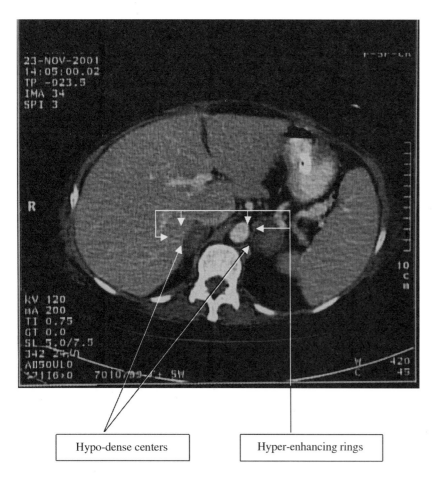

Hypo-dense centers

Hyper-enhancing rings

FIGURE 12.1. Computed tomography of the abdomen showing a hyperenhancing ring around a low-density center. These findings were compatible with acute bilateral adrenal hemorrhage.

cortisol may not be as pronounced if the baseline cortisol level was already high. This is particularly relevant in intensive care unit patients whose adrenal glands have been maximally stimulated due to the severe stress of their illness. During the Cortrosyn stimulation test, peak cortisol levels of at least 18 to 20 μg/dL typically indicate adequate adrenal function (1). This patient's Cortrosyn stimulation test revealed a baseline cortisol of 2.5 μg/dL, cortisol at 30 minutes of 3.0 μg/dL, and 60-minute cortisol of 3.0 μg/dL. Both the peak serum cortisol and rise in cortisol (delta) are markedly abnormal and diagnostic of adrenal insufficiency.

A single *random plasma cortisol level* can be useful to assess adrenal insufficiency in critically ill patients. A random cortisol level of 18 μg/dL or more is considered adequate adrenal function in patients under severe stress. A random cortisol level of less than 5 μg/dL is diagnostic for adrenal insufficiency (1). Levels between 5 and 18 μg/dL are indeterminate results and require further testing. This patient had a basal cortisol level of 2.5 μg/dL, which is diagnostic of adrenal insufficiency.

The *CT scan* has greatly enhanced our ability to detect adrenal hemorrhage. Prior to CT scanning, cases of bilateral massive adrenal hemorrhage were often diagnosed postmortem. Rarely, cases were diagnosed during operations such as exploratory laparotomy. CT scans are now widely available and can rapidly show anatomic changes consistent with BMAH (2). This patient's CT scan showed a hyperenhancing ring around a low-density center, findings compatible with acute bilateral adrenal hemorrhage (Fig. 12.1).

BMAH is diagnosed by demonstrating anatomic evidence for bilateral adrenal hemorrhage and biochemical proof of adrenal insufficiency (*choice C*). In this case, both a Cortrosyn stimulation test and adrenal CT scan were performed and were consistent with BMAH.

Which of the following can occur in patients with primary adrenal insufficiency?

A. Electrolyte abnormalities
B. Hypotension
C. Mental status changes
D. Abdominal pain
E. All of the above

Electrolyte abnormalities, particularly hyponatremia and hyperkalemia, are commonly seen in the setting of primary adrenal insufficiency. Hyperkalemia is caused by aldosterone deficiency, which decreases potassium secretion in the distal renal tubules. Hyponatremia results from several mechanisms, most notably renal salt wasting from aldosterone deficiency and antidiuretic hormone (ADH) secretion triggered by volume depletion (3). Diagnosing adrenal insufficiency solely based on electrolyte abnormalities is difficult, as many patients have comorbid conditions that can produce similar laboratory findings. Hyponatremia can develop in patients with congestive heart failure, hepatic

insufficiency, hypothyroidism, or increased ADH secretion in response to surgery or pain. Hyperkalemia may occur in patients with renal failure or in patients on medications such as angiotensin-converting enzyme (ACE) inhibitors or spironolactone. Clinicians must recognize that these electrolyte changes are not always seen in adrenal insufficiency, and their absence does not rule out the disorder.

Hypotension is commonly seen in primary adrenal insufficiency. The hypotension can be severe, with systolic blood pressure under 90 mm Hg, and may not respond to catecholamines (4). Hypotension may develop due to volume depletion from aldosterone deficiency or from the loss of direct peripheral vasoconstriction associated with glucocorticoid deficiency.

Mental status changes can occur in primary adrenal insufficiency due to hyponatremia and hypotension. Serum sodium levels under 120 mEq/L can precipitate seizures and confusion. Mental status changes can be exacerbated by the critically ill state that accompanies most patients in intensive care units.

Gastrointestinal symptoms are frequently noted in patients with primary adrenal insufficiency. Patients may complain of abdominal pain, cramping, nausea, vomiting, or diarrhea (2). Patients who develop BMAH may complain of significant abdominal pain. The pain can be diffuse and can radiate to the back. About two-thirds of patients with BMAH have abdominal pain upon presentation (2).

All of the above can occur in primary adrenal insufficiency. Because of the nonspecific nature of these symptoms, clinicians must have a high index of suspicion in order to diagnose adrenal insufficiency. In this case, the patient had hypotension and abdominal pain; however, both findings were initially attributed to more common postsurgical complications. Her electrolytes were initially normal, and her mental status was appropriate for a critically ill patient. Therefore the diagnosis of adrenal insufficiency was difficult to reach in this patient, as her symptoms were nonspecific.

Which of the following is not a risk factor for developing BMAH?

A. Postoperative state
B. Coagulopathy
C. Thromboembolic disease
D. Diabetes
E. Sepsis

The *postoperative state* has been described as a risk factor for BMAH. While any surgery can predispose patients to developing BMAH, open-heart and joint replacement surgeries are most commonly associated with BMAH (2).

Coagulopathy is associated with increased risk of BMAH. The use of heparin, either unfractionated or low molecular weight, appears to be a risk factor for developing BMAH, especially when administered for more than 6 days (2,5).

Heparin-induced thrombocytopenia may have a role in BMAH, although the mechanism is unclear (5). Thrombocytopenia is also a risk factor for BMAH, with one analysis showing an adjusted odds ratio of 14.6 for patients with thrombocytopenia versus those with normal platelets (5).

Thromboembolic disease is associated with increased risk of developing BMAH. Reports in the literature have described an increased risk for adrenal hemorrhage in association with both venous and arterial thromboses. Patients prone to thromboembolic events, such as those with antiphospholipid antibody syndrome, should be considered at increased risk for BMAH. This patient developed distal lower-extremity DVTs but was not systemically anticoagulated.

Sepsis has been reported in about one-third of patients with BMAH (2).Various bacterial, viral, and parasitic infections throughout the body have been associated with BMAH.

BMAH has also been linked with conditions such as coronary artery disease, myocardial infarction, congestive heart failure, and pregnancy (2). Diabetes mellitus has not been associated with an increased risk of BMAH (5).

The exact mechanism of BMAH is not entirely understood, but ACTH may play a role (6). Stress on the body leads to increased corticotropin secretion, which results in increased adrenal blood flow. In animals, chronic stimulation of the adrenals with ACTH has been shown to result in degeneration, focal necrosis, and hemorrhage of the adrenal cortices. While the adrenal glands receive blood flow from three branches of the renal arteries, only one central adrenal vein drains the adrenal sinusoids. Impaired drainage of the adrenals creates increased blood pressure inside the gland and may lead to hemorrhage.

This patient had multiple potential risk factors for BMAH, including her postoperative state, an intraabdominal infection, and deep venous thrombosis. Her persistent abdominal pain may have been secondary to adrenal hemorrhage, and her drop in hematocrit on POD 5 may have reflected the magnitude of hemorrhage.

TREATMENT OF BILATERAL MASSIVE ADRENAL HEMORRHAGE

Prompt treatment of patients with BMAH is critical, since the condition is fatal if untreated. Although obtaining a CT scan and performing a Cortrosyn stimulation test is the appropriate diagnostic approach, glucocorticoid therapy should not be withheld due to the severity of the disease and the considerable potential for morbidity and mortality (7). There may be a considerable delay while awaiting a CT scan and the results of a Cortrosyn stimulation test. During this time, administration of glucocorticoids treats adrenal insufficiency until a definitive diagnosis is established.

Most of the glucocorticoid preparations, including hydrocortisone, interfere with cortisol assays. Therefore when BMAH is suspected, a glucocorticoid that does not interfere with subsequent cortisol measurement, such as dexamethasone, should be started. Once the diagnosis of BMAH has been established, dexamethasone may be changed to hydrocortisone with gradual tapering as the patient improves. Another management strategy is to draw blood for a random cortisol level, start stress doses of hydrocortisone, and obtain a CT of the adrenals. If the random cortisol level is not diagnostic of adrenal insufficiency (less than 5 µg/dL), a Cortrosyn stimulation test can be performed once the patient is clinically stable and off hydrocortisone for 24 hours.

Which of the following statements regarding the long-term management of patients with BMAH is correct?

A. **Glucocorticoid therapy is needed only during acute illnesses.**
B. **Patients should be discharged on maintenance doses of oral glucocorticoids and mineralocorticoids.**
C. **Patients do not need mineralocorticoid therapy.**
D. **Adrenal function is likely to recover over 4 to 6 months with no further need for glucocorticoids.**

Long-term treatment of patients with BMAH focuses on management of their primary adrenal insufficiency. Most patients do not recover their adrenal function and will require life-long steroid coverage (2). This is likely secondary to atrophy of adrenal glands, which is usually evident within 1 year on follow-up CT scans (2).

The dose of glucocorticoids should be gradually tapered to a maintenance dose to minimize side effects as the patient clinically improves. As little as 15 to 20 mg of hydrocortisone per day has been reported to provide adequate replacement therapy (4). Because of the physiologic diurnal secretion of cortisol, the majority of the dose should be given in the morning. A simple maintenance dose of hydrocortisone includes 12.5 to 15 mg in the morning and 2.5 to 5 mg in the evening.

In contrast to secondary adrenal insufficiency, patients with primary adrenal insufficiency, including BMAH, also require mineralocorticoid therapy due to aldosterone deficiency. Fludrocortisone, 0.05 to 0.2 mg orally once per day, provides adequate mineralocorticoid replacement (4). Therefore, choice B is the correct management strategy.

CONCLUSION

After the CT scan was found to be compatible with bilateral adrenal hemorrhage, the patient was started on intravenous dexamethasone 2 mg every 6 hours. After the Cortrosyn stimulation test performed on the same day confirmed the diagnosis of adrenal insufficiency, dexamethasone was switched to intravenous hydrocortisone 50 mg every 8 hours. The dexamethasone was gradually tapered as the patient improved clinically, with stabilization of her blood pressure and normalization of her potassium. After approximately 3 weeks in the ICU, the patient was transferred to a regular nursing floor in stable condition. The patient was started on fludrocortisone 0.1 mg once a day, and the hydrocortisone was decreased to less than 100 mg per day. She was discharged home in good condition after 5 weeks in the hospital.

REFERENCES

1. Grinspoon SK, Biller BM. Clinical review 62: laboratory assessment of adrenal insufficiency. *J Clin Endocrinol Metab* 1994;79: 923–931.

2. Rao RH. Bilateral massive adrenal hemorrhage. *Med Clin North Am* 1995;79:107–129.

3. Orth DN, Kovacs WJ. The adrenal cortex. In: Wilson JD, Foster DW, Kronenberg HM, et al., eds. *Williams textbook of endocrinology,* 9th ed. Philadelphia: WB Saunders, 1998:517–664.

4. Oelkers W. Adrenal insufficiency. *N Engl J Med* 1996;335: 1206–1212.

5. Kovacs KA, Lam YM, Pater JL. Bilateral massive adrenal hemorrhage: assessment of putative risk factors by the case-control method. *Medicine* 2001;80:45–53.

6. Rao RH, Vagnucci AH, Amico JA. Bilateral massive adrenal hemorrhage: early recognition and treatment. *Ann Intern Med* 1989; 110:227–235.

7. Vasa FR, Molitch ME. Endocrine problems in the chronically critically ill patient. *Clin Chest Med* 2001;22:193–208.

13

MUSCLE SPASMS IN A YOUNG MAN WITH SHORT STATURE, MILD MENTAL RETARDATION, AND BRACHYDACTYLY

TIMIR S. BAMAN
MARIO SKUGOR
ALEJANDRO MORALES
DANIEL J. BROTMAN

CASE PRESENTATION

A 26-year-old white man presented to the emergency department with muscle spasms and episodic paralysis. He had felt well until 6 months earlier, when he began to develop progressive fatigue and what he described as "freezing-up spells" upon mild exertion. During these episodes, he noticed facial paralysis and occasional spasms of the right leg. The episodes would spontaneously remit after several seconds. He noted no precipitating factors other than physical exertion.

Past medical history was notable for cataracts and learning disabilities throughout his schooling. He was not taking any prescription medications. He denied tobacco, alcohol, and illicit drug use. The patient knew of no relatives with neuromuscular or endocrine diseases. Review of systems was negative except for erectile dysfunction and chronic constipation. He denied fevers, weight loss, or seizure history.

Physical examination revealed a short, stocky young man in no distress. He was 5 feet, 2 inches tall (157.5 cm) and weighed 174 pounds (79.1 kg) (Fig. 13.1). He had round facies (Fig. 13.2) and brachydactyly (short, stubby fingers; Fig. 13.3). Vital signs were normal. The thyroid was normal to palpation. Heart, lung, and abdominal examinations were unremarkable. Neurologic examination was nonfocal, but spinal reflexes were markedly hyperactive. Percussion of the facial nerve produced facial spasm (Chvostek sign), and he developed forearm spasm after inflation of a blood pressure cuff around the arm for 2 minutes (Trousseau sign). Muscle bulk and tone were normal, but there was mild tenderness of the thighs and arms with palpation. The skin was dry and coarse.

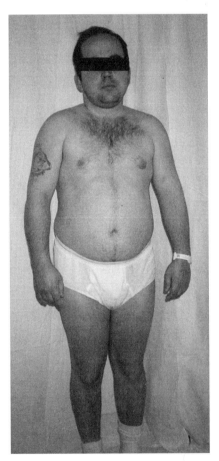

FIGURE 13.1. Photograph of this 26-year-old man with muscle spasms demonstrating short stature and stocky build.

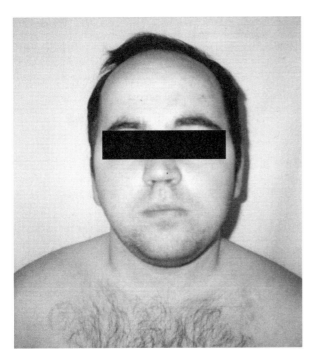

FIGURE 13.2. Photograph of this patient demonstrating round facies.

QUESTIONS/DISCUSSION

All of the following are part of the differential diagnosis in this patient except:

A. **Hypothyroidism**
B. **Hypocalcemia**
C. **"Hungry bone" syndrome**
D. **Hypomagnesemia**
E. **Familial hypocalciuric hypercalcemia**

Hypothyroidism should be considered in this patient. Muscle spasms, fatigue, constipation, and dry, coarse skin are all consistent with the diagnosis of hypothyroidism. However, hyperreflexia is not seen in this condition. Deep tendon reflexes in hypothyroidism typically exhibit a delayed relaxation phase ("hung-up" reflexes) (1).

Familial hypocalciuric hypercalcemia is usually asymptomatic, but some patients develop clinical manifestations of hypercalcemia, such as fatigue, weakness, polydipsia, polyuria, and cognitive disturbances. This condition is associated with high plasma calcium levels and normal parathyroid hormone (PTH) levels. The underlying mechanism is disturbance of the calcium "set point," and parathyroidectomy does not correct the hypercalcemia. Urinary calcium excretion is low, especially for the degree of hypercalcemia (2). Stiffness and muscle spasms are not features of this condition and it is not in the differential diagnosis for this patient.

The "hungry bone syndrome" is a hypocalcemic period occurring immediately after surgical cure of primary or secondary hyperparathyroidism in patients who developed marked hyperparathyroid skeletal disease. It results from the rapid deposition of calcium and phosphate into the bone. Many patients have a transient hypocalcemic episode after parathyroid surgery, but only those requiring parenteral administration of calcium for symptomatic hypocalcemia are said to have "hungry bone syndrome" (3). This patient could not have the "hungry bone syndrome" since he had no history of recent neck surgery.

Hypomagnesemia can cause tetany in the absence of hypocalcemia, but in most cases, hypomagnesemia is associated with hypocalcemia. Clinical signs of hypocalcemia may be very resistant to treatment until hypomagnesemia is corrected (4).

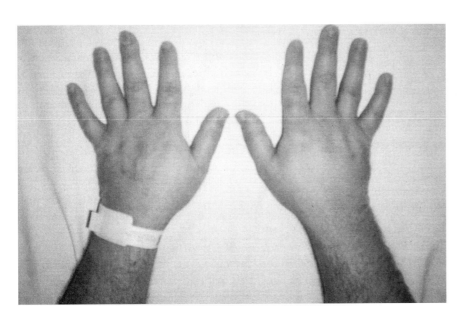

FIGURE 13.3. Photograph of this patient's hands demonstrating brachydactyly.

TABLE 13.1. CAUSES OF HYPOCALCEMIA

Hypoparathyroidism	Postsurgical
	Autoimmune
	Congenital
	Radiation-induced
	Infiltrative diseases
	Hungry bone syndrome
Vitamin D deficiency	Dietary deficiency
	Lack of sun exposure
	Malabsorptive syndromes
	Liver insufficiency
	Renal disease
Parathyroid resistance syndromes	Pseudohypoparathyroidism types 1a, 1b, 1c, and 2
Vitamin D resistance	Receptor-mediated
	Enzymatic synthesis defects
Medications	Bisphosphonates
	Phosphate
	Calcitonin
	Foscarnet
	Pentamidine
	Ketoconazole
	Antineoplastic medications
	Phenytoin
	Phenobarbital
Miscellaneous	Acute pancreatitis
	Massive citrated blood transfusions
	Massive tumor lysis
	Toxic shock syndrome
	Rhabdomyolysis
	Hypomagnesemia

TABLE 13.2. ADMISSION LABORATORY VALUES

Test	Result
Sodium	141 mmol/L
Potassium	4.0 mmol/L
Chloride	99 mmol/L
Bicarbonate	28 mmol/L
BUN	16 mg/dL
Creatinine	0.9 mg/dL
Glucose	71 mg/dL
Calcium	5.4 mg/dL
Phosphorus	6.3 mg/dL
Magnesium	2.1 mg/dL
Albumin	4.2 g/dL
CK	666 U/L
TSH	4.14 μU/mL

BUN, blood urea nitrogen; CK, creatine kinase; TSH, thyroid-stimulating hormone.

 Hypocalcemia must be considered in this patient. Hypocalcemia may be caused by a variety of conditions (Table 13.1). Symptomatic hypocalcemia may present with mild symptoms such as perioral paresthesias, myalgias, clumsiness, muscle spasms, and cramps, but it may also result in more serious manifestations, including seizures, cognitive impairment, movement disorders (mainly parkinsonism), psychiatric manifestations (anxiety, depression, and psychosis), papilledema, congestive heart failure, and arrhythmias (5). The presence of Chvostek and Trousseau signs is supportive of hypocalcemia. Chvostek sign may be seen in 10% to 15% of normal individuals (6), but Trousseau sign is much more specific and points strongly to hypocalcemia as a cause of symptoms in this patient.

The laboratory findings in Table 13.2 are consistent with all of the following disease processes except:

A. Hypoparathyroidism
B. Intravenous administration of phosphate
C. Administration of vitamin D in pharmacologic quantities
D. Administration of phosphate-containing enemas
E. Pseudohypoparathyroidism

Hypoparathyroidism fits this laboratory profile perfectly. Lack of parathyroid hormone leads to decreased renal phosphate excretion and diminished renal conversion of 25(OH) vitamin D to 1,25(OH)$_2$ vitamin D. This, in turn, leads to diminished renal reabsorption of calcium and intestinal calcium absorption. Hyperphosphatemia and hypocalcemia may ensue (7). Release of calcium and phosphate from the bone is diminished in this condition. Mild rhabdomyolysis with elevated muscle enzymes may occur.

Intravenous administration of phosphate (in doses of 1 to 2 g) (8) and administration of phosphate-containing enemas (through paracellular absorption in the colon) may lead to hyperphosphatemia (9). The most important short-term consequences of hyperphosphatemia are hypocalcemia and tetany. Long-term consequences of hyperphosphatemia such as soft-tissue calcification and secondary hyperparathyroidism are most commonly seen in patients with renal insufficiency and impaired renal phosphate excretion.

Administration of vitamin D in pharmacologic doses can lead to the development of hyperphosphatemia. This is mediated by the suppression of PTH secretion due to hypercalcemia and renal failure that is also induced by hypercalcemia. This patient does not have hypercalcemia or renal failure. Thus, this answer is not correct.

Pseudohypoparathyroidism fits this metabolic picture. Biochemically, resistance to PTH action represents hypoparathyroidism (hypocalcemia, with its clinical symptoms and signs, and hyperphosphatemia). However, PTH levels are elevated. Administration of exogenous PTH does not induce phosphaturic or calcemic effects in these patients (10).

The patient was treated with intravenous calcium gluconate and magnesium. This increased his plasma calcium level to 6.4 mg/dL with rapid resolution of his symptoms. The intact PTH level was 377 pg/mL (normal is 10 to 60 pg/mL).

On further questioning of the patient and family members, it was discovered that he had previously been diagnosed with pseudohypoparathyroidism (PHPT) but had not been compliant with therapy. His body habitus and intellectual difficulties in association with pseudohypoparathyroidism suggest that he has type 1a PHPT. This condition is also called Albright hereditary osteodystrophy (11) and consists of PHPT and characteristic skeletal features: short stature, round facies, and brachydactyly. Obesity, subcutaneous calcifications, and mild cognitive impairment are also common. Cataracts may result from chronic hypocalcemia.

Which one of the following therapeutic measures is most appropriate for the long-term treatment of this patient?

A. Total parathyroidectomy followed by calcium supplementation
B. Administration of intestinal phosphate binders
C. Vitamin D and calcium supplementation
D. Partial (three and a half glands) parathyroidectomy
E. Administration of pharmacologic doses of human recombinant PTH

Total parathyroidectomy has no role in the treatment of patients with hyperparathyroidism or hypoparathyroidism. The elevated PTH level in this patient is secondary to hypocalcemia and hyperphosphatemia and is not the cause of his disease. Removal of all parathyroid tissue in any patient will cause permanent hypoparathyroidism. This sometimes occurs after total thyroidectomy, radical neck dissection, and repeated surgeries for primary hyperparathyroidism. In these patients, calcium supplementation may not be sufficient to maintain eucalcemia, and vitamin D (or its analogs; Table 13.3) therapy is required in most patients (7).

Administration of phosphate binders such as aluminum hydroxide can improve hyperphosphatemia. However, this is rarely needed and generally does not correct hypocalcemia associated with PHPT (10). All serious consequences of hypoparathyroidism are mediated by hypocalcemia. Raising the plasma calcium level is of paramount importance in these patients.

The administration of vitamin D or vitamin D analogs together with calcium supplementation is a mainstay of treatment of PHPT and hypoparathyroidism. Patients with PHPT usually require smaller doses of these medications than those with hypoparathyroidism. In some patients, thiazide diuretics may be beneficial to diminish renal calcium excretion (12).

In contrast with postsurgical hypoparathyroidism (13), there are no reports of successful treatment of patients with pseudohypoparathyroidism using recombinant human PTH in any dose, presumably due to PTH resistance.

The patient was advised to take daily supplementation of calcium and vitamin D and to undergo close laboratory follow-up. He was also advised to go to the emergency room at the onset of any symptoms suggestive of hypocalcemia.

Which of the following is a desirable plasma calcium range for patients on vitamin D and calcium supplementation for hypoparathyroidism and pseudohypoparathyroidism?

A. 6.0 to 7.0 mg/dL
B. 7.0 to 8.5 mg/dL
C. 8.5 to 9.5 mg/dL
D. 9.5 to 10.5 mg/dL
E. 10.5 to 11.0 mg/dL

Symptoms of hypocalcemia are very unpleasant and may be life-threatening. Before the availability of vitamin D preparations, death from seizures and tetany was not uncommon. Patients with hypoparathyroidism should maintain a plasma calcium in the low normal range (8.5 to 9.5 mg/dL). However, levels below the normal range are acceptable if the patient remains asymptomatic. Calcium levels are best adjusted by changes in the vitamin D dose, using caution to avoid hypercalcemia from excess vitamin D.

The risk of hypercalcemia is much higher if calcium is maintained in the upper normal range. These patients also have a propensity for high urinary calcium excretion, leading to nephrolithiasis and nephrocalcinosis. Monitoring of plasma calcium levels is very important, and should be done initially every 2 to 3 days if short-acting vitamin D preparations are used (calcitriol), or weekly if long-acting forms are used. Once a stable calcium level is achieved, serum levels may be checked indefinitely at 3- to 6-month intervals to detect incipient vitamin D toxicity.

TABLE 13.3. AVAILABLE FORMS OF VITAMIN D

Form of Vitamin D	Daily Dose	Time to Effect
Calcitriol	0.25–2.25 μg	3–7 days
Dihydrotachysterol	0.2–2.4 mg	1–2 weeks
Alfacalcidol	1–3 μg	1–2 weeks
Calcidiol	25–225 μg	2–4 weeks
Ergocalciferol	1–5 mg (1 μg = 40 IU)	4–8 weeks

REFERENCES

1. Hueston WJ. Treatment of hypothyroidism. *Am Fam Physician* 2001;64:1717–1724.
2. Marx SJ. Familial hypocalciuric hypercalcemia. In: Favus MJ, ed. *Primer on the metabolic bone diseases and disorders of mineral metabolism,* 4th ed. Philadelphia: Lippincott Williams & Wilkins, 1999:195–198.

3. Bilezikian JP. Primary hyperparathyroidism. In: Favus MJ, ed. *Primer on the metabolic bone diseases and disorders of mineral metabolism,* 4th ed. Philadelphia: Lippincott Williams & Wilkins, 1999:187–195.

4. Zimmet P, Breidahl HD, Nayler WG. Plasma ionized calcium in hypomagnesemia. *Br Med J* 1968;1:622–623.

5. Tohme JF, Bilezikian JP. Hypocalcemic emergencies. *Endocrinol Metab Clin North Am* 1993;22:363–375.

6. Shane E. Hypocalcemia. In: Favus MJ, ed. *Primer on the metabolic bone diseases and disorders of mineral metabolism,* 4th ed. Philadelphia: Lippincott Williams & Wilkins, 1999:223–226.

7. Goltzman D, Cole DEC. Hypoparathyroidism. In: Favus MJ, ed. *Primer on the metabolic bone diseases and disorders of mineral metabolism,* 4th ed. Philadelphia: Lippincott Williams & Wilkins, 1999:226–230.

8. Hruska KA, Lederer ED. Hyperphosphatemia and hypophosphatemia. In: Favus MJ, ed. *Primer on the metabolic bone diseases and disorders of mineral metabolism,* 4th ed. Philadelphia: Lippincott Williams & Wilkins, 1999: 245–253.

9. Hu MS, Kayne LH, Jamgotchian N, et al. Paracellular phosphate absorption in rat colon: a mechanism for enema-induced hyperphosphatemia. *Miner Electrolyte Metab* 1997;23:7–12.

10. Levine MA. Parathyroid hormone resistance syndromes. In: Favus MJ, ed. *Primer on the metabolic bone diseases and disorders of mineral metabolism,* 4th ed. Philadelphia: Lippincott Williams & Wilkins, 1999:230–235.

11. Porter RH, Cox BG, Heaney D, et al. Treatment of hypoparathyroid patients with chlorthalidone. *N Engl J Med* 1978;298:577–581.

12. Albright F, Burnett CH, Smith PH, et al. Pseudohypoparathyroidism: example of "Seabright-Bantam syndrome": report of 3 cases. *Endocrinology* 1942;30:922–932.

13. Winer KK, Yanovski JA, Cutler GB Jr. Synthetic human parathyroid hormone 1-34 vs calcitriol and calcium in the treatment of hypoparathyroidism. *JAMA* 1996;276:631–636.

14

A 36-YEAR-OLD MAN WITH POLYDIPSIA, POLYURIA, AND NAUSEA

MARTIN E. LASCANO
RICHARD S. LANG

CASE PRESENTATION

A 36-year-old previously healthy man presented to the emergency department complaining of 2 weeks of increased thirst, frequent urination up to 10 times per day, and nausea. He had also experienced a nonproductive cough, sore throat, and nasal congestion during the same period. On the day of admission, he had two episodes of vomiting. He denied fever, chills, headache, visual changes, dyspnea, chest pain, palpitations, abdominal pain, diarrhea, dysuria, and vertigo.

The patient had been consuming about 2 gallons of fluid daily, primarily water, beer, soda, and orange juice. He noted decreased appetite for the previous 10 days, with most of his oral intake consisting of fluids, fast food, and candy. He had lost an undetermined amount of weight during this time. He admitted to consuming 12 to 20 beers daily for the prior 7 years. His last drink was on the morning of this presentation. He further admitted to using crack cocaine and marijuana, with his last use 2 days prior. He smoked up to one pack of cigarettes per day for the previous 20 years.

The patient's diabetic sister had observed his symptoms and obtained a finger-stick blood sugar that registered "HIGH." In addition to his sister, the patient's father and another sister had type 2 diabetes mellitus (DM).

Physical examination revealed a thin, mildly agitated patient who was awake, alert, and appropriately oriented. He was afebrile, with a heart rate of 86 beats per minute, respiratory rate of 18 per minute, and blood pressure of 141/84 mm Hg. Upon standing, his heart rate increased to 105 beats per minute and blood pressure decreased to 112/60 mm Hg. Oral mucosa was dry. His neck was supple without jugular venous distension. Lungs were clear to auscultation. Cardiac examination revealed no murmurs or gallops. His abdomen was soft and nontender, without organomegaly. The skin was warm and dry without any rashes or lesions. There was no lymphadenopathy. Neurologic examination did not reveal any focal abnormalities.

A urinalysis revealed a glucose level of greater than 1,000 mg/dL, 1+ ketones, and negative leukocyte esterase and nitrites. Electrolytes included sodium, 113 mmol/L; potassium, 5.5 mmol/L; chloride, 76 mmol/L; bicarbonate, 19 mmol/L; blood urea nitrogen, 15 mg/dL; creatinine, 0.8 mg/dL; and glucose, 1,489 mg/dL. Complete blood count revealed white blood cell count, 5.2 K/μL; hemoglobin, 13.9 g/dL; hematocrit, 44.8%; and platelets, 236 K/μL. Serum ketones measured positive in small amounts, and β-hydroxybutyrate was 0.3 mmol/L (normal, 0.0 to 0.3 mmol/L). Serum amylase and lipase were normal. Chest x-ray did not show any signs of acute disease.

QUESTIONS/DISCUSSION

This patient most likely has new-onset DM with diabetic ketoacidosis (DKA).

A. True
B. False

The clinical presentation of this patient is typical for new-onset diabetes. He fulfills the diagnostic criteria set by the American Diabetes Association and the World Health Organization (Table 14.1) (1). Diabetes can initially present in the form of either of its two most serious acute metabolic complications: diabetic ketoacidosis (DKA) and hyperglycemic hyperosmolar syndrome (HHS).

TABLE 14.1. CRITERIA FOR THE DIAGNOSIS OF DIABETES MELLITUS

Diagnosis of diabetes mellitus requires one of the following:
  Random plasma glucose ≥200 mg/dL with symptoms of diabetes mellitus (polyuria, polydipsia, polyphagia, rapid weight loss)
  Fasting plasma glucose ≥126 mg/dL (documented on more than one occasion)
  Plasma glucose ≥200 mg/dL, 2 h after a 75-g, oral glucose load

DKA is characterized by a marked catabolic disturbance in the metabolism of carbohydrates, protein, and fat. Its hallmark features are hyperglycemia (usually less than 600 mg/dL), increased anion-gap metabolic acidosis, and ketosis (2). DKA typically develops over less than 24 hours, and the patient may present without any prior symptoms (3). The degree of hyperglycemia is variable in these patients, with approximately 15% of patients having glucose values of less than 350 mg/dL (euglycemic DKA) (4).

In contrast, HHS can develop more slowly, over the course of several days to greater than 1 week. Its most common laboratory features include blood glucose levels of greater than 600 mg/dL, serum osmolality of 320 mOsm/L or more, and prerenal azotemia. Mild acidosis and ketosis may be present, but they are not typically the predominant features (5). Lactic acidosis due to infection or other causes may cause mild elevation of the anion gap. However, in pure HHS, the pH is greater than 7.3 and bicarbonate concentration is greater than 15 mmol/L (3). Values less than these should prompt suspicion of a mixed DKA and HHS syndrome.

Clinically, DKA and HHS have significant overlap. However, patients with HHS typically have more dramatic evidence of volume depletion (4). This patient demonstrated clear signs of volume depletion on physical examination, including dry mucosa, orthostatic tachycardia, and orthostatic hypotension. Volume depletion is a key component of the diagnosis of HHS. Although many patients in DKA are hypovolemic, evidence of volume depletion may not be as readily apparent in these patients (2). The presence of only mild amounts of serum and urine ketones and the markedly elevated blood glucose favor the diagnosis of HHS.

Further supporting the diagnosis of HHS is this patient's calculated effective plasma osmolality of 320 mOsm/L. This value is calculated using the following formula: $[2 \times (Na + K)] + (glucose/18)$. This measurement is important in patients with HHS because it defines the degree of hyperosmolality more accurately than the measured osmolality reported by the laboratory does (4,6). The calculated effective osmolality includes sodium, potassium, and glucose, while excluding urea and compounds such as alcohol that affect measured osmolality but are not osmotically active, since they permeate freely across membranes.

Both HHS and DKA can present with significant neurologic symptoms. In this patient's case, the lack of mental status changes was likely due to the mild degree of hyperosmolality, as he was able to maintain oral fluid intake (mainly free water) during the days before his presentation. The magnitude of hyperosmolality correlates well with the degree of change in mental status in these patients (2,6). Lethargy and confusion typically develop when serum osmolality exceeds 320 to 330 mOsm/L; coma is seen with values greater than 340 mOsm/L. Up to 20% to 25% of patients with HHS present with coma (7).

The pathogenesis of HHS is less clear than that of DKA. However, both disorders are thought to develop as a result of relative or partial insulin deficiency coupled with elevation of counterregulatory hormones, including glucagon, cortisol, and growth hormone (2,4). These hormonal alterations cause hyperglycemia by causing decreased utilization of glucose by muscle, fat, and liver, and increased hepatic and renal production of glucose. The lack of significant ketogenesis and subsequent acidosis in HHS is attributed to plasma insulin concentrations that are adequate to prevent lipolysis but inadequate to facilitate glucose uptake by peripheral tissues (3). Glycosuria ensues with obligatory water loss, as well as losses of sodium, potassium, and other electrolytes. As hypovolemia progresses, renal insufficiency develops, which limits the ability of the kidney to excrete glucose. This renal insufficiency worsens the hyperglycemia, and severe hyperosmolality develops, which can cause changes in mental status and coma.

Which of the following is/are potential precipitants of HHS in this patient?

A. **Infection**
B. **Diet**
C. **Substance abuse**
D. **New-onset DM**
E. **All of the above**

Table 14.2 lists the common precipitating factors of HHS and DKA. Infection is usually identified as the most common precipitant of both entities (3). This patient experienced symptoms consistent with an upper respiratory

TABLE 14.2. COMMON PRECIPITATING FACTORS OF DIABETIC KETOACIDOSIS AND HYPERGLYCEMIC HYPEROSMOLAR SYNDROME

New-onset diabetes mellitus (DM)
Poorly controlled DM (noncompliance with diet)
Discontinuation of therapy in DM (mainly in type 1 DM)
Inadequate fluid intake (mainly in type 2 DM)
Infection
Stroke
Acute pancreatitis
Myocardial infarction
Severe burns
Trauma
Renal failure
Medications
   Corticosteroids
   Thiazide diuretics
   Sympathomimetic agents
   Phenytoin
   Hyperalimentation
Substance abuse
   Alcohol
   Cocaine
Psychologic stressors

infection that coincided with his other symptoms. Even minor infections may precipitate HHS and DKA, especially when other potential precipitants are present. New-onset DM is a considerable risk factor for the development of DKA. New-onset diabetes less commonly precipitates HHS, although elderly patients who are unaware of their symptoms and unable to access fluid freely are at increased risk for HHS. Discontinuation of treatment in both type 1 and 2 diabetics may precipitate HHS and DKA, especially when combined with noncompliance with dietary recommendations. This patient reported consumption of beverages and foods high in carbohydrates, which likely contributed to the worsening of his symptoms. In addition, he had a recent history of use of crack cocaine and continued use of alcohol, both of which have been implicated in the development of HHS (8). All potential precipitants of DKA and HHS should be addressed and treated early in the course of treatment.

What type of intravenous fluid replacement is appropriate for this patient?

A. **Isotonic saline (0.9% NaCl)**
B. **Half isotonic saline (0.45% NaCl)**
C. **Half isotonic saline (0.45% NaCl) with potassium chloride**
D. **Ringer lactate**

The mainstay of the treatment of HHS is fluid replacement. These patients typically have a total body water (TBW) deficit of 20% to 25%, which represents approximately 12% of body weight. An average 70-kg patient with HHS has a fluid deficit of approximately 9 L (9). To determine appropriate fluid replacement, the corrected sodium should be calculated by adding 1.6 mmol/L for every 100-mg/dL increase in glucose above 100 mg/dL. This patient had a corrected serum sodium of 135 mmol/L. This patient had signs of hypovolemia, including orthostasis, a situation that warrants aggressive initial fluid replacement with normal saline (0.9% NaCl).

The goal of fluid replacement in HHS should be to correct about 50% of the estimated fluid deficit within the first 12 hours and the remainder of the deficit over the next 24 hours, by which time oral fluid intake may be appropriate (2). On average, 1 to 2 L of normal saline should be infused during the first hour, with the subsequent choice of fluids based on the hydration status, serum electrolytes, and urine output. Since the fluid deficit in HHS has occurred over a period of days to weeks, clinicians need to balance the need for volume repletion with the dangers of reversing the hyperosmolar state too quickly (5). Overly rapid correction of a hyperosmolar state can cause neurologic deterioration (3). The development of cerebral edema is a rare but frequently fatal complication associated with the treatment of HHS and DKA. Cerebral edema occurs almost exclusively in children with DKA (10).

While treating HHS, serum electrolytes, glucose, BUN, and creatinine should be monitored every 2 to 4 hours. Arterial blood gases are generally unnecessary unless metabolic acidosis is suspected from the patient's condition or from the anion gap in the initial set of electrolytes.

Potassium replacement should not be started with the initial intravenous fluids unless the potassium concentration is less than 4 mmol/L (4). However, clinicians need to recognize that potassium stores are frequently depleted in these patients, despite high or normal serum concentrations. Potassium concentration should be maintained between 4 and 5 mmol/L. Once renal function is stable, 20 to 40 mEq/L of potassium should be added to each liter of intravenous fluid infused.

Phosphate replacement has failed to show any beneficial effect in clinical outcomes in DKA (11). No studies reporting the effects of phosphate replacement in HHS have been reported. However, if serum phosphate concentrations are below 1.0 mg/dL, 20 to 30 mEq/L of potassium phosphate should be added to each liter of fluid to prevent potential complications of hypophosphatemia, such as muscle weakness and respiratory depression.

Bicarbonate use in DKA is controversial, with no clear benefit shown when it is administered in patients with a pH greater than 6.9 (12). In HHS, bicarbonate is clearly indicated only when life-threatening acidosis (pH < 6.9) is present due to an additional cause such as lactic acidosis.

Which of the following initial insulin regimens is appropriate for this 70-kg patient?

A. **Regular insulin, 10 U, intravenous bolus**
B. **Regular insulin, 10 U, subcutaneous**
C. **NPH insulin, 10 U, subcutaneous**
D. **Regular insulin, 4 to 7 U/hr, intravenous drip**
E. **Regular insulin, 10 U, intravenous bolus, followed by 4 to 7 U/hr, intravenous drip**

In HHS, adequate fluid replacement alone will significantly reduce hyperglycemia by correcting hypovolemia and enhancing the renal excretion of glucose. Nonetheless, insulin is usually necessary to correct hyperglycemia further. Typically, an intravenous bolus of regular insulin of 0.15 U/kg is administered before starting an intravenous drip of regular insulin at a rate of 0.05 to 0.1 U/kg/hr. Intravenous administration of insulin is preferred in these patients because low perfusion pressures can lead to erratic absorption and distribution of subcutaneous insulin (2).

Patients with HHS tend to require less insulin than patients with DKA do because they still produce some endogenous insulin. Nonetheless, it is initially important to monitor blood sugars hourly to follow the drop in plasma glucose concentration. Various algorithms to adjust the rate of insulin infusion are used (8). Typically, the expected hourly decrease in plasma glucose concentration is 50 to 75 mg/dL. If the patient is receiving appropriate hydration and the glucose is decreasing less than expected, the insulin drip may be doubled hourly until the desired steady decline is achieved.

Once the plasma glucose concentration reaches 250 to 300 mg/dL, the rate of insulin infusion should be decreased by 50%, and 5% to 10% dextrose in water could be started to avoid hypoglycemia. In DKA, the infusion of insulin and fluids containing dextrose is continued to inhibit further ketosis. Since ketosis is not the issue in HHS, once osmolality returns to normal, mental status changes resolve, and the patient can tolerate oral intake, a multiple-dose schedule of subcutaneous insulin administration should be started. This should use a combination of short- or rapid-acting and intermediate- or long-acting insulin. It is important to note that the intravenous insulin drip should be continued 1 to 2 hours after the subcutaneous regimen is begun to prevent recurrent hyperglycemia.

In known diabetics, insulin or oral treatment may be restarted at prior doses and adjusted to achieve good control. In newly diagnosed diabetics, an insulin regimen of multidose subcutaneous injections with a combination of short- or rapid-acting and intermediate- or long-acting insulin is appropriate. In type 2 diabetics, a trial of oral agents combined with dietary therapy and close follow-up is another possible treatment option. Newly diagnosed diabetics need to receive diabetic teaching, nutritional counseling, and close follow-up to prevent further acute complications of DM.

Case Conclusion

The patient received 2 L of 0.9% NaCl over 1 hour and 10 U of regular insulin as an intravenous bolus. An intravenous drip of regular insulin at 7 U/hr was started. He was transferred to a regular nursing floor, where he continued to receive intravenous fluid replacement with 0.9% NaCl with hourly capillary glucose checks. Six hours after arrival, his chemistries revealed sodium, 133 mmol/L; potassium, 3.5 mmol/L; bicarbonate, 24 mmol/L; blood urea nitrogen, 15 mg/dL; creatinine, 0.7 mg/dL; phosphorus, 2.3 mg/dL; and glucose, 476 mg/dL. Twenty mEq/L of potassium was added to each liter of fluids, and once his serum glucose concentration was below 300 mg/dL, the rate of insulin infusion was halved.

Twelve hours after admission, the patient's nausea had resolved, and he was able to tolerate oral intake. Oral potassium supplementation was given, feedings were restarted, and a regimen of multidose subcutaneous insulin administration was started, overlapping with intravenous insulin infusion for 90 minutes.

Alcohol and drug counseling, diabetic teaching, and nutrition instruction were provided. The patient was started on an oral hypoglycemic agent. Upon discharge, he was asymptomatic and follow-up was arranged for 1 week.

CONCLUSION

HHS represents an emergency that requires prompt diagnosis and implementation of therapy to prevent significant morbidity and mortality. The cornerstone of its management is the correction of volume depletion and hyperosmolality with intravenous fluids. Insulin administration and electrolyte replacement are also vital components of treatment. Potential precipitating factors should be sought, addressed, and corrected early in the course of therapy. Following recovery, prevention of further episodes should become the main goal, with institution of appropriate pharmacologic treatment, diabetic teaching, and nutrition instruction all essential components.

REFERENCES

 1. Report of the Expert Committee on the Diagnosis and Classification of Diabetes Mellitus. *Diabetes Care* 2000;23(Suppl 1):S4.
 2. Magee MF, Bhatt BA. Management of decompensated diabetes: diabetic ketoacidosis and hyperglycemic hyperosmolar syndrome. *Crit Care Clin* 2001;17:75–106.
 3. Hyperglycemic crises in patients with diabetes mellitus. *Diabetes Care* 2001;24:1988–1996.
 4. Delaney MF, Zisman A, Kettyle WM. Diabetic ketoacidosis and hyperglycemic hyperosmolar nonketotic syndrome. *Endocrinol Metab Clin North Am* 2000;29:683–705.
 5. Powers AC. Diabetes mellitus. In: Braunwald E, Fauci AS, Kasper DL, et al., eds. *Harrison's principles of internal medicine,* 15th ed. New York: McGraw-Hill, 2001:2109–2137.
 6. Siperstein MD. Diabetic ketoacidosis and hyperosmolar coma. *Endocrinol Metab Clin North Am* 1992;21:415–432.
 7. Ellemann K, Soerensen JN, Pedersen L, et al. Epidemiology and treatment of diabetic ketoacidosis in a community population. *Diabetes Care* 1984;7:528–532.
 8. Umpierrez GE, Kelly JP, Navarrete JE, et al. Hyperglycemic crises in urban blacks. *Arch Intern Med* 1997;157:669–675.
 9. Ennis ED, Stahl EJ, Kreisberg RA. The hyperosmolar hyperglycemic syndrome. *Diabetes Rev* 1994;2:115–126.
10. Matz R. How big is the risk of cerebral edema in adults with DKA? *J Crit Illn* 1996;11:768–772.
11. Fisher JN, Kitabchi AE. A randomized study of phosphate therapy in the treatment of diabetic ketoacidosis. *J Clin Endocrinol Metab* 1984;57:177–180.
12. Barnes HV, Cohen RD, Kitabchi AE, et al. When is bicarbonate appropriate in treating metabolic acidosis including diabetic ketoacidosis? In: Gitnick G, Barnes HV, Duffy TP, et al., eds. *Debates in medicine.* Chicago: Yearbook, 1990:172.

15

LEG PAIN AND ANXIETY IN A 31-YEAR-OLD WOMAN WITH CROHN DISEASE

ASHISH ATREJA
CYNTHIA C. ABACAN

CASE PRESENTATION

A 31-year-old woman was admitted with 6 months of intermittent abdominal pain and leg spasms. She had also noted increasing right leg pain for a few weeks before admission. The leg pain had increased such that she was virtually bedridden for the 2 weeks before admission. The leg spasms were precipitated by any movement of the lower extremities. Review of systems was remarkable for increased irritability, labile mood, and scalp pruritus. Her past medical history was significant for Crohn disease, with multiple bowel resections secondary to obstruction and adhesions. Her last surgery was 3 years earlier and involved the resection of 120 cm of ileum. Since that time, her weight decreased from 160 pounds to 128 pounds. On presentation, the patient's medications included a multivitamin, calcium 500 mg/day, ibuprofen, fluoxetine, and a fentanyl patch. The remainder of her history, including other surgical, social, and family history, was unrevealing.

On physical examination, she was afebrile, with a pulse of 99 beats per minute, respiratory rate of 22 per minute, and blood pressure 140/69 mm Hg. Head and neck examination showed conjunctival pallor and excoriations on the scalp. Her pulmonary and cardiac examinations were normal. Abdominal examination revealed normal bowel sounds without tenderness or organomegaly. Neurologic examination was nonfocal. Musculoskeletal examination was significant for tenderness over the ribs bilaterally and severe pain on movement of the right hip with markedly decreased range of motion.

Initial laboratory studies revealed serum calcium of 5.1 mg/dL, phosphorus of 2.3 mg/dL, magnesium of 1.5 mg/dL, and creatinine of 0.5 mg/dL. Her albumin was 3.7 g/dL, and alkaline phosphatase was 498 U/L. Transaminases, bilirubin, amylase, and lipase were all normal. Her hemoglobin was 10.3 g/dL with a mean corpuscular volume of 110 fL.

QUESTIONS/DISCUSSION

Which of the following is the most likely cause for this patient's hypocalcemia?

A. **Hypoalbuminemia**
B. **Pancreatitis**
C. **Hypoparathyroidism**
D. **Magnesium deficiency**
E. **Osteomalacia**

The most common cause of low total serum calcium is hypoalbuminemia. Since calcium is approximately 50% protein bound, the free calcium level will fluctuate based on serum albumin. Therefore, the level of metabolically active calcium can be measured by checking a serum ionized calcium level or by adjusting the calcium based on the albumin. Serum calcium corrects by a factor of 0.8 mg/dL for each 1 g/dL decrease in serum albumin [calculated calcium = measured serum calcium + 0.8 (4 − serum albumin)]. This patient's albumin was 3.7 g/dL. Adjusting for albumin, her serum calcium increased minimally, to 5.34 mg/dL. Hypoalbuminemia does not explain this patient's hypocalcemia. Her measured ionized calcium was found to be 0.7 mmol/L (normal, 1.08 to 1.30 mmol/L).

Acute pancreatitis can result in hypocalcemia by causing calcium soaps to precipitate in the abdominal cavity. Serum calcium less than 8 mg/dL is one of the criteria to predict the severity of acute pancreatitis (1). Patients with acute pancreatitis usually present with upper abdominal pain, nausea, and vomiting in the presence of elevated pancreatic enzymes. This patient did not present with acute symptoms, nor did she have elevated amylase and lipase.

Patients with hypoparathyroidism can also develop hypocalcemia. The most common acquired cause of decreased parathyroid hormone (PTH) secretion is surgery, especially thyroid surgery or radical neck surgery for head and neck cancer. Other causes of acquired hypoparathyroidism include irradiation, infiltrative diseases of the parathyroid glands, and human immunodeficiency virus (HIV) infection (2). This patient did not have any history of head and neck surgery or irradiation. Her age at presentation and the absence of a family history are atypical for congenital hypoparathyroidism. In addition, serum phosphorus is typically normal or elevated in hypoparathyroidism. However, hypoparathyroidism remains a possibility and should be excluded with appropriate laboratory evaluation.

Magnesium depletion can lead to functional hypoparathyroidism due to increased PTH resistance and decreased PTH secretion. However, this occurs only with severe magnesium depletion (serum magnesium concentrations below 0.8 mg/dL). This patient did have mild hypomagnesemia, but not to a degree to explain her hypocalcemia.

Osteomalacia is a disorder of bone matrix mineralization in adults (3). Patients often present with diffuse bone and muscle pains and may have increased irritability and anxiety. In contrast to osteoporosis, various laboratory abnormalities may be present, depending on the underlying etiology. This patient presented with many features consistent with osteomalacia, including muscle spasms, pain, hypocalcemia, hypophosphatemia, and elevated alkaline phosphatase. Based on this information, osteomalacia is the most likely explanation for this patient's hypocalcemia.

Other causes of hypocalcemia include acute and chronic hyperphosphatemia, acute respiratory alkalosis, and intravenous complexing with citrate or ethylenediamine tetraacetic acid (EDTA) (as in multiple blood transfusions). Acute hyperphosphatemia may occur in rhabdomyolysis, tumor lysis syndrome, and acute renal failure. Chronic hyperphosphatemia is nearly always due to chronic renal failure. This patient did not have any predisposing conditions for acute hyperphosphatemia, and her serum phosphorus was low. Moreover, her normal blood urea nitrogen and creatinine suggested an etiology of hypocalcemia other than chronic renal failure.

Which of the following statements regarding laboratory tests in metabolic bone disease is false?

A. **Serum calcium is typically normal in patients with osteoporosis.**
B. **Alkaline phosphatase is typically elevated in osteoporosis.**
C. **Serum phosphorus is typically normal in patients with Paget disease.**
D. **Patients with hyperparathyroidism often develop hypercalcemia.**

Osteomalacia is one of several disorders defined as part of the spectrum of metabolic bone disease. Metabolic bone disease describes those disorders that result in low bone density and strength. Other associated conditions include osteoporosis, hyperparathyroidism, Paget disease, and conditions secondary to chronic renal failure and chronic liver failure. These conditions can be differentiated on the basis of various laboratory abnormalities and radiographic features (Table 15.1).

Osteoporosis is defined as a low bone mass that results in fragile bone structure. An increased risk of fracture is associated with osteoporosis as a consequence of deterioration in bone structure. Osteoporosis is a clinical diagnosis made on the basis of a combination of risk factors for osteoporosis, clinical history, radiographic changes, and bone densitometry. Serum calcium, phosphate, and alkaline phosphatase are typically normal in osteoporosis. No serologic test is presently available to diagnose osteoporosis. However, several markers of bone turnover are available that may assist in establishing the diagnosis or screening for the disease (4). These include urine assays for N-telopeptides (NTX), free pyridinolines (Pyr), free deoxypyridinoline (Dpyr), and C-telopeptides (CTX). These biochemical markers of bone resorption can be used clinically to predict the risk of osteoporosis-related fractures and to assess the response of an osteoporotic patient to antiresorptive therapy.

Osteitis fibrosa cystica (cystic bone destruction) is a pathologic condition associated with hyperparathyroidism (5). Primary hyperparathyroidism is diagnosed by demonstrating hypercalcemia in the presence of normal to elevated parathyroid hormone levels. Some patients require parathyroidectomy based on the level of hypercalcemia and the severity of their symptoms.

Paget disease (osteitis deformans) is a disorder of excessive bone resorption. It is often an incidental finding on a radiograph. Serum calcium and phosphorus levels are usually within normal limits. However, alkaline phosphatase may be elevated, suggesting high bone turnover in these patients. There is also increased urinary excretion of hydroxyproline-containing peptides (C- and N-telopeptides). Many patients are asymptomatic and do not require therapy. Bisphosphonates have been used with success in some patients with severe pain.

Osteomalacia does not have a pathognomonic clinical finding. Since it represents a bone mineralization defect, it had traditionally been diagnosed by bone biopsy. However, a thorough history and physical examination in combina-

TABLE 15.1. LABORATORY ABNORMALITIES IN METABOLIC BONE DISEASES

Disease	Serum Calcium	Serum Phosphorus	Alkaline Phosphatase
Osteomalacia	↓→	↓→	↑
Osteoporosis	→	→	→
Paget disease	→	→	↑→
Hyperparathyroidism	↑	↓→	↑→

↓, decreased; ↑, increased; →, within normal range.

tion with noninvasive tests, such as serum calcium, phosphorus, alkaline phosphatase, and radiographs, may be sufficient for diagnosing patients with a compatible clinical presentation. A retrospective study by Bingham et al. (6) on biopsy-proven osteomalacia found no benefit for the use of PTH as a screening test; however, this study did describe measuring $1,25(OH)_2D_3$ levels as potentially useful.

This patient had hypocalcemia, hypophosphatemia, and an elevated alkaline phosphatase. Plain radiographs showed multiple fractures of the ribs, a recent fracture of the right inferior pubic ramus, and a healing fracture of the right proximal femur. A bone scan revealed multiple areas of increased uptake in the ribs bilaterally, thoracic vertebrae, left ischial tuberosity, and right proximal femur.

What is the most likely mechanism of osteomalacia in this patient?

A. **Impaired intake and/or absorption of calcium**
B. **Impaired vitamin D-25-hydroxylase activity**
C. **Impaired 25(OH)D-1-α-hydroxylase activity**
D. **Impaired target organ response to vitamin D**

Although the mechanism of osteomalacia in patients with inflammatory bowel disease (IBD) is not fully understood, the most likely explanation for osteomalacia in this patient relates to impaired calcium intake and/or absorption. There is an association between osteomalacia and vitamin D deficiency (7). This deficiency could result from a malabsorptive state as a consequence of IBD. Patients with malabsorption typically have hypophosphatemia, low to normal serum calcium, and decreased levels of 25-hydroxy vitamin D. Secondary hyperparathyroidism also frequently occurs since hypocalcemia is a potent stimulus for parathyroid hormone secretion.

1,25-Dihydroxyvitamin D $[1,25(OH)_2D_3$, calcitriol] is the active form of vitamin D. Vitamin D is primarily obtained from exposure to sunlight or through diet as cholecalciferol. In the liver, cholecalciferol is metabolized to 25-hydroxyvitamin D $[25(OH)D_3]$ by vitamin D-25-hydroxylase. Then $25(OH)D_3$ is converted in the kidneys to $1,25(OH)_2D_3$ by 25-hydroxy-D-1-α-hydroxylase. Hepatic or renal disease may cause impaired metabolic activation of vitamin D. In addition, some patients may have impaired target organ response to vitamin D, as is seen in hereditary vitamin D-resistant rickets (Table 15.2).

The mechanisms of osteomalacia can be distinguished with a complete history and appropriate laboratory testing. Decreased vitamin D_2 (25-hydroxyvitamin D) levels occur with inadequate intake or absorption. In contrast, patients with defects in hepatic or renal metabolism have decreased levels of vitamin D_3 and normal vitamin D_2 levels. Patients with hereditary vitamin D-resistant rickets have normal or elevated levels of vitamin D_3 and vitamin D_2. This patient had a vitamin D_2 level of less than 3 ng/mL (normal, 8.9 to 46.7 ng/mL), suggesting defective intake or absorption. She

TABLE 15.2. CAUSES OF OSTEOMALACIA

Deficient intake or production
  Dietary
  Inadequate sunlight exposure
Decreased absorption
  Small intestinal malabsorption
  Gastrectomy
  Hepatobiliary disease
  Chronic pancreatic deficiency
Defective metabolism
  Cirrhosis
  Anticonvulsants
  Chronic renal failure
  Tumor-associated osteomalacia
Defective target organ response
  Hereditary vitamin D–resistant rickets
Miscellaneous
  Hypophosphatemia
  Hypercalcemia
  Acidosis
  Fanconi syndrome
  Total parenteral nutrition

also had a PTH level of 651 pg/mL (normal, 10 to 60 pg/mL), consistent with secondary hyperparathyroidism as a result of severe hypocalcemia.

This patient had several conditions predisposing her to osteomalacia. She could have developed malabsorption as a result of extensive inflammatory bowel disease or multiple bowel resections causing short gut syndrome. The presence of an intact ileocolic valve provides some protection against developing bacterial overgrowth syndrome, although this could still have contributed to her malabsorption. In addition to reduced absorption, the patient may have had decreased endogenous production of vitamin D as a result of reduced exposure to sunlight from spending the majority of her time indoors over the preceding 3 years.

The management of osteomalacia aims at correcting the underlying cause. Replacement of calcium, phosphorus, and vitamin D is necessary to achieve bone healing, as evidenced by improvement in bone mineral density and urinary calcium excretion. Close monitoring of serum calcium levels is also required to monitor adequacy of replacement. Vitamin D is available in several forms. Calcidiol is a product of 25-hydroxylation of cholecalciferol in the liver, and calcitriol is produced in the kidneys by α-hydroxylation of calcidiol. Both of these have a faster onset of action and a shorter half-life than cholecalciferol. Patients who receive calcitriol have a higher prevalence of hypercalcemia; therefore, frequent monitoring of serum calcium levels is necessary. Either calcidiol or calcitriol is suitable for patients with liver disease, but calcitriol is a better alternative for patients with renal insufficiency, since they have impaired synthesis of calcitriol. Patients with malabsorption syndromes should receive parenteral vitamin D or high-dose oral vitamin D. In addition, patients should take 1 to 1.5 g of supplemental calcium per day.

Hospital Course

The patient received a bolus of intravenous calcium and a continuous calcium infusion. She was also started on intramuscular vitamin D_3 and B_{12}. Her pain, spasms, and anxiety improved considerably over the next 2 to 3 days. She was also found to have deficiencies in vitamin A, vitamin B_{12}, selenium, zinc, and chromium. She was discharged home on oral calcidiol, a multivitamin containing trace elements, and high-dose oral cobalamin. In addition, the patient was scheduled to receive weekly intramuscular injections of vitamin D (50,000 U) for 1 month. At follow-up 3 months later, the patient was asymptomatic. At that time, she had normal serum calcium, vitamin D_2, and vitamin B_{12}. Her hemoglobin and alkaline phosphatase had also improved to a near-normal range.

CONCLUSION

Metabolic bone disease predisposes patients to spontaneous fractures and carries great public health significance because of its potential morbidity and mortality. Many of these diseases can be diagnosed early and treated before the onset of major complications. Osteomalacia is a metabolic bone disease that is frequently difficult to diagnose early, since patients typically present with nonspecific symptoms. However, it is readily reversible once appropriate therapy is instituted. Therefore, awareness of the risk factors and laboratory abnormalities associated with osteomalacia can help clinicians make an early diagnosis and prevent significant morbidity and, in rare cases, mortality.

REFERENCES

1. Corfield AP, Cooper MJ, Williamson RC, et al. Prediction of severity in acute pancreatitis: prospective comparison of three prognostic indices. *Lancet* 1985;24:403–407.
2. Lehmann R, Leuzinger B, Salomon F. Symptomatic hypoparathyroidism in acquired immunodeficiency syndrome. *Horm Res* 1994;42:295–299.
3. Holick F, Krane S. Introduction to bone and mineral metabolism. In: Braunwald E, Fauci AS, Kasper DL, et al., eds. *Harrison's principles of internal medicine,* 15th ed. New York: McGraw-Hill, 2001:2192–2205.
4. Woitge HW, Seibel, MJ. Biochemical markers to survey bone turnover. *Rheum Dis Clin North Am* 2001;27:49–80.
5. Khan A, Bilezikian J. Primary hyperparathyroidism: pathophysiology and impact on bone. *CMAJ* 2000;163:184–187.
6. Bingham CT, Fitzpatrick LA. Noninvasive testing in the diagnosis of osteomalacia. *Am J Med* 1993;95:519–523.
7. Vogelsang H, Ferenci P, Woloszczuk W, et al. Bone disease in vitamin D-deficient patients with Crohn's disease. *Dig Dis Sci* 1989;34:1094–1099.

16

A 41-YEAR-OLD WOMAN WITH THINNING HAIR

MARK EVERETT ROSE
JOEL WEISBLAT
CHRISTIAN NASR

CASE PRESENTATION

A 41-year-old woman presented to the outpatient clinic with the question: "Do I have a thyroid problem?" The patient reported that her hair had been thinning during the previous 2 years. She also reported intermittent palpitations that lasted "a few seconds." The palpitations were not associated with chest pain, shortness of breath, nausea, or vomiting. She denied any change in energy level, throat fullness or pain, dysphagia, or change in voice. The patient reported no prior illnesses or prior physical examination. She had never received ionizing radiation to the neck or chest. The patient worked as a medical technologist. She denied prior history of alcohol, tobacco, or caffeine use. The patient had a cousin with an "underactive thyroid." There was no family history of thyroid malignancy.

Physical examination revealed blood pressure of 120/85 mm Hg, pulse 80 beats per minute and regular, and respiratory rate of 16 per minute. Extraocular movements were intact; pupils were equal, round, and reactive to light. Exophthalmos was not present. There was no cervical lymphadenopathy. There was a 2.5-cm smooth, firm, nontender nodule in the lower pole of the left thyroid lobe. The isthmus and right thyroid lobe were normal to palpation. The cardiac, pulmonary, and abdominal examinations were all normal. She had 5/5 strength in all muscle groups. Reflexes were 2+ throughout. She did not have a tremor.

Which of the following is the appropriate first test to evaluate the patient's thyroid nodule?

A. **Thyroid ultrasound**
B. **Fine-needle aspiration biopsy (FNAB)**
C. **Computed tomography (CT) of the neck**
D. **Thyroid stimulating hormone (TSH)**
E. **Radionuclide scan**
F. **Thyroglobulin level**

Fine-needle aspiration biopsy (FNAB) is considered the preferred initial diagnostic test to evaluate a solitary thyroid nodule (1). FNAB has a sensitivity of 83% and a specificity of 92% for thyroid carcinoma, with a diagnostic accuracy of 95% (2). The sensitivity and specificity of FNAB vary somewhat, depending on the operator. In experienced hands, FNAB has a false-negative rate of 5% and a false-positive rate of 1%. Nondiagnostic cytology rates range from 5% to 21%, with an average of 15% (3).

Thyroid ultrasound can identify thyroid size and the presence of thyroid nodules, but it cannot differentiate a malignant nodule from a benign one (4). There is ongoing debate about the utility of serial ultrasounds to evaluate nodules of less than 1 cm or nonpalpable nodules (5). Certain features suggest malignancy, including the presence of a hypoechoic lesion, poorly defined margins, or punctate calcifications (6).

CT and magnetic resonance imaging (MRI) of the neck can help in the evaluation of a goiter with a substernal component. However, neither imaging modality is preferred for the evaluation of a solitary thyroid nodule.

A radionuclide scan helps distinguish a hyperfunctioning nodule from a hypofunctioning nodule. Since neither result can completely rule out the presence of thyroid malignancy, the radionuclide scan is not considered the initial diagnostic test of choice. It is an appropriate next step if the TSH is undetectable. In this case, an autonomously functioning nodule that takes up iodine exclusively and suppresses the rest of the gland is almost never malignant. A scan is also indicated in certain situations, including determining the functional status of a nodule in Grave disease or multinodular goiter.

A thyroglobulin level helps in the serial evaluation of a patient who is status post complete thyroidectomy for thyroid malignancy; however, it is neither sensitive nor specific for the initial evaluation of a solitary thyroid nodule.

TSH aids in determining the presence of a hyperthyroid, euthyroid, or hypothyroid state. Since thyroid cancer can present in any of the three thyroid states, TSH is not helpful in determining the malignant potential of a solitary thyroid nodule (7). One exception is the presence of an undetectable TSH, in which case a radionuclide scan may be done.

A FNAB was done. The cytology was consistent with a hypercellular follicular nodule with atypia.

What is the appropriate next step in the management of this nodule?

A. **Serial ultrasounds and thyroglobulin levels**
B. **Thyroid lobectomy and isthmectomy with intraoperative frozen sections**
C. **Radioactive iodine (^{131}I) scan to determine if the nodule is hot or cold**
D. **Bone scan to look for thyroid metastases**

Although FNAB is a good tool for diagnosing papillary thyroid carcinoma, it does not differentiate benign and malignant follicular neoplasms. The current approach when a FNAB suggests a follicular neoplasm is thyroid lobectomy with isthmectomy and intraoperative frozen sections (8). If an intraoperative frozen section is consistent with minimally invasive follicular carcinoma and the tumor is unifocal without vascular invasion or extension outside the thyroid capsule, there are two treatment options. One option is TSH suppression with levothyroxine without completion thyroidectomy. The other option is to proceed with total thyroidectomy and radioactive iodine ablation. Since randomized trials have not been performed to compare the various approaches, debate continues regarding optimal management of minimally invasive follicular carcinoma. The options should be discussed with the patient.

In cases where invasive follicular carcinoma is found on frozen section, total thyroidectomy with radioactive iodine ablation and levothyroxine suppression therapy is the current standard of care. Pasieka et al. (9) found that patients who undergo completion thyroidectomy for well-differentiated follicular carcinoma have malignancy in the contralateral lobe about half of the time. Therefore, those who undergo completion thyroidectomy also receive subsequent radioactive iodine. Consequently, they are at risk for complications of surgery, notably injury to the recurrent laryngeal nerve and hypoparathyroidism, as well as the side effects of radioactive iodine.

A left-sided thyroid lobectomy and isthmectomy with intraoperative frozen sections was done. The frozen sections showed a hypercellular follicular lesion. It was determined that the right thyroid lobe would remain, with further surgery deferred pending the results of the permanent pathologic section. The permanent section showed a 1.9 cm minimally invasive follicular cell carcinoma. The options

were discussed with the patient, and she underwent a completion thyroidectomy with postoperative radioiodine ablation. Levothyroxine therapy was begun.

In a patient with follicular carcinoma who is status post near total thyroidectomy and postoperative radioiodine ablation, which of the following is appropriate postoperative follow-up?

A. **Serial TSH levels only**
B. **Serial thyroglobulin and TSH levels, serial total body iodine scans, and focused history and physical examinations**
C. **Serial history and physical examinations only**
D. **Serial bone scans to evaluate for metastatic disease**

Measurement of serial thyroglobulin and TSH levels, with serial total body iodine scans and focused history and physical examination, is the standard follow-up for patients who are status post near total thyroidectomy and postoperative radioiodine ablation (10). In this patient, serial total body iodine scans were negative for remnants of thyroid tissue in the thyroid bed or metastatic thyroid tissue. In addition, focused history and physical examinations were performed. The patient denied any dysphagia, hoarseness, dyspnea, or musculoskeletal symptoms. Physical examination did not reveal lymphadenopathy or other evidence of recurrent disease. Thyroglobulin levels remained undetectable with levothyroxine suppression.

Which of the following is a complication of radioactive iodine ablation?

A. **Radiation sickness**
B. **Transient amenorrhea within the first year of therapy**
C. **Dose-dependent sterility in men**
D. **Increased risk of bladder cancer and leukemia**
E. **All of the above**

Although this patient had not experienced any specific complications of radioactive iodine, primary care physicians need to be aware of potential complications. Acutely, patients can develop radiation sickness, which is self-limited and begins within 24 hours of treatment. Symptoms of radiation sickness include nausea, vomiting, and headache. In addition, 20% of patients will develop radiation thyroiditis, characterized by neck and ear pain, thyroid swelling and pain, and transient thyrotoxicosis if they have a significant thyroid remnant. Late complications of treatment include transient amenorrhea in 25% of women and a dose-dependent increase in miscarriage rates for the first year after therapy. Men are at risk for reduced sperm motility and permanent sterility, depending on the dose of iodine. Consequently, sperm banking is recommended for men who are planning on fathering children. There is a four in 10,000 increased annual risk for bladder cancer and five in 1,000 increased annual risk for leukemia in those who have been treated with radioactive iodine (11).

Which of the following statements is false regarding thyroid malignancies?

A. **Papillary thyroid carcinoma is the most common thyroid malignancy.**
B. **Patients with anaplastic thyroid carcinoma rarely survive more than 1 year.**
C. **Work-up of medullary carcinoma includes genetic screening of first-degree relatives.**
D. **Patients with medullary carcinoma require screening for pheochromocytoma only if they present with symptoms consistent with pheochromocytoma.**

Papillary carcinoma is the most common form of thyroid malignancy, accounting for 75% of all cases. Papillary carcinoma, like follicular carcinoma, is a differentiated carcinoma. Standard management of papillary cancer includes total thyroidectomy with postoperative radioactive iodine ablation, levothyroxine suppression, and appropriate follow-up.

Anaplastic carcinoma is the least common and most aggressive thyroid malignancy. Sugitani et al. recently reported that acute symptoms, tumor greater than 5 cm, distant metastases, and leukocytosis greater than 10 K/µL have been associated with poorer prognosis and survival rate at 6 months (12). Current therapies are essentially palliative; patients rarely live past 1 year.

Medullary carcinoma is due to a germline mutation in the RET protooncogene in approximately 20% of patients (13). Medullary thyroid carcinoma can be associated with multiple endocrine neoplasia (MEN) type IIa, MEN type IIb, and familial medullary thyroid carcinoma. Therefore, an important part of the initial diagnostic evaluation of medullary thyroid carcinoma includes a complete family history. Since MEN is an autosomal dominant condition, genetic screening for medullary thyroid cancer should be screened for in first-degree relatives when clustering is evident.

Regardless of presenting symptoms, patients with medullary carcinoma should be screened for pheochromocytoma with 24-hour urinary metanephrines and catecholamines. Screening for pheochromocytoma is especially crucial because if a pheochromocytoma is present, it needs to be resected before resection of the medullary thyroid carcinoma. Treatment of medullary thyroid carcinoma requires a total thyroidectomy with potential central neck dissection to remove all disease. Follow-up differs from papillary and follicular carcinoma in that serum calcitonin levels are an important marker of disease recurrence (13). Like any thyroid cancer, prognosis improves with early detection.

CONCLUSION

The primary care physician is frequently the physician who initially discovers a solitary thyroid nodule. Although fewer than 10% are malignant, prognosis depends on the early detection and treatment of the disease. Consequently, it is important that primary care physicians recognize and employ the appropriate evaluation of solitary thyroid nodules.

REFERENCES

1. Grant CS, Hay ID, Gough IR, et al. Long-term follow-up of patients with benign thyroid fine-needle aspiration cytologic diagnoses. *Surgery* 1989;106:980–986.
2. Gharib H, Goellner JR. Fine-needle aspiration biopsy of the thyroid: an appraisal. *Ann Intern Med* 1993;118:282–289.
3. Gharib H, Goellner JR, Johnson DA. Fine-needle aspiration cytology of the thyroid: a 12-year experience with 11,000 biopsies. *Clin Lab Med* 1993;13:699–709.
4. Hegedus L. Thyroid ultrasound. *Endocrinol Metab Clin North Am* 2001;30:339–360.
5. Asanuma K, Kobayashi S, Shingu K, et al. The rate of tumour growth does not distinguish between malignant and benign thyroid nodules. *Eur J Surg* 2001;167:102–105.
6. Burguera B, Gharib H. Thyroid incidentalomas: prevalence, diagnosis, significance, and management. *Endocrinol Metab Clin North Am* 2000;29:187–203.
7. Kraimps JL, Bouin-Pineau MH, Mathonnet M, et al. Multicentre study of thyroid nodules in patients with Graves' disease. *Br J Surg* 2000;87:1111–1113.
8. Mazzaferri EL, Kloos RT. Current approaches to primary therapy for papillary and follicular thyroid cancer. *J Clin Endocrinol Metab* 2001;86:1447–1463.
9. Pasieka JL, Thompson NW, McLeod MK, et al. The incidence of bilateral well-differentiated thyroid cancer found at completion thyroidectomy. *World J Surg* 1992;16:711–716.
10. Singer PA, Cooper DS, Daniels GH, et al. Treatment guidelines for patients with thyroid nodules and well-differentiated thyroid cancer. *Arch Intern Med* 1996;156:2165–2172.
11. Edmonds CJ, Smith T. The long-term hazards of the treatment of thyroid cancer with radioiodine. *Br J Radiol* 1986;59:45–51.
12. Sugitani I, Kasai N, Fujimoto Y, et al. Prognostic factors and therapeutic strategy for anaplastic carcinoma of the thyroid. *World J Surg* 2001;25:617–622.
13. Heshmati HM, Gharib H, van Heerden JA, et al. Advances and controversies in the diagnosis and management of medullary thyroid carcinoma. *Am J Med* 1997;103:60–69.

17

A 38-YEAR-OLD WOMAN WITH SEVERE HEADACHE

KATHERINE KEITH
JESSE T. JACOB
AMIR H. HAMRAHIAN

CASE PRESENTATION

A 38-year-old woman presented to the emergency department with a 1.5-day history of severe headache, nausea, and vomiting. The headache was gradual in onset. She described it as "a hammering in the back of her head" and "wires being pressed into her skull." The pain radiated to her neck but was not associated with neck stiffness. The headache was unlike any she had previously experienced. She could not hold down any fluids, and had episodes of nonbilious, nonbloody emesis. She had a fever of 39.1°C the previous day. Upon presentation, she noted worsening photophobia, which had developed over the previous month. She denied any other visual changes or neurologic symptoms. On review of systems, the patient noted diarrhea for 2 to 3 months, but had not had a bowel movement in the prior 2 days. Other than chronic right-upper-quadrant abdominal pain, she had no other gastrointestinal complaints. She denied any symptoms of an upper respiratory illness or recent sick contacts.

The patient's past medical history was significant for a long-standing history of difficult-to-control migraines, recently diagnosed Grave hyperthyroidism, chronic right-upper-quadrant abdominal pain of unclear etiology, anemia secondary to heavy, irregular menses from uterine fibroids, and anxiety disorder. She had undergone a nondiagnostic laparotomy 4 years earlier for the chronic abdominal pain. She was taking sertraline and lorazepam for anxiety. She denied the use of tobacco, alcohol, or illicit drugs.

Grave disease was diagnosed 1 month before admission. She first noted symptoms 3 to 4 months before diagnosis, which, upon admission, included fatigue, insomnia, diarrhea, tremors, myalgias, palpitations, mood swings, heat intolerance, mild photophobia, and difficulty climbing stairs. She had lost 30 pounds during the 3 to 4 weeks before presentation. The patient had received radioactive iodine (^{131}I) therapy with 26 mCi of ^{131}I 2 days before this admission. Before receiving ^{131}I, the patient had been treated with extended-release metoprolol 50 mg twice a day. Outpatient thyroid function testing included thyroid stimulating hormone (TSH) of less than 0.004 μU/mL, T4 of 45.2 μg/dL, T3 of 453 ng/dL, T4 uptake of 0.8, and free thyroxine index (FTI) of 56.5 μg/dL. Four-hour ^{131}I uptake was 58.8%, with a predicted 24-hour uptake of 62.8%.

QUESTIONS/DISCUSSION

Which of the following is/are potential etiologies of this patient's symptoms?

A. Migraine
B. Meningitis
C. Subarachnoid hemorrhage
D. Thyroid storm
E. All of the above

All of the preceding need to be considered in the differential diagnosis of this patient's symptoms. Bacterial meningitis, thyroid storm, and subarachnoid hemorrhage are life-threatening conditions; therefore, prompt diagnosis is imperative.

Migraines are generally described as throbbing, unilateral headaches that are often associated with photophobia, phonophobia, nausea, and vomiting. The onset is variable but is generally not sudden. Classic migraines are associated with an aura, which is a feeling or symptom that the patient comes to recognize as heralding the onset of the headache. Auras are usually visual but may be auditory, gustatory, or any of a number of other neurologic symptoms. Less frequently, patients temporarily experience more frightening neurologic symptoms, such as numbness or weakness. The headache may have predictable precipitants, including menstruation or certain foods. Patients usually have a history of similar headaches and/or a family history of migraines. Fever is not typically associated. Although not all of this patient's symptoms are typical of migraines, migraines could explain her presentation.

The triad of fever, neck stiffness, and mental status change suggests meningitis (1). Bacterial meningitis may be difficult to differentiate from viral meningitis based on signs and symptoms alone, unless the patient is in shock or has a typical meningococcal rash, in which case a bacterial cause is overwhelmingly probable. Both bacterial and viral meningitis are associated with severe headache, photophobia, nausea, and vomiting, all of which this patient was experiencing. Fever is usually present, although a patient in shock may be hypothermic. Bacterial meningitis can be fatal within a few hours. If meningitis is suspected, a lumbar puncture (LP) for cerebrospinal fluid (CSF) evaluation is necessary. If there is a question of increased intracranial pressure (ICP) or if focal neurologic findings are present on physical examination, computed tomography (CT) of the head should precede an LP.

Headaches associated with subarachnoid hemorrhage are usually described as sudden in onset, like a "thunderclap," and the worst headache of the patient's life. Such headaches are also often associated with photophobia, nausea, and vomiting. Fever may be present, and nuchal rigidity frequently develops (2). Since the source of bleeding is arterial, signs of increased ICP may quickly develop, including a decreased level of consciousness, papilledema, decerebrate posturing, and the triad of bradycardia, decreased respiratory rate, and third nerve palsy (2). Death may occur within minutes to hours if definitive surgical treatment is not performed. Given the greater likelihood of increased ICP in these patients, a noncontrast CT of the head should be the first diagnostic test. If CT does not reveal bleeding or evidence of increased ICP, an LP should be performed to evaluate for blood or xanthochromia in the CSF (2).

Thyroid storm is a severe and life-threatening form of thyrotoxicosis, carrying a mortality rate of 20% to 50% (3). Thyroid storm needs to be considered in any patient with a goiter and/or history of hyperthyroidism who presents with fever, tachycardia, and/or mental status changes, including agitation, delirium, psychosis, extreme lethargy, or coma (3). Other common symptoms include nausea, vomiting, and diarrhea. These symptoms represent an exaggeration of the usual symptoms of hyperthyroidism (4).

Case Continued. Physical examination revealed a tremulous woman in mild distress. Her temperature was 37.5°C; pulse, 105 beats per minute; respiratory rate, 36 per minute; blood pressure, 142/59 mm Hg; and oxygen saturation, 97% on room air. Extraocular movements were intact. There was no obvious proptosis, but the patient noted diplopia on visual field examination. Funduscopic examination revealed crisp disc margins. A tender, diffusely enlarged thyroid, estimated to weigh at least 80 g, without discrete nodules was noted. A prominent bruit was heard over the thyroid. Jugular venous distension was present to the angle of the jaw. The neck was

supple with full range of motion and without nuchal rigidity. Cardiac examination revealed tachycardia, third and fourth heart sounds, and a grade II/VI diastolic murmur at the left sternal border. Her lungs were clear, and the abdominal examination was remarkable only for tenderness to palpation in the right upper quadrant. No extremity edema was noted. Neurologic examination was significant for hyperreflexia and proximal muscle weakness. No rash or skin discoloration was present.

Laboratory data on admission revealed normal electrolytes, blood urea nitrogen, creatinine, and complete blood count, except for hemoglobin of 9.2 g/dL and hematocrit of 27.8%. Repeat thyroid function tests (TFTs) revealed TSH of 0.92 μU/mL, T4 of 34.6 μg/dL, T3 of 547 ng/dL, and T4 uptake of 0.2. The free thyroxine index could not be calculated.

The most likely diagnosis for this patient is thyroid storm. She had a precipitant history of recently diagnosed hyperthyroidism and administration of RAI 2 days before presentation in the presence of exaggerated signs and symptoms of hyperthyroidism. In addition, her physical examination was significant for tachycardia and signs of congestive heart failure (third and fourth heart sounds and jugular venous distension). As a result of these findings and the laboratory data, thyroid storm was diagnosed. Given the high likelihood of this diagnosis, neither a CT of the head nor a lumbar puncture was performed in this patient.

Which of the following is not considered a diagnostic criterion for thyroid storm?

A. **Nausea and vomiting**
B. **Tachycardia**
C. **Tremor**
D. **Fever**
E. **Pulmonary edema**

Burch and Wartofsky (3) have outlined criteria for the diagnosis and assessment of thyroid storm (Table 17.1). The six criteria are divided into thermoregulatory dysfunction, central nervous system (CNS) effects, gastrointestinal (GI)/hepatic dysfunction, cardiovascular dysfunction, congestive heart failure (CHF), atrial fibrillation, and precipitant history (3). Specific findings within each of these categories are assessed point values, and a cumulative score is determined that assists clinicians in assessing the severity of thyroid storm. The maximum possible score is 130. A score of 45 or greater highly suggests thyroid storm, whereas a score of 25 to 44 suggests impending storm, and a score of 25 or less makes thyroid storm unlikely (3).

The criteria utilized by Burch and Wartofsky assign greater point values for progressively higher temperatures. Central nervous system criteria range from mild (agitation) to moderate (delirium, psychosis, and extreme lethargy) to severe (seizure and coma). Tremor by itself is not one of the neurologic criteria. Moderate gastrointestinal effects include diarrhea, nausea/vomiting, and abdom-

TABLE 17.1. DIAGNOSTIC CRITERIA FOR THYROID STORM

	Point Value
Thermoregulatory Dysfunction	
Temperature (°F)	
99–99.9	5
100–100.9	10
101–101.9	15
102–102.9	20
103–103.9	25
104.0	30
Central Nervous System Effects	
Absent	0
Mild	10
Agitation	
Moderate	20
Delirium	
Psychosis	
Extreme lethargy	
Severe	30
Seizure	
Coma	
Gastrointestinal–Hepatic Dysfunction	
Absent	0
Moderate	10
Diarrhea	
Nausea/vomiting	
Abdominal pain	
Severe	20
Unexplained jaundice	
Cardiovascular Dysfunction	
Tachycardia	
90–109	5
110–119	10
120–129	15
130–139	20
140	25
Congestive Heart Failure	
Absent	0
Mild	5
Pedal edema	
Moderate	10
Bibasilar rales	
Severe	15
Pulmonary edema	
Atrial Fibrillation	
Absent	0
Present	10
Precipitant History	
Negative	0
Positive	10

From Burch HB, Wartofsky L. Life-threatening thyrotoxicosis: thyroid storm. *Endocrinol Metab Clin North Am* 1993;22:263–277, with permission.

inal pain, whereas severe gastrointestinal effects include unexplained jaundice. Cardiovascular dysfunction is quantified according to the degree of tachycardia. Congestive heart failure ranges from mild (pedal edema) to moderate (bibasilar rales) to severe (pulmonary edema). Atrial fibrillation is classified as either absent or present. The final criterion is evidence of any precipitant history (3). Precipitants of thyroid storm include thyroid or nonthyroid surgery, trauma, infection, and, as in this case, an iodine load (5).

Based on this patient's symptoms and diagnostic studies, which of the following management strategies is not appropriate?

A. Ablation with ^{131}I (RAI)
B. Thyroidectomy
C. β-blocker and a thionamide (propylthiouracil or methimazole)
D. Lugol solution
E. Corticosteroids

^{131}I ablation is contraindicated in this patient because of the severity of her presenting symptoms and her TFTs. ^{131}I quickly becomes concentrated within the thyroid gland, causing tissue damage and release of preformed thyroid hormone into the circulation. As a result, the symptoms of hyperthyroidism may initially worsen. In a patient with symptoms suggestive of severe hyperthyroidism, ^{131}I may induce thyroid storm (5). Pretreatment with a thionamide and β-blocker is indicated for patients with severe hyperthyroidism, the elderly, or patients with underlying heart disease. ^{131}I is also contraindicated in pregnant patients, patients who are breast-feeding, and patients with active ophthalmopathy. RAI may worsen Grave ophthalmopathy (6).

Thyroidectomy is utilized in special circumstances. Indications for thyroidectomy include a goiter causing compression of underlying structures; a very large goiter that is unlikely to shrink adequately upon becoming euthyroid, thus creating a cosmetic problem; or the presence of a coexisting nodule. Rarely, a patient who is fearful of radioactivity or cannot tolerate other therapies may also benefit from surgery (7).

β-Blockers, such as metoprolol, attenuate the hyperadrenergic response and can decrease symptoms. Propylthiouracil (PTU) acts by inhibiting both the peripheral conversion of T4 to T3 and the oxidation of iodine in the thyroid. Methimazole, which acts by only the latter mechanism, may also be useful since it decreases thyroid hormone synthesis within hours of administration. These agents may induce remission when taken for up to 2 years, but permanent remission is achieved in only 20% to 30% of patients. They are more frequently used to achieve euthyroid states before ablation or surgery (7).

Lugol solution, supersaturated potassium iodide, or iopanoic acid (an oral contrast agent) contains iodine and inhibits peripheral conversion of T4 to T3. Lugol solution is generally avoided as primary therapy because of the possibility of inducing resistant hyperthyroidism. However, together with methimazole and a β-blocker, Lugol solution may quickly ameliorate symptoms. It may also be used in patients who are allergic to thionamides (7).

Corticosteroids inhibit the peripheral conversion of T4 to T3, as well as the release of hormones from the gland in Grave hyperthyroidism. Steroids are generally reserved for patients with severe hyperthyroidism. Convincing evidence demonstrating the efficacy of corticosteroids is lacking (4).

This patient had a mild form of thyroid storm. Based on Burch and Wartofsky's criteria, her score was 55. During hospitalization, the dose of metoprolol was increased, decreasing her heart rate into the 80s by the time of discharge. She was also started on intravenous dexamethasone 2 mg every 6 hours and discharged on tapering doses of prednisone. Initial treatment with ketorolac and promethazine only provided temporary mild relief of her headache, nausea, and vomiting. Administration of prochlorperazine per rectum relieved her headache and nausea. She was discharged 2 days after admission without headache, nausea, vomiting, fever, or signs of heart failure.

CONCLUSION

Thyroid storm can have devastating, even fatal, consequences if not promptly treated. The symptoms of thyroid storm can closely resemble those associated with several common conditions. Clinicians need to recognize and understand the precipitants and manifestations of thyroid storm in order to make a prompt diagnosis and begin appropriate treatment.

REFERENCES

1. Attia J, Hatala R, Cook DJ, et al. The rational clinical examination. Does this adult patient have acute meningitis? *JAMA* 1999; 282:175–181.
2. Edlow JA, Caplan LR. Avoiding pitfalls in the diagnosis of subarachnoid hemorrhage. *N Engl J Med* 2000;342:29–36.
3. Burch HB, Wartofsky L. Life-threatening thyrotoxicosis: thyroid storm. *Endocrinol Metab Clin North Am* 1993;22:263–277.
4. Ross DS. Treatment of thyroid storm. UpToDate Online, November 19, 2001, *www.uptodate.com*, Version 10.3.
5. Weetman AP. Controversy in thyroid disease. *J R Coll Physicians Lond* 2000;34:374–380.
6. Woeber KA. Update on the management of hyperthyroidism and hypothyroidism. *Arch Fam Med* 2000;9:743–747.
7. Ross DS. Treatment of Graves' hyperthyroidism. UpToDate Online, August 29, 2001, *www.uptodate.com*, Version 10.3.

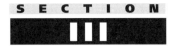

SECTION

III

GASTROENTEROLOGY

18

A 57-YEAR-OLD MAN WITH NEW-ONSET ASCITES

RONY M. ABOU-JAWDE
GABRIEL BOU MERHI
TAREK MEKHAIL
WILLIAM D. CAREY

CASE PRESENTATION

A 57-year-old man presented with increasing abdominal girth, lower-extremity edema, and generalized weakness. He had been well until 3 months before presentation, at which time these symptoms gradually developed. He also complained of diffuse crampy abdominal pain and dyspnea on exertion but denied orthopnea or paroxysmal nocturnal dyspnea. The patient denied any fever, night sweats, chest pain, palpitations, nausea, vomiting, melena, rectal bleeding, or change in urine output. He had no previous history of blood transfusion, alcohol intake, or exposure to tuberculosis. He had quit smoking 20 years earlier. He reported no family history of malignancy, hematologic disorders, or liver disease.

On physical examination, the patient was afebrile with normal vital signs and in no acute distress. There was no scleral icterus. His heart and lung examinations were unremarkable. His abdomen was tensely distended with a positive fluid wave, and superficial venous collaterals were present. The liver was not palpable; however, there was evidence of massive splenomegaly with a spleen tip palpable 15 cm below the left costal margin. Extremities showed 2+ pedal edema with good peripheral pulses.

Laboratory studies revealed a white blood cell count of 10.39 K/μL, with 12% metamyelocytes, 3% blasts, and 5% nucleated red blood cells. The hemoglobin was 9.2 g/dL, and the platelet count was 113,000/μL. A peripheral blood smear showed neutrophilic leukocytosis, leukoerythroblastic changes, and thrombocytopenia. His electrolytes, renal function, and hepatic profile were normal. Viral hepatitis serologies were negative. His urinalysis was negative for proteinuria. An echocardiogram showed normal left and right ventricular function, without valvular pathology. His chest x-ray (CXR) did not show bony, mediastinal, or parenchymal pathology. No pleural effusion was present. Abdominal ultrasound showed patent hepatic vasculature (portal, hepatic, and splenic veins), large-volume ascites, a normal liver texture and size, and an enlarged spleen.

QUESTIONS/DISCUSSION

Based on the preceding, what is the most likely cause of this patient's ascites?

A. Heart failure
B. Liver failure (cirrhosis)
C. Renal failure
D. None of the above

Heart failure and renal failure are very unlikely to be the cause of this patient's ascites, given the presence of normal renal function, an unremarkable urinalysis, normal echocardiogram, and a normal CXR. In contrast, cirrhosis is difficult to exclude at this point. In order to further evaluate the ascites, a paracentesis was done, with removal of 6 L of clear fluid.

Which of the following ascitic fluid findings is helpful in differentiating portal hypertension-associated ascites from nonportal hypertension-associated ascites?

A. Serum-ascites albumin gradient (SAAG)
B. Absolute neutrophil count
C. Ascitic fluid culture
D. Ascitic fluid lactate dehydrogenase (LDH)

Peritoneal fluid analysis may help to determine if the ascites is due to portal hypertension, if the ascitic fluid is infected, and if the ascites is reflective of an unusual presentation of an underlying disease, such as a malignancy. Table 18.1 summarizes the results of this patient's ascitic fluid analysis. Ascitic fluid cytology is shown in Fig. 18.1.

TABLE 18.1. ASCITIC FLUID ANALYSIS

- Red blood cells: 3,900/mL
- White blood cells: 900/mL (neutrophils, 15%; lymphocytes, 35%; monocytes, 42%; reactive cells, 5%)
- Lactate dehydrogenase (LDH): 454 U/L; total protein, 2.8 g/dL; albumin, 1.2 g/dL
- Serum ascites albumin gradient (SAAG): 1.7
- Cytology: negative for malignant cells; multinucleated giant cells consistent with megakaryocytes (Fig. 18.1)
- Cultures (bacterial, fungal, and mycobacterial): negative

TABLE 18.2. CLASSIFICATION OF ASCITES

Portal Hypertension-Related (SAAG >1.1)	Nonportal Hypertension-Related (SAAG <1.1)
Sinusoidal	TB peritonitis
Cirrhosis	Ruptured viscous peritonitis
Spontaneous bacterial peritonitis	Peritoneal carcinomatosis
Hepatitis	Pancreatitis
Liver metastasis	Vasculitis
Hepatocellular carcinoma	
Postsinusoidal	
Constrictive pericarditis	
Right-sided heart failure	
Budd–Chiari	
Venoocclusive disease	
Tricuspid insufficiency	
Presinusoidal	
Portal vein thrombosis	
Splenic vein thrombosis	
Schistosomiasis	

SAAG, serum ascites albumin gradient.

Table 18.2 summarizes the classification of ascites. The serum-ascites albumin gradient, or SAAG, is very helpful in differentiating the different causes of ascites. It is calculated by subtracting the ascitic albumin concentration from the serum albumin concentration. In this patient, the serum albumin was 2.9 g/dL and the ascitic albumin was 1.2 g/dL. Hence the SAAG was 1.7. Based on the elevated SAAG, portal hypertension-induced ascites was considered the likely etiology.

Further work-up included computed tomography (CT scan) of the abdomen, which revealed ascites, splenomegaly, and evidence of mesenteric stranding and peritoneal nodularity, consistent with peritoneal carcinomatosis (Fig. 18.2). Transjugular liver biopsy with pressure measurements revealed the following: right atrial systolic pressure, 12 mm Hg; inferior vena cava, 14 mm Hg; right hepatic venous pressure, 12 mm Hg; wedge hepatic venous pressure, 20 mm Hg; and a corrected wedge/gradient (wedge hepatic venous pressure minus right hepatic venous pressure), 8 mm Hg. These findings are consistent with mild portal hypertension. The right hepatic vein was widely patent. Liver biopsy revealed normal hepatic parenchyma without

evidence of fibrosis. Clusters of cells infiltrating the sinusoids, compatible with extramedullary hematopoiesis, were present.

These additional tests effectively ruled out cirrhosis, spontaneous bacterial peritonitis, hepatitis, and liver metastases as causes of the portal hypertension-induced ascites. Bone marrow aspirate and biopsy done to evaluate the anemia and thrombocytopenia were diagnostic for myelofibrosis.

FIGURE 18.1. Ascitic fluid cytology. Within a mixed cellular background of granulocytes, monocytes, and lymphocytes, there were occasional typical **(left)** and atypical **(right)** megakaryocytes (Wright–Giemsa, original magnification 100×).

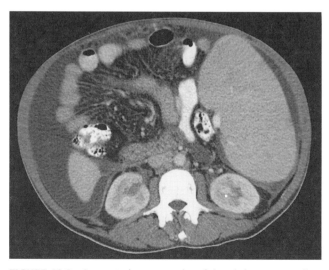

FIGURE 18.2. Computed tomography of the abdomen revealing splenomegaly, ascites, mesenteric stranding, and peritoneal nodularity. The liver appears normal in texture.

Myelofibrosis

Myelofibrosis, also known as agnogenic myeloid metaplasia, is a disorder of unknown etiology involving multipotent hematopoietic stem cells. Common features of myelofibrosis include bone marrow fibrosis, splenomegaly, extramedullary hematopoiesis, and myeloid metaplasia with a leukoerythroblastic blood smear. Most patients are asymptomatic in the early phases of the disease and are diagnosed as part of an evaluation for splenomegaly incidentally detected on physical examination. Some may present with hematologic manifestations, abdominal symptoms related to the mass effect of an enlarged spleen (1), or symptoms of a hypercatabolic state, such as weight loss, fatigue, night sweats, and low-grade fever (2).

Approximately 10% of patients with myelofibrosis present with ascites. A similar percentage also present with portal hypertension and evidence of esophageal varices (3). Some reports have indicated that myelofibrosis may present as ascites secondary to seeding of the peritoneum by myelometaplastic cells (1).

Multiple etiologies and mechanisms have been proposed to explain the development of portal hypertension and ascites in the setting of myelofibrosis (Table 18.3). One contributing factor for portal hypertension can be increased blood flow through the portal system, known as "forward hypertension." (1). Increased blood flow may be due to splenomegaly, with flow in the splenic vein increasing to 3,000 mL/min, up from the normal rate of 100 mL/min (4). Portal pressures measured before and after splenectomy confirm increased splenic blood flow in extramedullary hematopoiesis (5,6). However, ascites may occur even in splenectomized patients with myelofibrosis (7). Portal hypertension secondary to portal vein or hepatic vein thrombosis (Budd–Chiari syndrome) occurs in some patients with myelofibrosis (8).

Extensive portal zone infiltration by primitive hematopoietic cells might cause intrahepatic perisinusoidal obstruction and contribute to portal hypertension. In cases described, the wedge hepatic venous pressure was normal, but intrasplenic pressure was increased (9).

Rarely, widespread thrombotic occlusions can cause obliterative portal venopathy secondary to smaller portal vein involvement. This venopathy eventually leads to a nodular regenerative hyperplasia, causing increased portal outflow resistance and sinusoidal hypertension (10).

Myelofibrosis is characterized by extramedullary hematopoiesis, mostly in the reticuloendothelial organs, such as the spleen, liver, and lymph nodes (11). However, organs such as the kidneys, pancreas, adrenal glands, heart, retroperitoneum, stomach, epididymis, gallbladder, ovaries, skin, and pleura and omentum can also be involved (12). Ectopic implants in the peritoneum may result in the development of ascites. The occurrence of such a condition is rare, and ascites from extramedullary hematopoiesis is even rarer as the initial presentation of myelofibrosis (1,13). Some reports have suggested that peritoneal involvement could result from minute spontaneous splenic ruptures (7). Others described these foci as "metastatic lesions," causing ascites due to obstruction of lymphatic ducts by extramedullary foci or due to increased permeability of the capillaries (1). Silverman et al. have suggested that the most likely mechanism of ascites formation is desquamation of the myeloid and megakaryocytic cells into the peritoneum (11). Megakaryocytes are rarely found in the peritoneum or in the ascitic fluid and are highly suggestive of peritoneal extramedullary hematopoiesis (7). In one study examining almost 5,000 peritoneal and pleural fluid samples, only five samples (0.1%) had megakaryocytes, of which three had myelofibrosis, one had lymphoma, and one had chronic myelogenous leukemia (7). Accordingly, cytologic analysis should be performed in all cases of ascites and myelofibrosis.

Based on the multiple possible pathophysiologic mechanisms and etiologies responsible for ascites in extramedullary hematopoiesis, it is crucial to determine the factors contributing to the ascites in myelofibrosis in order to treat appropriately.

Which of the following is/are potentially appropriate treatments for ascites from extramedullary hematopoiesis?

A. Splenectomy
B. Chemotherapy
C. Radiation
D. Serial paracenteses
E. All of the above

Several treatment options are available to treat myelofibrosis and its complications (Table 18.4). Most of the treatment is supportive and ultimately palliative. Serial paracenteses are often required for relief of symptoms due to rapid fluid accumulation. Splenectomy, in good surgical candidates, can be used for refractory anemia and relief from symptomatic splenomegaly and portal hypertension, but this modality is typically not very effective (14). Some investigators have even attributed a more aggressive clinical course of myelofibrosis with splenectomy (2). Alkylating agents such as hydroxyurea or busulfan can be used for

TABLE 18.3. POTENTIAL ETIOLOGIES OF MYELOFIBROSIS CAUSING PORTAL HYPERTENSION

Proposed Etiologies	Proposed Mechanisms
"Forward hypertension"	Increased blood flow due to splenomegaly
Portal or hepatic vein thrombosis	Increased splanchnic blood flow resistance
Intrahepatic perisinusoidal obstruction	Portal zone infiltration due to EMH

EMH, extramedullary hematopoiesis.

TABLE 18.4. TREATMENT MODALITIES FOR MYELOFIBROSIS AND ITS COMPLICATIONS

Treatment Options	Indications	Outcomes/Comments
Splenectomy	RA, PHT, splenomegaly	Possibly more aggressive
Alkylating agents	Hematologic/ascites control	MF
Radiation	Nonhepatosplenic EMH	Not effective
Leveen shunt	Intractable ascites	Cytopenia, no survival benefit
Intraperitoneal cytarabine (Ara-C)	EMH-induced ascites	Old procedure
		Case reports

EMH, extramedullary hematopoiesis; PHT, portal hypertension; MF, myelofibrosis; RA, refractory anemia.

hematologic control of disease, for symptom control, and for prevention of ascites, but none of these agents has been consistently effective (1,15).

Hematopoietic tissues in bone marrow or at extramedullary sites are highly sensitive to radiation therapy. Radiation therapy may be very useful in treating symptomatic, nonhepatosplenic extramedullary hematopoiesis, such as in patients with spinal cord compression or with pleural or peritoneal involvement (2,7,15–17). In one study of 23 patients with myelofibrosis and myeloid metaplasia, splenic irradiation resulted in transient reduction in splenic size in more than 90% of patients for a mean duration of 6 months; however, 26% developed severe myelosuppression (2). Sixty-two percent of patients treated with radiotherapy for symptomatic hepatomegaly, with or without ascites, became cytopenic, with two patients dying. An objective response did not always occur, although most patients had subjective relief. However, this relief lasted only for a median of 3 months, without a survival benefit (2). This study did not evaluate the role of radiotherapy in earlier stages of myelofibrosis with peritoneal implants and secondary ascites. Presently, no specific treatment has shown a sustained response and favorable effect on survival for patients with ascites secondary to myelofibrosis.

CONCLUSION

This patient presented with new-onset ascites, which is an unusual initial manifestation of myelofibrosis. There was no evidence of cardiac or renal disease. Cytologic analysis of the ascitic fluid revealed megakaryocytes, suggesting extramedullary hematopoiesis. The elevated SAAG was suggestive of portal hypertension-induced ascites. However, the mild degree of hepatic wedge pressure elevation could not adequately explain the severity of the patient's ascites. CT of the abdomen was consistent with peritoneal nodularity and suggestive of peritoneal carcinomatosis (EMH deposits). Liver biopsy confirmed the presence of extramedullary hematopoiesis, and bone marrow biopsy revealed myelofibrosis. The patient was treated conserva-

tively with diuretics and frequent abdominal paracenteses for symptom relief.

This case demonstrates several important features in the approach to patients with ascites. Not all ascites develops as a result of cirrhosis, heart failure, or renal failure. Patients with new-onset ascites need a paracentesis, with specific fluid analysis and calculation of the SAAG to categorize the ascites for diagnostic and management purposes. Less common causes of ascites, such as extramedullary hematopoiesis, need to remain part of the differential diagnosis in patients presenting with ascites.

REFERENCES

1. Hung SC, Huang ML, Liu SM, et al. Massive ascites caused by peritoneal extramedullary hematopoiesis as the initial manifestation of myelofibrosis. *Am J Med Sci* 1999;318:198–200.
2. Tefferi A, Jimenez T, Gray LA, et al. Radiation therapy for symptomatic hepatomegaly in myelofibrosis with myeloid metaplasia. *Eur J Haematol* 2001;66:37–42.
3. Ward HP, Block MH. The natural history of agnogenic myeloid metaplasia (AMM) and a critical evaluation of its relationship with the myeloproliferative syndrome. *Medicine* 1971;50:357–420.
4. Dudley FJ, Cebon J, Ireton HJ. A 70-year-old man with portal hypertension. *Aust N Z J Med* 1985;15:461–467.
5. Sullivan A, Rheinlander H, Weintraub LR. Esophageal varices in agnogenic myeloid metaplasia: disappearing after splenectomy: a case report. *Gastroenterology* 1974;66:429–432.
6. Schwartz SI. Myeloproliferative disorders. *Ann Surg* 1975;182:464–471.
7. Oren I, Goldman A, Haddad N, et al. Ascites and pleural effusion secondary to extramedullary hematopoiesis. *Am J Med Sci* 1999;318:286–288.
8. Aufses AH Jr. Bleeding varices associated with hematologic disorders. *Arch Surg* 1960;80:655–659.
9. Shaldon S, Sherlock S. Portal hypertension in the myeloproliferative syndrome and the reticuloses. *Am J Med* 1962;32:758–764.
10. Wanless IR, Godwin TA, Allen F, et al. Nodular regenerative hyperplasia of the liver in hematologic disorders: a possible response to obliterative portal venopathy. A morphometric study of nine cases with a hypothesis on the pathogenesis. *Medicine* 1980;50:367–379.
11. Silverman JF. Extramedullary hematopoietic ascitic fluid cytology in myelofibrosis. *Am J Clin Pathol* 1985;84:125–128.
12. Pitcock JA, Reinhard EH, Justin BW, et al. A clinical and patho-

logical study of seventy cases of myelofibrosis. *Ann Intern Med* 1962;57:73–84.

13. Stahl RL, Hoppstein L, Davidson TG. Intraperitoneal chemotherapy with cytosine arabinoside in agnogenic myelofibrosis with myeloid metaplasia and ascites due to peritoneal extramedullary hematopoiesis. *Am J Hematol* 1993;43:156–157.

14. Glew RH, Haese WH, McIntyre PA. Myeloid metaplasia with myelofibrosis. The clinical spectrum of extramedullary hematopoiesis and tumor formation. *Johns Hopkins Med J* 1973;132:253–270.

15. Patel NM, Kurtides ES. Ascites in agnogenic myeloid metaplasia: association with peritoneal implant of myeloid tissue and therapy. *Cancer* 1982;50:1189–1190.

16. Crawford DC, Nightingale S, Bates D, et al. Spinal cord compression by extramedullary haematopoiesis in myelofibrosis. *Postgrad Med J* 1984;60:62–63.

17. Jacobs P, Wood L, Robson S. Refractory ascites in the chronic myeloproliferative syndrome: a case report. *Am J Hematol* 1991; 37:128–129.

19

A 73-YEAR-OLD MAN WITH FEVER AND JAUNDICE

MOHAMMED S. GHANAMAH
AARON BRZEZINSKI

CASE PRESENTATION

A 73-year-old man presented to the emergency department with right-upper-quadrant pain, fever, chills, and jaundice. The patient developed severe, sharp, and constant pain 1 day before presentation. The pain did not radiate. He did not recall anything that specifically made the pain better or worse. The pain was associated with fever up to 38.1°C and chills. There was associated nausea without vomiting. Over this same period, he also noticed that his urine was darker than usual. The patient also noticed a yellowish discoloration of his skin and eyes. He denied any weight loss.

His past medical history included obesity, obstructive sleep apnea, chronic atrial fibrillation, and osteoporosis. Past surgical history included bilateral knee replacements and an inguinal hernia repair. The patient's medications on admission included furosemide, warfarin, and oxycodone as needed for pain. He denied alcohol intake or intravenous drug use. There was no history of previous blood transfusion.

On physical examination, the patient was in pain and fully oriented. His vital signs included a temperature of 39°C orally, blood pressure of 100/60 mm Hg, pulse of 90 beats per minute, and respiratory rate of 22 per minute. His skin and sclerae were icteric. Pulmonary and cardiac examinations were normal. Abdominal examination revealed right-upper-quadrant tenderness to deep palpation, without rebound or rigidity. Murphy sign was negative, and there was no hepatosplenomegaly or palpable masses.

QUESTIONS/DISCUSSION

Which of the following diagnoses is least likely in this patient?

A. **Acute cholecystitis**
B. **Acute pancreatitis**
C. **Acute viral hepatitis**
D. **Peptic ulcer disease**
E. **Acute cholangitis**

Patients with acute cholecystitis typically complain of right-upper-quadrant or epigastric pain. The pain may radiate to the right shoulder or back. Associated complaints may include nausea, vomiting, and anorexia. Mild elevations in bilirubin may be seen (1). Although acute attacks are classically precipitated by large or fatty meals, many patients will not report a distinct association between food intake and episodes of cholecystitis (1).

Patients with acute pancreatitis frequently have an abrupt onset of severe, unrelenting epigastric pain that radiates to the back. The pain is usually associated with vomiting and retching. Patients can develop mild jaundice. The most common causes of acute pancreatitis are cholelithiasis and heavy alcohol intake. In 1% to 2% of patients, bluish discoloration is present in the flank (Grey Turner sign) or periumbilical area (Cullen sign), indicating hemorrhagic pancreatitis. The serum amylase and lipase rise early and can remain elevated for several days after the acute attack.

The presentation of acute viral hepatitis may be acute or insidious, often starting with symptoms of anorexia, nausea and vomiting, malaise, arthralgias, myalgias, headache, and upper respiratory symptoms. These symptoms may precede the onset of jaundice by 1 to 2 weeks. The liver becomes enlarged and tender, and patients can develop right-upper-quadrant pain. Serum transaminases increase by varying degrees during the prodromal phase and typically precede the rise in bilirubin. Transaminases can peak at levels ranging from 400 U/L to greater than 4,000 U/L. These levels are usually reached when patients are icteric and diminish progressively as patients recover from acute hepatitis (2).

Patients with peptic ulcer disease typically present with abdominal pain. The pain is usually located in the epigastrium and is variably described as an aching, burning, or gnawing sensation. Varying degrees of nausea and vomiting are common. The presentation is typically not acute unless a complication such as bleeding, perforation, or obstruction has occurred. Jaundice is not an associated feature of peptic ulcer disease, making it the least likely diagnosis in this patient.

Acute cholangitis typically develops as a result of biliary obstruction, which is usually partial. The main causes of biliary obstruction are choledocholithiasis, biliary stricture, and neoplasm. With obstruction, ductal pressure rises, and bacteria proliferate and migrate into the systemic circulation via the hepatic sinusoids. The symptoms of cholangitis, referred to as Charcot triad, are right-upper-quadrant pain, jaundice, and fever. Typical laboratory findings include leukocytosis, hyperbilirubinemia, and an elevated alkaline phosphatase. Serum aminotransferases may be elevated, which might reflect microabscess formation in the liver. Suppurative cholangitis represents the most severe form of cholangitis, in which confusion and shock are also present.

This patient's initial laboratory studies showed a white blood cell count of 3.24 K/μL, hematocrit of 39%, and platelets of 147 K/μL. Hepatic panel revealed albumin, 3.8 g/dL; aspartate aminotransferase (AST), 308 U/L; alanine aminotransferase (ALT), 101 U/L; alkaline phosphatase, 290 U/L; total bilirubin, 3.2 mg/dL; and direct bilirubin, 2.2 mg/dL. Renal function, electrolytes, amylase, and lipase were all normal.

All of the following are potentially appropriate initial therapeutic or diagnostic strategies in this patient except:

A. **Intravenous antibiotics**
B. **Right-upper-quadrant ultrasound**
C. **Endoscopic retrograde cholangiopancreatography (ERCP)**
D. **Magnetic resonance cholangiopancreatography (MRCP)**

This patient's hepatic profile is most consistent with biliary obstruction. Based on the hepatic profile and pancreatic enzymes, both acute viral hepatitis and acute pancreatitis are far less likely. In a patient with fever and evidence of biliary obstruction, clinicians must have a high index of suspicion for acute cholangitis. Initial management of these patients should include blood cultures, followed by prompt administration of intravenous antibiotics. Broad-spectrum antibiotics that cover Gram-negative bacteria, such as *Escherichia coli*, *Klebsiella* species, *Pseudomonas* species, and anaerobes should be started. Anaerobic coverage is particularly indicated in patients who have undergone previous biliary surgery. Biliary cultures are positive in approximately 75% of patients (2).

For patients with evidence of biliary obstruction, a right-upper-quadrant ultrasound is an appropriate initial imaging study to look for common bile duct (CBD) dilatation and the presence of cholelithiasis and/or choledocholithiasis. The sensitivity of ultrasound for detecting dilated bile ducts and biliary obstruction varies from 55% to 91%. Moreover, ultrasound may be negative when small stones are present in the bile duct (3).

Endoscopic retrograde cholangiopancreatography (ERCP) can confirm the diagnosis by showing CBD obstruction. ERCP is 80% to 100% sensitive and 85% to 100% specific for the detection of CBD stones (4). ERCP can also be therapeutic when a sphincterotomy, stone extraction, or stent insertion is performed. Eighty percent of patients will respond to initial management with intravenous fluids and antibiotics. In those cases, biliary drainage can be performed on an elective basis. However, if biliary sepsis is suspected clinically, pro-

ceeding immediately to ERCP without an ultrasound may be an appropriate approach. Unless the obstruction is relieved, the patient may remain at risk for significant morbidity and even mortality.

ERCP is not a procedure devoid of complications. The most common complication is acute pancreatitis, which occurs in about 25% of patients undergoing ERCP (2). Post-ERCP pancreatitis is usually mild and self-limited, but it does occasionally result in significant morbidity. Bleeding occurs following 1% of endoscopic sphincterotomies (2). Other rare complications include infection and perforation. Despite these risks, ERCP remains a safe procedure for treating retained common bile duct stones.

Magnetic resonance cholangiopancreatography (MRCP) is a more recent addition to the tools available to evaluate for CBD stones. MRCP can provide detailed imaging of the gallbladder and biliary and pancreatic ducts. MRCP is particularly useful in those patients who are post cholecystectomy or in whom ERCP was unsuccessful or failed to define ductal abnormalities completely. In the presence of a dilated CBD, MRCP is 90% to 95% concordant with ERCP in diagnosing CBD stones greater than 4 mm in diameter (4,5). Unlike ERCP, MRCP does not provide the opportunity for drainage. MRCP is not an appropriate initial test to assess for biliary tract disease, especially in those patients with cholangitis.

Case Continued

After blood cultures were drawn, the patient was started on intravenous piperacillin/tazobactam and gentamicin for empiric treatment of acute cholangitis. Right-upper-quadrant ultrasound showed biliary sludge and multiple gallstones, without evidence of ductal dilatation. There was no sonographic evidence of acute cholecystitis (negative sonographic Murphy sign and no pericholecystic fluid).

Given the patient's clinical status, an ERCP was performed the day after admission. It revealed a 5-mm distal CBD stone just proximal to the ampulla, resulting in complete obstruction without biliary or contrast flow. The extrahepatic tree was mildly dilated. A biliary sphincterotomy was performed, with extraction of the stone obstructing the distal CBD and reestablishment of biliary flow.

The patient's jaundice resolved gradually following the ERCP, and the serum bilirubin normalized over the subsequent 3 days. Two days into the hospitalization, two of two sets of blood cultures came back positive for *Klebsiella pneumoniae*.

CONCLUSION

Cholangitis is a potentially life-threatening condition. Early recognition and immediate treatment of pyogenic cholangitis are essential. Mainstays of appropriate treatment include intravenous antibiotics and the prompt establishment of drainage of the biliary tract. In cases of suspected biliary sepsis, clinicians need to recognize the role of emergent biliary decompression with ERCP.

REFERENCES

1. Diethelm AG, Stanley RJ, Robbin ML. The acute abdomen. In: Sabiston DC Jr, editor. *Textbook of surgery,* 15th ed. Philadelphia: WB Saunders, 1997:825–846.

2. Topazian M. Gastrointestinal endoscopy. In: Braunwald E, Fauci AS, Kasper DL, et al., eds. *Harrison's principles of internal medicine,* 15th ed. New York: McGraw-Hill, 2001:1635–1642.

3. Salem S, Vas W. Ultrasonography in evaluation of the jaundiced patient. *J Can Assoc Radiol* 1981;32:30–34.

4. Chan YL, Chan AC, Lam WW, et al. Choledocholithiasis: comparison of MR cholangiography and endoscopic retrograde cholangiography. *Radiology* 1996;200:85–89.

5. Soto JA, Yucel EK, Barish MA, et al. MR cholangiopancreatography after unsuccessful or incomplete ERCP. *Radiology* 1996;199: 91–98.

20

A 34-YEAR-OLD WOMAN WITH RASH, WEIGHT LOSS, AND RIGHT-UPPER-QUADRANT PAIN

GABRIEL BOU MERHI
RONY M. ABOU-JAWDE
RONALD ADAMS

CASE PRESENTATION

A previously healthy 34-year-old black woman presented with a year history of malaise, hair loss, facial rash, bilateral distal-lower-extremity numbness and burning, weight loss, and abdominal pain. Loss of hair occurred in the right temporooccipital area. These areas of alopecia increased in number and size over the next few months. Antifungal creams and subcutaneous glucocorticoid injections were prescribed without improvement. Several months later, she noted red, tender, raised skin lesions around her lips. Painless dark patches replaced these lesions 3 weeks after their appearance. The patient also noted an 80-pound unintentional weight loss over the preceding year. She was admitted to the hospital for further evaluation. She was not taking any medications.

On physical examination, she was afebrile with perioral lesions (Fig. 20.1) and patchy alopecia. Cardiac and pul-monary examinations were normal. Abdominal examination revealed severe right-upper-quadrant tenderness to palpation, negative Murphy sign, normal bowel sounds, and no hepatosplenomegaly. Neurologic examination showed normal deep tendon reflexes in all extremities, normal sensory responses, and no motor weakness. The rest of the examination was normal.

Laboratory studies revealed normal complete blood count, electrolytes, renal function, calcium, albumin, and coagulation parameters. Her hepatic panel included aspartate aminotransferase, 75 U/L; alanine aminotransferase, 16 U/L; alkaline phosphatase, 331 U/L; and γ-glutamyltranspeptidase, 580 U/L. C-reactive protein was elevated at 5.0 mg/dL.

Fungus was not isolated from the scalp cultures. Antinuclear antibody (ANA), cytomegalovirus (CMV) titers, Epstein–Barr virus (EBV) titers, viral hepatitis panel, and human immunodeficiency virus (HIV)-1 serology were all negative. She was anergic on skin testing. Chest x-ray (CXR) was normal. Right-upper-quadrant ultrasound showed a normal biliary tree, without cholelithiasis; the liver was not well visualized.

QUESTIONS/DISCUSSION

Which of the following diagnoses is least likely to explain this patient's symptom complex?

A. Systemic lupus erythematosus (SLE)
B. Sarcoidosis
C. Malignancy
D. Viral hepatitis
E. Tuberculosis

■ *SLE:* Many of this patient's symptoms are consistent with a diagnosis of SLE, including the cutaneous manifestations and malaise. However, the negative ANA makes SLE less likely; the ANA is a highly sensitive test for the diagnosis of SLE (1).

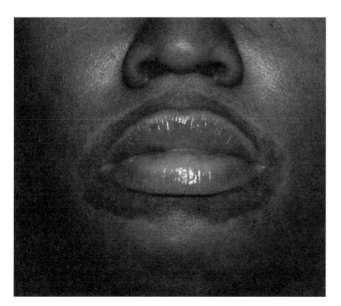

FIGURE 20.1. This patient has indurated blue-purple, swollen shiny lesions, which are consistent with lupus pernio.

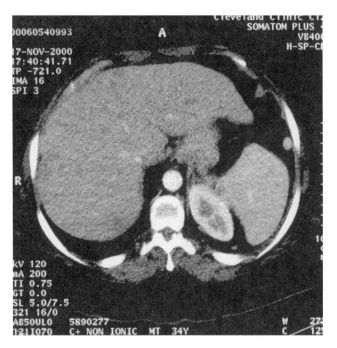

FIGURE 20.2. Computed tomogram of the abdomen showing heterogeneous micronodular appearance of the liver and spleen. These findings were thought to be consistent with cirrhosis, infiltrative liver disease, or neoplasia.

■ *Viral hepatitis:* This is least likely, given the negative hepatitis panel and the normal ALT, which is usually elevated in acute viral hepatitis.
■ *Tuberculosis:* The absence of any history of tuberculosis exposure and the normal CXR render the diagnosis of

tuberculosis less likely. However, given this patient's symptom complex, including weight loss, tuberculosis cannot be excluded completely at this point.

The two leading diagnoses considered at this point were malignancy (namely, lymphoma and primary or metastatic liver malignancies) and sarcoidosis.

Further work-up included computed tomography (CT) of her abdomen to evaluate her abdominal pain. The CT scan revealed a heterogeneous micronodular appearance of the liver and spleen consistent with cirrhosis, an infiltrative process (especially granulomatous disease), or neoplasia (Fig. 20.2).

The next step was a liver biopsy to identify the lesions seen on CT scan. The biopsy showed multiple nonnecrotizing granulomas (Fig. 20.3), and trichrome stains of the hepatic tissue did not show any organisms.

Which of the following is/are associated with granulomatous hepatic disease?

A. **Sarcoidosis**
B. **Tuberculosis**
C. **Hodgkin disease**
D. **Ingestion of mineral oil**
E. **All of the above**

Hepatic granulomas can be seen in conjunction with various disease processes and ingestions, including all the preceding choices. Certain histologic features on liver biopsy can help differentiate the various etiologies of granulomatous hepatic disease (Table 20.1) (2).

The clinical and pathologic picture is consistent with sarcoidosis. In addition, the patient's age, race, and elevated

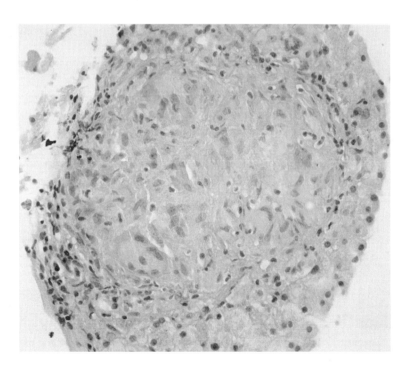

FIGURE 20.3. Liver biopsy showing multiple nonnecrotizing granulomas.

TABLE 20.1. DIFFERENTIAL DIAGNOSIS OF HEPATIC GRANULOMAS BASED ON HISTOLOGY

Histopathology	Examples
Noncaseating	Sarcoidosis
Caseating	Tuberculosis
Fibrin ring	Hodgkin disease, cytomegalovirus, toxoplasmosis, hepatitis A
Lipogranulomas	Patients who ingest mineral oil

Data from Maddrey WC. Granulomas of the liver. In: Schiff ER, Sorrell MF, Maddrey WC, eds. *Schiff's diseases of the liver.* 8th edition. Philadelphia: Lippincott–Raven Publishers, 1999:1571–1585.

TABLE 20.2. FREQUENCY OF ORGAN INVOLVEMENT IN SYSTEMIC SARCOIDOSIS

Lungs	90%
Lymph nodes (Intrathoracic)	75% to 90%
Liver	60% to 90%
Spleen	50% to 60%
Musculoskeletal (joint involvement)	25% to 50%
Bone marrow	15% to 40%
Skin	25%
Eyes	25%
Parotid gland	<10%
Nervous system	5%
Heart	5%

Data from Crystal R. Sarcoidosis. In: Braunwald E, Fauci AS, Kasper DL, et al., ed. *Harrison's principles of internal medicine.* 15th edition. New York: McGraw-Hill, 2000:1969–1974.

angiotensin-converting enzyme (ACE) level of 80 U/L (normal, 3 to 48 U/L) all support this diagnosis.

Manifestations of Sarcoidosis

Sarcoidosis is a multisystem chronic disease of unknown etiology. Pathologically, accumulations of T-lymphocytes, mononuclear phagocytes, and noncaseating granulomas, as well as derangement of normal tissue architecture, are present in the affected organs. The diagnosis of sarcoidosis is usually made by a combination of clinical, radiographic, and histologic findings. The prevalence in the United States is between 10 and 40 per 100,000 people (3). Blacks are disproportionately affected, with blacks 10 to 17 times more likely to develop the disease than whites.

Which of the following organ systems is least likely to be involved in sarcoidosis?

A. Lungs
B. Skin
C. Lymph nodes
D. Nervous system
E. Kidneys

The lungs and lymph nodes are the most commonly affected organ systems (Table 20.2) (4). In about 50% of cases of sarcoidosis, organs other than the lungs and lymph nodes are involved, with involvement of the liver, spleen, and bone marrow the most common sites (Table 20.2). Renal involvement in sarcoidosis is least common among the preceding choices.

Hepatic Sarcoidosis

Symptoms and functional derangement due to liver involvement are uncommon. Between 10% and 40% of patients with hepatic sarcoidosis have hepatomegaly and/or biochemical evidence of liver involvement, with elevations of alkaline phosphatase and γ-glutamyl transpeptidase the most common abnormalities on the hepatic profile (Table 20.3) (5).

Cutaneous Sarcoidosis

Cutaneous sarcoidosis occurs in 25% of cases, with lupus pernio a common manifestation. Indurated blue-purple, swollen shiny lesions that typically involve the nose, cheeks, ears, lips, fingers, and knees characterize lupus pernio. Lupus pernio is seen more frequently in black patients with sarcoidosis and may reflect more aggressive disease (6). Among the most common cutaneous manifestations of sarcoidosis are subcutaneous nodules and erythema nodosum. Erythema nodosum typically presents as tender, erythematous lesions located on the distal lower extremities.

Nervous System Sarcoidosis

Both the central and peripheral nervous systems can be affected. Central nervous system involvement can manifest as chronic meningitis and hypothalamic or pituitary dysfunction. With peripheral nervous system involvement, sarcoidosis usually presents as unilateral facial nerve paralysis or peripheral neuropathy with a "socklike" distribution. Bilateral lower-extremity numbness, tingling, and pain are typical presenting complaints (7).

TABLE 20.3. CLINICAL FINDINGS IN PATIENTS WITH HEPATIC SARCOIDOSIS

Clinical Sign	Frequency
Hepatomegaly	10% to 40%
Splenomegaly	10% to 30%
Fever and arthralgia	50% to 60%
Increased liver enzymes[a]	20% to 40%

[a]Alkaline phosphatase, gamma glutamyl transpeptidase.
Data from Mueller S, Boehme MW, Hofmann WJ, et al. Extrapulmonary sarcoidosis primarily diagnosed in the liver. *Scand J Gastroenterol* 2000;35:1003–1008.

Glucocorticoids and Sarcoidosis

Glucocorticoids are a mainstay in the treatment of pulmonary sarcoidosis. As a treatment for hepatic sarcoidosis, glucocorticoids, in a few cases, have improved liver function tests over 6 to 8 weeks (8).

Management

Systemic sarcoidosis was diagnosed, and prednisone at a dose of 25 mg twice a day was initiated. The patient's alopecia and systemic symptoms improved significantly, and the aspartate aminotransferase normalized. Prednisone was tapered over 2 months, and the patient remained only on gabapentin 100 mg three times a day for neuropathic pain.

CONCLUSION

This patient was ill for more than 1 year with hepatic, splenic, dermatologic, neurologic, and constitutional manifestations of chronic sarcoidosis. The absence of pulmonary symptoms and the normal chest x-ray may have contributed to a delay in diagnosis and treatment. Despite extensive investigation, no other cause for granulomatous hepatitis (Fig. 20.3) was discovered.

The combination of alopecia, facial rash, liver enzyme derangement, and constitutional symptoms should prompt evaluation for systemic illnesses like sarcoidosis, SLE, and malignancy. Although the pattern of inflammation seen on the liver biopsy is not specific for sarcoidosis, the clinical illness, the results of laboratory and histologic testing, and the response to treatment with systemic glucocorticoids suggest sarcoidosis as the likeliest diagnosis. This patient demonstrates the less common picture of systemic sarcoidosis without nodal or pulmonary involvement.

REFERENCES

1. Tan EM, Cohen AS, Fries JF, et al. The 1982 revised criteria for the classification of systemic lupus erythematosus. *Arthritis Rheum* 1982;25:1271–1277.
2. Maddrey WC. Granulomas of the liver. In: Schiff ER, Sorrell MF, Maddrey WC, eds. *Schiff's diseases of the liver,* 8th ed. Philadelphia: Lippincott Williams & Wilkins, 1999:1571–1585.
3. Henke CE, Henke G, Elveback LR, et al. The epidemiology of sarcoidosis in Rochester, Minnesota: a population-based study of incidence and survival. *Am J Epidemiol* 1986;123:840–845.
4. Crystal R. Sarcoidosis. In: Braunwald E, Fauci AS, Kasper DL, et al., eds. *Harrison's principles of internal medicine,* 15th ed. New York: McGraw-Hill, 2001:1969–1974.
5. Mueller S, Boehme MW, Hofmann WJ, et al. Extrapulmonary sarcoidosis primarily diagnosed in the liver. *Scand J Gastroenterol* 2000;35:1003–1008.
6. Mana J, Marcoval J, Graells J, et al. Cutaneous involvement in sarcoidosis: relationship to systemic disease. *Arch Dermatol* 1997;133:882–888.
7. Sharma OP. Cardiac and neurologic dysfunction in sarcoidosis. *Clin Chest Med* 1997;18:813–825.
8. Nores JM, Chesneau MC, Charlier JP, et al. A case of hepatic sarcoidosis: review of the literature. *Ann Gastroenterol Hepatol (Paris)* 1987;23:257–260.

21

A 73-YEAR-OLD MAN WITH RECURRENT GASTROINTESTINAL BLEEDING

SALEH A. ISMAIL
DARWIN L. CONWELL

CASE PRESENTATION

A 73-year-old man with a history of recurrent lower gastrointestinal (GI) bleeding presented to the emergency department with two episodes of bright red blood per rectum. Upon presentation, he did not have hematemesis but did note mild abdominal pain. He also noted feeling lightheaded but denied chest pain, palpitations, or shortness of breath.

The patient's past medical history is significant for coronary artery disease, hypertension, and hyperlipidemia. He underwent coronary artery bypass grafting surgery 3 years earlier. He also had a 4-year history of recurrent lower GI bleeding. One month before this presentation, the patient was hospitalized and required 2 units of packed red blood cells, which was the first time the patient required transfusion. During that hospitalization, the patient had a normal esophagogastroduodenoscopy (EGD) and a colonoscopy, which revealed one polyp. The polyp was removed and found to be a tubular adenoma. The colonoscopy also revealed diverticulosis and vascular ectasia, both of which had been seen on prior colonoscopies. The patient denied any history of liver disease, bleeding disorders, or alcohol abuse.

On presentation, the patient's medications included metoprolol, atorvastatin, aspirin 325 mg once a day, and famotidine. The patient denied the use of other nonsteroidal antiinflammatory drugs.

Physical examination revealed an elderly man in no acute distress. His temperature was 36.1°C. His blood pressure in the supine position was 85/58 mm Hg, and his pulse was 101 beats per minute. Upon standing, his blood pressure fell to 78/50 mm Hg, and his pulse rose to 112 beats per minute. Cardiac examination revealed tachycardia without murmurs. Lungs were clear. Abdominal examination revealed no tenderness or distension, with normal bowel sounds. There was no organomegaly. Rectal examination revealed bright maroon-colored stool without any masses. There was no lower-extremity edema. Examination of the skin did not reveal palmar erythema or spider angiomata.

Admission laboratory testing revealed a hemoglobin of 8.3 g/dL, hematocrit of 24.2%, and platelet count of 225 K/μL. The patient's electrolytes were normal. Blood urea nitrogen was 23 mg/dL, and the creatinine was 0.8 mg/dL. Liver function tests were normal. His coagulation parameters were normal. A type and crossmatch was also performed.

QUESTIONS/DISCUSSION

All of the following factors place patients with GI bleeding at increased risk for adverse outcomes except:

A. **Systolic blood pressure less than 100 mm Hg**
B. **History of GI bleeding**
C. **Ongoing bleeding**
D. **Increased prothrombin time**
E. **Comorbid conditions**

Patients with acute gastrointestinal bleeding can be stratified into low- and high-risk groups for the likelihood of developing adverse events during hospitalization. Patients considered at high risk are those with comorbid conditions, decreased serum albumin, increased prothrombin time, and elevated serum bilirubin (1–3). Others use the BLEED criteria in classifying patients as at high or low risk (2,3). These criteria include the presence of ongoing *b*leeding, *l*ow systolic blood pressure (below 100 mm Hg, excluding orthostatic readings), *e*levated prothrombin time (greater than 1.2 times the control value), *e*rratic mental status, and presence of unstable comorbid *d*isease. Patients are considered at high risk if they have at least one of these criteria. In these studies, a history of prior GI bleeding was not found to place patients at increased risk of adverse outcomes (2,3).

Determining those patients at increased risk will help direct initial management and decisions regarding disposition (intensive care unit, monitored unit, regular unit, or outpatient management). Low-risk patients have lower mortality rates, lower rates of rebleeding, shorter hospitalizations, and reduced transfusion requirements (2,3). These patients can typically be managed in settings other than an intensive care unit (ICU). Higher-risk patients are typically managed in either an ICU or monitored setting.

Based on his history, physical examination, and initial laboratory tests, this patient was considered at high risk. His blood pressure responded to initial volume resuscitation, and he was admitted to a monitored unit. A nasogastric aspirate revealed bilious material without blood or coffee-ground material.

Following initial evaluation and resuscitation, which of the following tests is most appropriate to evaluate this patient's bleeding?

A. **Colonoscopy**
B. **EGD with push enteroscopy**
C. **Arteriogram**
D. **Technetium-99m red blood cell scan**

Hematochezia is the passage of maroon or red blood or blood clots per rectum. Both upper and lower GI bleeding can produce hematochezia, although lower GI bleeding produces hematochezia more frequently. Upper GI bleeding needs to be rapid to produce hematochezia. Table 21.1 summarizes one study that identified the sources of bleeding in 80 patients with hematochezia (4). Eleven percent had an upper GI source of bleeding (duodenal ulcer, gastric ulcer, and varices) and 9% had small bowel sources of hematochezia (Crohn ileitis, vascular ectasia, Meckel diverticulum, and tumor) (4,5). Of the 74% of patients with colonic lesions, angiodysplasia, diverticula, polyps, and cancer were the most common causes of hematochezia. The

TABLE 21.1. DIAGNOSIS FOR 80 PATIENTS WITH SEVERE HEMATOCHEZIA

Lesion Site	Number of Patients (%)
Colonic (total)	59 (74%)
Angiodysplasia	24 (30%)
Diverticulosis	13 (17%)
Polyp or cancer	9 (11%)
Focal colitis or ulcers	7 (9%)
Rectal lesions	3 (4%)
Bleeding polyp stalk	2 (2%)
Endometriosis	1 (1%)
Upper gastrointestinal	9 (11%)
Small bowel	7 (9%)
No site found	5 (6%)

Adapted from Jensen DM. Diagnosis and treatment of severe hematochezia: the role of urgent colonoscopy after purge. *Gastroenterology* 1988;95:1569–1574.

remaining 6% of patients did not have an identifiable source of bleeding.

Certain historical features may favor particular diagnoses. In a young adult presenting with hematochezia, an evaluation for a Meckel diverticulum is more appropriate than it would be in an elderly patient. Diverticulosis and angiodysplasia are the most common causes of hematochezia in elderly patients. Bleeding from cancerous lesions tends to be low-grade and recurrent. Symptoms of fever, abdominal pain, and diarrhea favor colitis, which could be due to inflammatory bowel disease, infection, or ischemia (5). In this patient, the presence of documented diverticulosis and vascular ectasia favored a lower GI source.

The American College of Gastroenterology has issued practice guidelines outlining the approach to patients with hematochezia (1). These patients need to have a nasogastric lavage to evaluate for the presence of upper GI bleeding. A nasogastric aspirate with copious amounts of bile and negative for blood makes an upper GI bleed less likely. EGD should be the first test performed if nasogastric aspiration reveals coffee-ground material or bright red blood. EGD should also be considered if a nasogastric lavage does not yield bilious fluid, since a closed pylorus can mask duodenal bleeding, especially in hemodynamically unstable patients with hematochezia.

If nasogastric lavage does not reveal evidence of upper GI bleeding, a colonoscopy should be the first test. Colonoscopy has considerable potential diagnostic and therapeutic advantages. It can help localize a bleeding source, allow for collection of pathologic specimens, and provide effective hemostasis. In volume-resuscitated patients, colonoscopy is generally a safe procedure with few complications. The optimum timing of colonoscopy is affected by the clinical setting; colonoscopy should be performed as soon as possible in patients with continuous hematochezia. Otherwise, colonoscopy can be delayed to allow for bowel preparation, which may increase the yield of colonoscopy (6–9). Colonoscopy is the appropriate initial test in this patient, who had a nasogastric aspirate negative for blood.

If colonoscopy is unrevealing because of the severity of bleeding, an arteriogram is an appropriate follow-up test. Arteriography requires active blood loss of at least 0.5 mL/min in order to detect a bleeding site. The procedure is 100% specific, but its sensitivity is variable, depending largely upon the pattern of bleeding. Arteriography is more sensitive when bleeding is acute and continuous; it is less useful in cases where bleeding is intermittent (10,11). Advantages of the procedure include the ability to localize anatomically the source of bleeding and the ability to perform therapeutic intervention with embolization and vasopressin.

Technetium-99m-labeled red blood cell scans are rarely used as an initial test in patients with gastrointestinal bleeding. A tagged red cell scan can detect bleeding at a rate as slow as 0.1 mL/minute (12). However, it is considerably less specific than arteriography. Tagged red cell scans can localize the source of bleeding to a particular region of the GI tract, but typically fail to define a precise anatomic location. Its diagnostic accuracy is widely variable. For this reason, tagged red cell scans are not the initial diagnostic test in patients with GI bleeding from an undetermined location (12).

Case Continued: This patient underwent a colonoscopy that revealed multiple angiodysplastic lesions in the cecum and ascending colon and scattered diverticulosis. A large arteriovenous malformation (AVM) was seen among the vascular lesions (Fig. 21.1). Slow bleeding was seen in the area of the angiodysplastic lesions. Epinephrine was injected to control bleeding, and argon plasma coagulation (APC) was performed to obliterate the arteriovenous malformation. Endoclips were applied to the AVM.

Which of the following statements regarding angiodysplasia of the GI tract is false?

A. **Angiodysplasia is the most common cause of hematochezia in patients more than 65 years of age.**
B. **Barium enema is useful for diagnosing angiodysplasia.**
C. **Angiodysplasia can occur in parts of the GI tract other than the colon.**

D. **The risk of bleeding associated with angiodysplasia increases with age.**

Angiodysplasia is the most common cause of hematochezia in patients more than 65 years of age. Angiodysplasia has been reported with greater frequency in patients with renal failure, von Willebrand disease, aortic stenosis, and cirrhosis of the liver. However, most cases of angiodysplasia are not associated with one of these conditions (13).

Pathologically, angiodysplasia represents ectasia of normal intestinal submucosal veins and overlying mucosal capillaries. The walls of these vessels consist of endothelial cells that lack smooth muscle. The lesions can be visualized with an endoscope, and the surrounding mucosa is typically normal, in contrast to a hemangioma. The lesions are flat or slightly elevated above the mucosal surface, red in color, and usually 2 to 10 mm in size. Angiodysplasia may be round, stellate, or sharply circumscribed with fernlike margins. A prominent feeding vessel may be present. Colonoscopy and angiography are the only effective ways to make the diagnosis. Barium enema is not a useful test for making the diagnosis of angiodysplasia. Most lesions are detected in the cecum and ascending colon, although they can occur throughout the colon. Angiodysplasia tends to become more extensive over time; as a result, the risk of bleeding tends to increase with age (13).

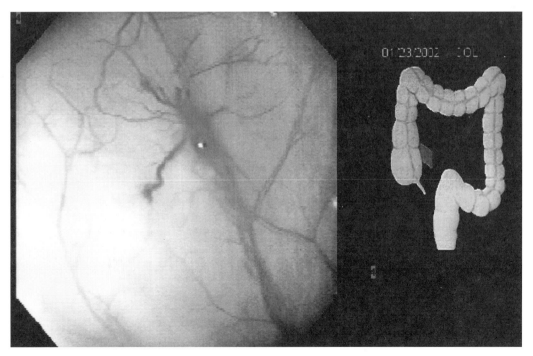

FIGURE 21.1. A large arteriovenous malformation visualized among multiple angiodysplastic lesions.

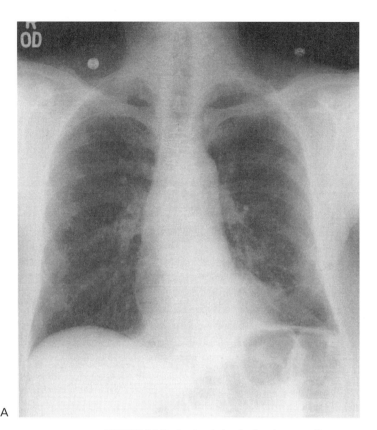
A

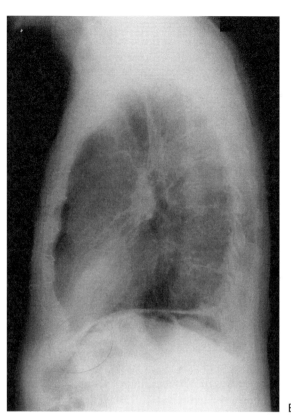
B

FIGURE 21.2. Acute abdominal series revealing pneumoperitoneum, which developed following treatment of the angiodysplastic lesion with argon plasma coagulation. **A:** Posterior–anterior view. **B:** Lateral view.

Bleeding from angiodysplasia tends to be episodic and self-limited. Patients usually present with painless hematochezia or melena. Lesions that are incidentally detected rarely bleed; treatment is unnecessary for these lesions. Since symptomatic patients tend to rebleed frequently, treatment of these lesions is indicated to decrease the rate of rebleeding (13,14).

The treatment of angiodysplasia includes endoscopic coagulation (with a bipolar probe or heater probe), injection sclerotherapy, and argon laser coagulation. Hormone therapy with conjugated estrogens may be useful in cases of refractory bleeding. Studies analyzing the effectiveness of hormone therapy have produced conflicting results (13).

Angiodysplasia can occur in other parts of the gastrointestinal tract, most often in the stomach and duodenum. Esophageal lesions are rare. The presence of upper GI or small bowel angiodysplasia should prompt an investigation of additional lower GI lesions, which occur in about 30% of cases (13).

Case Conclusion

Following treatment of the angiodysplastic lesion with APC, the patient was admitted for observation. A few hours later, the patient developed fever and mild abdominal pain. An acute abdominal series revealed pneumoperitoneum (Fig. 21.2). Since the patient did not have peritoneal signs and his abdominal pain was improving, he was managed conservatively. Over the subsequent 24 to 48 hours, the patient tolerated oral intake and had regular bowel movements. Hemoglobin and hematocrit on discharge were 10.4 g/dL and 30.8%, respectively, after a transfusion of 3 U of packed red blood cells. The patient was discharged home on iron supplements.

The pneumoperitoneum that developed was considered a complication of APC. APC is a noncontact thermal method introduced as an alternative to contact thermal coagulation (heater probe and bipolar cautery) and other noncontact methods. The advantage of APC photocoagulation is decreased tissue penetration and a decreased risk of perforation, ranging between 0.2% and 2.8% (15–17).

CONCLUSION

Gastrointestinal bleeding is a serious condition, with the potential for significant morbidity and mortality. Clinicians need to recognize which patients are at greatest risk for complications. A systematic approach, including a focused history and appropriate investigations, can be extremely helpful in determining the appropriate disposition and establishing a diagnosis. Certain causes of GI bleeding are more likely in certain age groups. Both EGD and colonoscopy are safe procedures, but clinicians also need to be aware of potential complications associated with these procedures.

REFERENCES

1. Zuccaro G Jr. Management of the adult patient with acute lower gastrointestinal bleeding. American College of Gastroenterology. *Am J Gastroenterol* 1998;93:1202–1208.
2. Kollef MH, Canfield DA, Zuckerman GR. Triage considerations for patients with acute gastrointestinal hemorrhage admitted to a medical intensive care unit. *Crit Care Med* 1995;23:1048–1054.
3. Kollef MH, O'Brien JD, Zuckerman GR, et al. BLEED: a classification tool to predict outcomes in patients with acute upper and lower gastrointestinal hemorrhage. *Crit Care Med* 1997;25:1125–1132.
4. Jensen DM, Machicado GA. Diagnosis and treatment of severe hematochezia: the role of urgent colonoscopy after purge. *Gastroenterology* 1988;95:1569–1574.
5. Zuckerman GR, Prakash C. Acute lower intestinal bleeding. Part II: etiology, therapy, and outcomes. *Gastrointest Endosc* 1999;49:228–238.
6. Wong JL, Dalton HR. Urgent endoscopy in lower gastrointestinal bleeding. *Gut* 2001;48:155–156.
7. Gostout CJ. The role of endoscopy in managing acute lower gastrointestinal bleeding. *N Engl J Med* 2000;342:125–127.
8. Rossini FP, Ferrari A, Spandre M, et al. Emergency colonoscopy. *World J Surg* 1989;13:190–192.
9. Jensen DM, Machicado GA, Jutabha R, et al. Urgent colonoscopy for the diagnosis and treatment of severe diverticular hemorrhage. *N Engl J Med* 2000;342:78–82.
10. Zuckerman DA, Bocchini TP, Birnbaum EH. Massive hemorrhage in the lower gastrointestinal tract in adults: diagnostic imaging and intervention. *Am J Roentgenol* 1993;161:703–711.
11. Gordon R, Ahl KL, Kerlan RK, et al. Selective arterial embolization for the control of lower gastrointestinal bleeding. *Am J Surg* 1997;174:24–28.
12. Dusold R, Burke K, Carpentier W, et al. The accuracy of technetium-99m-labeled red cell scintigraphy in localizing gastrointestinal bleeding. *Am J Gastroenterol* 1994;89:345–348.
13. Foutch PG. Angiodysplasia of the gastrointestinal tract. *Am J Gastroenterol* 1993;88:807–818.
14. McGuire HH Jr. Bleeding colonic diverticula: a reappraisal of natural history and management. *Ann Surg* 1994;220:653–656.
15. Conio M, Gostout CJ. Argon plasma coagulation (APC) in gastroenterology: experimental and clinical experiences. *Gastrointest Endosc Clin N Am* 1998;48:109–110.
16. Tan AC, Schellekens PP, Wahab P, et al. Pneumatosis intestinalis, retroperitonealis, and thoracalis after argon plasma coagulation. *Endoscopy* 1995;27:698–699.
17. Hoyer N, Thouet R, Zellweger U. Massive pneumoperitoneum after endoscopic argon plasma coagulation. *Endoscopy* 1998;30:S44–S45.

22

DIARRHEA AND DIFFUSE COLITIS IN A RENAL TRANSPLANT PATIENT

RONY M. ABOU-JAWDE
MATTHEW G. SMITH

CASE PRESENTATION

A 65-year-old man presented with a 2-day history of "explosive" diarrhea, with four to seven loose bowel movements a day. The patient denied fever, melena, hematochezia, nausea, or vomiting. However, he reported diffuse crampy abdominal pain, localized primarily in the left lower quadrant, with associated urgency and generalized weakness.

His past medical history was notable for a cadaveric renal transplant 6 months before this admission from a donor positive for cytomegalovirus (CMV). The patient was negative for CMV before transplant. His postoperative course was complicated by a left thoracotomy and pleurectomy for pulmonary aspergilloma/empyema. He received home intravenous antibiotics (HIVAT) with amphotericin B for approximately 3 weeks before presentation. The patient also had hypertension, hyperlipidemia, steroid-induced diabetes mellitus, chronic renal insufficiency (baseline creatinine of 3.5 to 4 mg/dL), and hypogammaglobulinemia.

His medications on presentation were sirolimus, prednisone, trimethoprim/sulfamethoxazole, esomeprazole, glimepiride, clotrimazole troche, albuterol, and amphotericin B.

On physical examination, he was afebrile with a heart rate of 102 beats per minute and regular, respiratory rate of 20 beats per minute, blood pressure of 107/70 mm Hg without orthostasis, and pulse oximetry of 95% on 2 L nasal cannula. The patient was in no acute distress. Head and neck examination was normal except for the presence of oral thrush. Heart and lung examinations were normal. Abdominal examination revealed distension and diffuse tenderness, greatest in the left upper quadrant, without masses, rebound, or guarding. The rectal examination revealed normal sphincter tone, no masses, and occult-blood negative stool.

APPROACH TO PATIENTS WITH ACUTE DIARRHEA

Most cases of acute diarrhea are self-limited irrespective of the etiology. However, further evaluation is warranted in cases of profuse diarrhea, bloody or mucoid diarrhea, fever, severe abdominal pain in patients more than 50 years of age, elderly patients (greater than 70 years of age), immunocompromised patients, or patients with symptoms for longer than 48 hours (1).

QUESTIONS/DISCUSSION

Which study would be least likely to help diagnose this patient's diarrhea?

A. Fecal leukocytes
B. Sigmoidoscopy/colonoscopy
C. Stool cultures
D. Stool for ova and parasites

Fecal leukocytes: The accuracy of fecal leukocytes in narrowing the differential diagnosis of acute diarrhea varies greatly. A metaanalysis found a peak sensitivity of 70% and a specificity of 50% (2). This variability has to do with specimen processing and operator experience. However, the presence of fecal leukocytes and occult blood can support the diagnosis of an infectious etiology in the context of a good medical history, although it cannot confirm a specific diagnosis. Therefore, even if fecal leukocytes were positive in this case, the underlying etiology needs to be identified to initiate appropriate treatment.

Sigmoidoscopy/colonoscopy: Sigmoidoscopy/colonoscopy is indicated in selected situations, such as differentiating inflammatory bowel disease from infectious diarrhea. These tests may also help with the diagnosis in immunocompromised patients at risk for opportunistic infections such as cytomegalovirus, or in ruling out ischemic colitis. In immunocompromised patients, a greater urgency often exists to establish a diagnosis, making sigmoidoscopy or colonoscopy a more useful tool in these patients.

Stool cultures: No consensus exists on ordering stool cultures. However, stool cultures are likely warranted in certain patient populations, such as immunocompromised patients, including human immunodeficiency virus (HIV) patients, patients with comorbidities such as diabetes mellitus and renal failure, or patients with known inflammatory bowel disease (to rule out infection versus a flare of the disease) (3,4).

Ova and parasites: Stool for ova and parasites is not always appropriate. It may be indicated in patients with chronic diarrhea, a history of travel to certain countries, exposure to infants in day care centers, a history of sexual encounters with homosexual men, AIDS and other immunocompromising diseases, waterborne outbreaks, or bloody diarrhea (1). Three specimens on consecutive days are usually sent, since parasite and ova excretion may be intermittent.

Case continued: The patient's metabolic profile showed sodium of 124 mmol/L, chloride of 96 mmol/L, blood urea nitrogen of 64 mg/dL, creatinine of 4.3 mg/dL, potassium of 5.1 mmol/L, and albumin of 2.3 g/dL. The white blood count was 36,440/μL, and hemoglobin was 14.3 g/dL.

The *Clostridium difficile* enzyme immunoassay (EIA) was negative for toxin A and B. Stool for ova and parasites was negative for *Giardia* and *Cryptosporidium.* Stool cultures were negative for *Campylobacter, Shigella,* and *Salmonella* species.

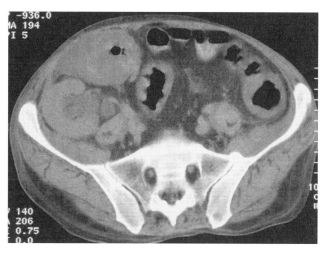

FIGURE 22.2. Computed tomography of the abdomen showing diffuse mural thickening of the entire colon, most suggestive of inflammatory bowel disease or pseudomembranous colitis.

CMV detection blood culture was positive with 120,293 copies/mL blood. Supine and upright views of the abdomen demonstrated "thumbprinting" along the transverse and right colon, compatible with a diffuse colitis. There was gaseous distension of small bowel loops in a pattern compatible with ileus (Fig. 22.1). Computed tomography (CT) of the abdomen with contrast showed diffuse mural thickening of the entire colon, most suggestive of inflammatory bowel disease or pseudomembranous colitis (Fig. 22.2).

At this point, what is the most likely diagnosis?

A. **Cytomegalovirus (CMV) colitis**
B. ***Clostridium difficile (C. difficile)* pseudomembranous colitis (PMC)**
C. **Bacterial colitis**
D. **Ischemic colitis**

With negative stool cultures, the common causes for *bacterial colitis* were far less likely. The lack of bloody diarrhea, the degree and nature of his symptoms, and the findings on the CT scan make *ischemic colitis* less likely but still possible at this point. The two remaining main differential diagnoses are CMV or *C. difficile* colitis.

Cytomegalovirus colitis: It is important to distinguish between CMV disease and CMV infection. Infection is present if one or more of the following is present: seroconversion with the appearance of anti-CMV IgM antibodies, fourfold increase in anti-CMV IgG titers, detection of CMV antigens in infected cells, or a positive viral load in the blood. In contrast, CMV disease requires clinical signs and symptoms, including fever, leukopenia, or organ involvement, such as hepatitis, pneumonitis, pancreatitis, or colitis (5,6). CMV colitis often presents with intractable diarrhea. Patients often experience diffuse abdominal pain and hematochezia, with tenesmus in CMV proctitis. CMV

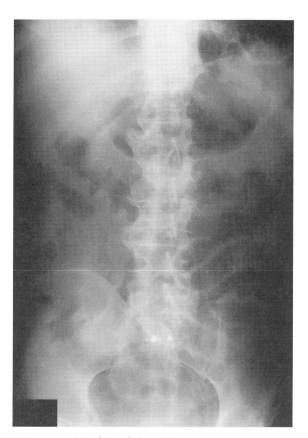

FIGURE 22.1. Plain film of the abdomen showing gaseous distension of loops of small bowel. This pattern is consistent with an ileus. There was also evidence of "thumbprinting" along the transverse and right colon, compatible with a diffuse colitis.

viremia is a predisposing factor for end organ involvement in CMV. Mucosal inflammation, tissue necrosis, vascular endothelial involvement, and cytomegalic cells with intracytoplasmic inclusions are characteristics of CMV colitis (7). This patient has CMV infection, but does not necessarily have CMV disease with CMV colitis.

Clostridium difficile: *C. difficile* is a spore-forming toxigenic bacterium that can cause diarrhea and colitis, usually after antibiotic use. The overall incidence of *C. difficile* has increased, becoming the fourth most common nosocomial disease reported to the Centers for Disease Control and Prevention (8). Diarrhea occurs in 5% to 39% of patients taking antibiotics, depending on the antibiotic (9). Most outpatient cases of antibiotic-induced diarrhea are a side effect of the medication, rather than due to *C. difficile*. Overall, PMC occurs in 10% of patients with antibiotic-associated diarrhea (9). Most cases of PMC develop in patients taking clindamycin, lincomycin, ampicillin, or cephalosporins. However, almost any antibiotic can cause PMC, including antifungals, antivirals, vancomycin, and metronidazole (10).

C. difficile diarrhea usually presents within 1 to 2 weeks of antibiotic administration, but symptoms may occur after 1 day or not until 6 weeks after antibiotics (11). Clinical presentation ranges from loose stools in mild cases to toxic megacolon or perforation in severe cases (11). Low-grade fever, diffuse crampy abdominal pain, dehydration, electrolyte depletion, hypoproteinemia, hemorrhage, sepsis, and pneumatosis coli are known complications of *C. difficile*–associated diarrhea (11). In general, the mortality from the disease ranges from 2% to 5% in the general population, to 10% to 20% in the elderly and debilitated patients, and to 30% to 80% in those with fulminant colitis or toxic megacolon (12). Risk factors for developing severe disease include old age, malignancy, uremia, chronic lung disease, immunosuppression, use of antiperistaltic drugs, hypoalbuminemia (less than 3 g/dL), hemoconcentration, and extremes of white counts (13). The differential diagnosis for *C. difficile* colitis is broad (Table 22.1) (13).

The clinical suspicion for PMC in this patient was high, mostly due to the CT scan findings, even with a

negative stool specimen for *C. difficile* toxins. To best resolve the issue and to avoid delaying treatment, a sigmoidoscopy was done. The sigmoidoscopy revealed severe PMC covering 80% of the bowel surface, starting at 10 cm of the rectosigmoid colon. Biopsies confirmed the presence of PMC.

Pathogenesis of C. difficile: Several steps must take place for *C. difficile*–associated diarrhea to occur. Among the crucial steps are the acquisition and germination of the spores, alteration in normal gut flora and/or mucosal immunity, and overgrowth of the *C. difficile*. The end result is toxin production, notably toxin A and B (14). The toxins interfere with protein synthesis in the mucosal cells, attract granulocytes, increase capillary permeability and induce more peristalsis (14). In severe cases, inflammation can involve deeper layers, leading to toxic dilation and perforation.

Which of the following laboratory tests is the appropriate initial diagnostic test for *C. difficile*?

A. Stool cultures
B. Stool cytotoxicity assays
C. Enzyme linked immunoassay (ELISA) for toxin A
D. ELISA for toxin A and B

As an initial diagnostic test, ELISA for both toxin A and B is the most appropriate test. Although stool cytotoxicity assays are considered the gold standard for diagnosing *C. difficile*, these tests are technically difficult, and results take up to 72 hours. ELISA for both toxin A and B provides sensitivity and specificity similar to those of the cytotoxicity assays. However, the ELISA is a faster and more convenient test. Testing for either toxin A or B alone reduces the sensitivity considerably (Table 22.2) (15).

Radiographic studies: Radiographic studies may assist in the diagnosis of *C. difficile*–associated diarrhea. Abdominal plain films may show paralytic ileus, dilated colon, or even "thumbprinting," as in this case. A CT scan may show diffusely thickened or edematous colonic mucosa and may identify disease localized to the right or proximal colon (16). A barium enema is not recommended because of an increased risk of perforation or megacolon (17).

Endoscopy: Findings on endoscopy may be normal in patients with mild disease but can quickly provide a diagnosis when findings are present. Flexible sigmoidoscopy will be diagnostic in more than 90% of patients, except when the disease presents only beyond the splenic flexure, in which case colonoscopy is required for diagnosis. Endoscopy is safe in patients without abdominal distention but can be dangerous and cause colonic perforation in patients with either severe disease or colonic dilatation. However, in experienced hands and with the use of minimal air insufflation, flexible sigmoidoscopy can provide the diagnosis early and allow rapid initiation of treatment before stool tests are available (18).

TABLE 22.1. DIFFERENTIAL DIAGNOSIS OF *CLOSTRIDIUM DIFFICILE*–ASSOCIATED DIARRHEA

Noninfectious	Infectious
Neutropenic enterocolitis (typhlitis)	*Campylobacter, Salmonella, Shigella* species
Crohn disease	*Escherichia coli*
Ulcerative colitis	*Listeria monocytogenes*
Chemical colitis (chemotherapy, gold)	Cytomegalovirus
Ischemic colitis	Staphylococcal enterocolitis (rare)

TABLE 22.2. DIAGNOSTIC TESTS FOR *CLOSTRIDIUM DIFFICILE*

Diagnostic Test	Comments
Stool culture	Demanding, low predictive value due to rate of asymptomatic carriers
Stool cytotoxicity assays (gold standard)	High specificity (99%) and sensitivity (94% to 100%). However, 5% with PMC will have negative tests.
ELISA for toxin A or B (two separate tests)	Less expensive, faster than cytotoxicity test. Sensitivity 75% to 85%, but can increase to 90% on repeating test on two or three separate stool specimens.
ELISA for toxin A and B (new)	Specificity (100%), and overall agreement (>98%) with the cytotoxicity assay.

ELISA, enzyme-linked immunosorbent assay; PMC, pseudomembranous colitis.
Data from Fekety R. Guidelines for the diagnosis and management of *Clostridium difficile*–associated diarrhea and colitis. American College of Gastroenterology, Practice Parameters Committee. *Am J Gastroenterol* 1997;92:739–750.

Which of the following is/are treatments for *C. difficile* PMC?

A. Supportive treatment
B. Oral/intravenous metronidazole
C. Oral vancomycin
D. Combination of metronidazole and vancomycin
E. All of the above

Supportive treatment: Patients with mild disease may benefit from conservative treatment, such as discontinuing or changing the offending antibiotic, rehydration, and isolation of the hospitalized patient. Narcotics and antimotility medications are contraindicated because they can induce severe colitis and toxic megacolon. Diarrhea will resolve in 15% to 23% of patients with this approach (13). When conservative treatment fails, antibiotics cannot be stopped, or in severe cases, specific antibiotic treatment is indicated.

Metronidazole: Oral metronidazole at a dose of 250 to 500 mg four times a day or 500 to 750 mg three times a day for 7 to 10 days is considered first-line antimicrobial therapy for PMC (13). Although vancomycin has similar response and relapse rates to metronidazole, metronidazole is considerably less expensive (13). Metronidazole is contraindicated in both children and pregnant women (13). Intravenous metronidazole is typically used when patients cannot take oral medications because of severe illness or gastrointestinal dysfunction.

Vancomycin: Oral vancomycin at doses of 125 mg four times a day for 7 to 14 days is reserved for instances in which the patient is not responding to metronidazole or is intolerant of metronidazole (13). Higher doses of vancomycin, 250 to 500 mg four times a day, are used to treat severely ill patients (13). Another drawback to regular use of vancomycin to treat *C. difficile* is the potential for the development of resistant organisms, such as vancomycin-resistant enterococci (13).

Other treatment options: Bacitracin has been shown to be less effective than vancomycin and metronidazole. Teico-

planin is used in Europe with comparable results to those of vancomycin but is not available in the United States. Cholestyramine can help decrease symptoms in mild disease, but when used alone has disappointing results. Since cholestyramine can bind vancomycin in the gut, it should not be coadministered with vancomycin (13). Surgery is needed only in 0.4% to 5% of patients, typically in critically ill patients. Indications for surgery include the presence of an acute abdomen, sepsis, multiorgan failure, hemorrhage, toxic dilatation, perforation, and/or deterioration despite adequate medical treatment (13). The procedure of choice is a subtotal colectomy.

CONCLUSION

In summary, this patient, who is status post renal transplant from a CMV-positive donor and receiving immunosuppression and amphotericin B, presented with acute diarrhea in the setting of CMV viremia. The initial etiology considered for the diarrhea was CMV colitis, especially with negative stool studies, including the *C. difficile* toxin. However, the diffuse colitis and colonic edema found on abdominal CT made CMV less likely and PMC more likely. Flexible sigmoidoscopy and colonic biopsy confirmed PMC. The patient was started on intravenous metronidazole and oral vancomycin, due to the severe nature of his disease, with marked improvement in his symptoms within 48 hours. In immunocompromised patients who present with acute diarrhea, clinicians need to pursue a diagnosis more aggressively than in the general population, as failure to make a prompt diagnosis could result in significant morbidity and mortality.

REFERENCES

1. DuPont HL. Guidelines on acute infectious diarrhea in adults. *Am J Gastroenterol* 1997;92:1962–1975.

2. Huicho L, Sanchez D, Contreras M, et al. Occult blood and fecal leukocytes as screening tests in childhood infectious diarrhea: an old problem revisited. *Pediatr Infect Dis J* 1993;12: 474–477.

3. Koplan JP, Fineberg HV, Ferraro MJ, et al. Value of stool cultures. *Lancet* 1980;2:413–416.

4. Rohner P, Pillet D, Pepey B, et al. Etiological agents of infectious diarrhea: implications for requests for microbial culture. *J Clin Microbiol* 1997;35:1427–1432.

5. Rubin RH. Infectious disease complications of renal transplantation. *Kidney Int* 1993;44:221–236.

6. Farrugia E, Schwab TR. Management and prevention of cytomegalovirus infection after renal transplantation. *Mayo Clin Proc* 1992;67:879–890.

7. Goodgame RW. Gastrointestinal cytomegalovirus disease. *Ann Intern Med* 1993;119:924–935.

8. Lyerly DM, Krivan HC, Wilkins TD. *Clostridium difficile:* its disease and toxins. *Clin Microbiol Rev* 1988;1:1–18.

9. McFarland LV. Epidemiology, risk factors and treatments for antibiotic-associated diarrhea. *Dig Dis* 1998;16:292–307.

10. Silva J, Fekety R, Werk C, et al. Inciting and etiologic agents of colitis. *Rev Infect Dis* 1984;6:S214–S221.

11. Tedesco FJ. Pseudomembranous colitis: pathogenesis and therapy. *Med Clin North Am* 1982;66:655–664.

12. Rubin MS, Bodenstein LE, Kent KC. Severe *Clostridium difficile* colitis. *Dis Colon Rectum* 1995;38:350–354.

13. Yassin SF, Young-Fadok TM, Zein NN, et al. *Clostridium difficile*-associated diarrhea and colitis. *Mayo Clin Proc* 2001;76: 725–730.

14. Pothoulakis C. Pathogenesis of *Clostridium difficile*-associated diarrhoea. *Eur J Gastroenterol Hepatol* 1996;8:1041–1047.

15. Fekety R. Guidelines for the diagnosis and management of *Clostridium difficile*-associated diarrhea and colitis. *Am J Gastroenterol* 1997;92:739–750.

16. Mylonakis E, Ryan ET, Calderwood SB, et al. *Clostridium difficile*–associated diarrhea: a review. *Arch Intern Med* 2001;161: 525–533.

17. Tedesco FJ, Stanley RJ, Alpers DH. Diagnostic features of clindamycin-associated pseudomembranous colitis. *N Engl J Med* 1974;290:841–843.

18. Gebhard RL, Gerding DN, Olson MM, et al. Clinical and endoscopic findings in patients early in the course of *Clostridium difficile*–associated pseudomembranous colitis. *Am J Med* 1985; 78:45–48.

23

A 59-YEAR-OLD MAN WITH CHRONIC DIARRHEA

ANTHONY K. LEUNG
ROBIN K. AVERY
MICHAEL B. LEHMAN

CASE PRESENTATION

A 59-year-old white man with a past medical history of hypothyroidism and mild mental retardation presented for evaluation of chronic diarrhea. The patient started to develop loose, watery diarrhea 18 months before presentation. The stools were not bloody and did not contain any mucus. His sister described the consistency of his stools as alternating between formed and semiformed. There was no associated abdominal cramping, fever, chills, or abdominal pain. He initially lost approximately 15 pounds with this episode. The family stopped all dairy products, which helped temporarily.

Fourteen months before presentation, the diarrhea returned. The patient's appetite remained good. He had no history of antibiotic usage, foreign travel, or identifiable sick contacts. He was seen by his family physician, and a complete blood count (CBC) at that time revealed a hemoglobin and hematocrit of 10.4 g/dL and 32.3%, respectively, with a mean corpuscular volume (MCV) of 66 fL. Iron supplementation was started. A trial of diphenoxylate/atropine improved the consistency of his stools somewhat.

Diarrhea persisted over the next several months. Before presenting to our institution, an extensive work-up, including computed tomography (CT) of the abdomen and pelvis, esophagogastroduodenoscopy (EGD) with distal duodenal biopsy, colonoscopy with random biopsies, small bowel series, and multiple serologies, was unrevealing.

QUESTIONS/DISCUSSION

All of the following statements regarding diarrhea are true except:

A. Chronic diarrhea is typically defined as diarrhea lasting longer than 4 weeks.

B. Acute diarrhea is usually infectious in origin.
C. Hyperthyroidism can cause diarrhea due to altered gastrointestinal (GI) motility.
D. Lactose intolerance causes secretory diarrhea.

In general, diarrhea can be defined as the abnormal passage of unformed stool and/or liquid and an increased frequency of passage of stool. The gastrointestinal (GI) tract handles approximately 9 L of fluid daily. Most of the fluid is reabsorbed in the large intestine. In a typical Western diet, stool that exceeds 200 g/day can be defined as diarrhea (1).

Clinicians need to inquire about specific historical features when evaluating patients with diarrhea. Relevant historical data include the duration of the diarrhea, the normal bowel habits of the patient, frequency of stools, diet, recent travel, and associated symptoms. The duration of the diarrhea is an especially important feature of the history because the differential diagnosis varies in part based on the duration of the diarrhea. Diarrhea that lasts longer than 4 weeks is considered chronic. Acute diarrhea is typically infectious in etiology and improves without specific therapy in many patients.

When evaluating patients with chronic diarrhea, clinicians need to consider a variety of potential etiologies. In general, chronic diarrhea can be categorized as secretory, osmotic, inflammatory, infectious, and dysmotility-related (1).

Secretory diarrhea develops due to an imbalance of fluid and electrolytes across the intestinal mucosal surface. Common causes of secretory diarrhea include medications, carcinoid, collagenous colitis, and celiac sprue. Clinically, secretory diarrhea persists even when a patient fasts.

In osmotic diarrhea, solutes are poorly absorbed across the mucosa and actively draw fluid into the intestinal lumen. Lactose intolerance is a common cause of osmotic diarrhea, not secretory diarrhea. Patients suffering from psychiatric illness, such as anorexia nervosa, often induce diarrhea by ingesting large quantities of laxatives.

Inflammatory diarrhea develops in patients with Crohn disease and ulcerative colitis. Patients often develop bloody diarrhea and are more likely to exhibit constitutional symptoms, such as fever, chills, and abdominal pain. Some other diseases that can produce inflammatory diarrhea are radiation colitis, diverticulitis, and ischemic colitis.

Infections cause acute diarrhea more often than they cause chronic diarrhea. Common pathogens causing acute diarrhea include *Escherichia coli, Salmonella, Shigella, Campylobacter,* Enterovirus, *Giardia, Cryptosporidium,* and *Cyclospora.* Infectious causes of chronic diarrhea include *Giardia,* mycobacterial infections, and Whipple disease.

Patients with diarrhea due to dysmotility have a considerably shorter transit time of intestinal contents. A common cause of this type of diarrhea is hyperthyroidism. Irritable bowel syndrome can also present with dysmotility; patients can experience symptoms shortly after the ingestion of food.

Case continued. Upon presentation to our institution, the patient denied anorexia, fever, chills, night sweats, pulmonary symptoms, rash, arthralgias, and neurologic symptoms. At that time, the patient had lost a total of 55 pounds. The patient's diarrhea did not resolve with dietary modifications or fasting.

Physical examination revealed a pleasant 59-year-old man. He was emaciated with evidence of bitemporal and buccal wasting. Cardiac and pulmonary examinations were normal. Abdominal examination was unremarkable except for the presence of mild ascites. Rectal examination revealed normal sphincter tone and guaiac-negative stool. There was no evidence of joint tenderness or swelling. Examination of the lower extremities revealed bilateral edema and hyper-keratotic, erythematous skin in the distal lower extremities. Neurologic examination was nonfocal.

Upon admission, laboratory testing revealed sodium of 142 mmol/L, potassium of 2.8 mmol/L, chloride of 116 mmol/L, bicarbonate of 13 mmol/L, blood urea nitrogen of 29 mg/dL, creatinine of 0.8 mg/dl, and glucose of 64 mg/dL. CBC revealed normocytic anemia (hemoglobin 9.8 g/dL) without leukocytosis. Thyroid function testing revealed evidence of mild hypothyroidism. EGD revealed diffuse white nodules throughout the second and third portions of the duodenum extending distally. Duodenal biopsies were consistent with Whipple disease, revealing an infiltrate of large macrophages with foamy cytoplasm surrounding empty spaces of varying sizes (Fig. 23.1). The macrophage cytoplasm contained inclusions of rods and granules that were periodic acid-Schiff (PAS) positive and diastase-resistant (Fig. 23.2).

Whipple Disease

The pathologist George Hoyt Whipple originally described the disease in 1907 in a 36-year-old missionary with arthritis, weight loss, nocturnal fever, and persistent diarrhea (2,3). For reasons not well understood, this disease predominantly affects white men in their fifth and sixth decades. A review of 664 patients with Whipple disease showed that 84% of those affected were men, with a mean age at diagnosis of 49 years (4). Thirty-five percent were farmers, and 66% had a history of occupational exposure to soil or animals. Genetic factors may play a role in the pathogenesis. Approximately 30% of affected patients are human leukocyte antigen B27 (HLA-B27)–positive. The exact

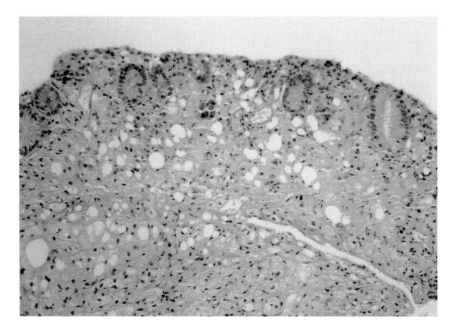

FIGURE 23.1. Low-power view of a hematoxylin and eosin (H&E) stained section from the patient's duodenal biopsy. Rounded, blunted villi and a lamina propria nearly devoid of inflammatory cells are present. Empty rounded spaces representing extracellular lipid are seen throughout the lamina propria.

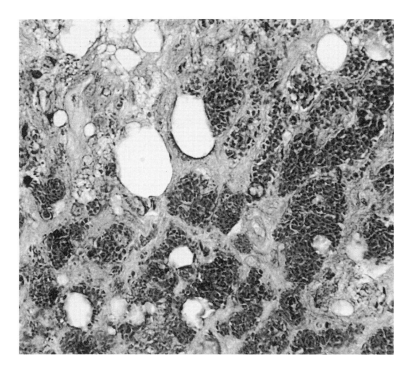

FIGURE 23.2. High-power view of a periodic acid–Schiff–stained section of the duodenal biopsy exhibiting the intense cytoplasmic staining of the macrophages in the lamina propria.

interaction between the genetics and the disease is not well defined. Whipple disease is rare, with 696 cases reported between 1907 and 1987 (5). The causative organism, a small Gram-positive bacillus named *Tropheryma whippelii* was not identified until 1992. An infectious cause of the disease had long been suspected, especially when affected individuals were treated successfully with antibiotics in 1952 (3,6).

All of the following are typical features of Whipple disease except:

A. **Weight loss**
B. **Constitutional symptoms such as fever and night sweats**
C. **Hyperpigmented skin**
D. **Neurologic symptoms**
E. **Renal involvement**

Whipple disease is a systemic disease that can affect the gastrointestinal tract, skin, central nervous system, eyes, heart, lungs, lymph nodes, liver, spleen, and bone marrow. Renal involvement is not typically associated with Whipple disease. The classic symptoms of this disease include weight loss, chronic diarrhea, abdominal pain, skin hyperpigmentation, and migratory arthralgias (7). However, patients can also present with chronic cough, lymphadenopathy, fever of unknown origin, endocarditis, constrictive pericarditis, and congestive heart failure (8). Clinicians need to consider Whipple endocarditis in a patient with blood-culture-negative endocarditis. Patients can also present with ophthalmologic manifestations, including uveitis (9).

Often overlooked, Whipple disease involving the central nervous system (CNS) can present with the most serious sequelae, including symptoms such as progressive dementia, memory loss, personality change, seizures, ophthalmoplegia, visual disturbances, and cranial nerve involvement (10). Approximately 20% of patients with Whipple disease present with only neurologic features. Magnetic resonance imaging (MRI) is superior to CT scan for detecting suspicious lesions in affected individuals; clinical response correlates well with MRI regression of CNS lesions (11).

Which of the following is/are appropriate tests to diagnose Whipple disease?

A. **Stool culture**
B. **EGD with small bowel biopsy**
C. **Polymerase chain reaction (PCR)**
D. **B and C**

Establishing a firm diagnosis of Whipple disease can be difficult. Technical difficulty in isolating the organism *in vitro*, especially in years past, has contributed to the difficulty with diagnosis. The disease can be diagnosed histologically with biopsies of organs commonly affected. EGD with biopsies of the distal duodenum or jejunum is the optimal method of diagnosis. The mucosal surface of the small intestine may appear flat, without widening of the villi. There also may be yellow-white plaques on the mucosa, representing accumulation of chyle in obstructed lymphatic channels. Similar white nodules were seen in the distal duodenum of this patient. The use of endoscopy can be supplemented by electron microscopy of the tissue or by

PCR amplification of *T. whippelii* DNA. Neither of these confirmatory tests was deemed necessary in this patient. Attempts at culture have not yielded consistent results.

PCR has become an integral part of diagnosis of Whipple disease. Researchers first isolated a 1,321-base sequence of ribosomal RNA from the 16S subunit of five patients with Whipple disease in 1992 (5). A study conducted by Ramzan et al. (12) designed to detect *T. whippelii* DNA from specimens from small bowel and lymph nodes found that PCR was highly sensitive and specific in detecting the disease, as well as in confirming suspicious cases.

Histologic sections of jejunal biopsies often suggest the diagnosis on standard hematoxylin and eosin staining. The villi are rounded or blunted. Extracellular lipid collections may be seen in the lamina propria, appearing as rounded empty spaces in the lamina propria and in distended lymphatic channels. The pathognomonic feature of Whipple disease is the presence of large macrophages with foamy, eosinophilic cytoplasm in the lamina propria of the jejunum (Fig. 23.1). These macrophages often distend the villi and displace the lymphocytes and plasma cells normally present. The cytoplasm of these foamy macrophages appears coarsely granular, and stains intensely with periodic acid–Schiff (PAS) (Fig. 23.2). Rarely, PAS-positive, Gram-positive bacilli may be seen in the extracellular space. While PAS-positive foamy macrophages, lipid vacuoles, and rounded, blunted villi were seen in this case, no organisms were seen in the extracellular space.

The pathologic differential diagnosis of Whipple disease includes *Mycobacterium avium intracellulare* (MAI) infection of the gastrointestinal tract. MAI typically occurs in immunocompromised patients who present with diarrhea and malabsorption. Pathologically, MAI can demonstrate infiltration of the lamina propria with PAS-positive macrophages. However, MAI stains positively for acid-fast bacilli, whereas *Tropheryma whippelii* does not. Stains for acid-fast bacilli were negative in this case.

Which of the following antibiotics is indicated for the long-term treatment of Whipple disease?

A. **Metronidazole**
B. **Trimethoprim/sulfamethoxazole**
C. **Ciprofloxacin**
D. **Clarithromycin**

Once uniformly fatal, Whipple disease has been treated successfully with antibiotics since 1952. A variety of different regimens have been used, including chloramphenicol, penicillin, penicillin plus streptomycin, tetracycline, ceftriaxone, and trimethoprim–sulfamethoxazole (6). Tetracycline had been first-line therapy for years (3). However, several retrospective studies demonstrated that patients treated with tetracycline had higher relapse rates, especially in CNS disease (13,14). Later studies demonstrated that trimethoprim–sulfamethoxazole was superior to tetracycline in pre-

venting relapse; trimethoprim–sulfamethoxazole has been a cornerstone of therapy since. Although trimethoprim–sulfamethoxazole is highly efficacious in preventing relapses, patients can still relapse on it. It has been postulated that the initial treatment should consist of an intravenous antibiotic with high CNS penetration, such as ceftriaxone 2 g once a day for 2 weeks, followed by a 1-year course of trimethoprim–sulfamethoxazole.

After appropriate treatment, the villi regain their normal shape, and the number of PAS-positive macrophages decreases. Inflammatory cells reappear in the lamina propria in normal proportions. The lipid collections and patchy accumulations of PAS-positive macrophages may persist indefinitely around intestinal crypts and dilated lymphatics.

CONCLUSION

After the diagnosis of Whipple disease was made, the patient received 2 weeks of ceftriaxone, followed by a year of trimethoprim–sulfamethoxazole. PCR for *Tropheryma whippelii* was negative. CT scan of the head was negative for any lesions suspicious for CNS involvement of Whipple disease. While in the hospital, the patient was started on total parenteral nutrition (TPN). He was discharged home with a Hickman catheter for TPN and antibiotic administration. In follow-up, the patient was doing well and had regained much of the weight he had lost. Repeat PCR remained negative.

REFERENCES

1. Ahlquist DA, Camilleri M. Diarrhea and constipation. In: Braunwald E, Fauci AS, Kasper DL, et al., eds. *Harrison's principles of internal medicine,* 15th ed. New York: McGraw-Hill, 2001: 241–252.
2. Fenollar F, Raoult D. Whipple's disease. *Clin Diagn Lab Immunol* 2001;8:1–8.
3. Dobbins WO 3rd. Whipple's disease: an historical perspective. *Q J Med* 1985;56:523–531.
4. Dobbins WO 3rd. *Whipple's disease.* Springfield, IL: Charles C Thomas, 1987.
5. Relman DA, Schmidt TM, MacDermott RP, et al. Identification of the uncultured bacillus of Whipple's disease. *N Engl J Med* 1992;327:293–301.
6. Paulley JW. A case of Whipple's disease (intestinal lipodystrophy). *Gastroenterology* 1952;22:128–133.
7. Marth T. Whipple's disease. In: Mandell GL, Bennett JE, Dolin R, eds. *Mandell, Douglas, and Bennett's principles and practice of infectious diseases,* 5th ed. Philadelphia: Churchill Livingstone, 2000:1171–1174.
8. Dobbins WO 3rd. The diagnosis of Whipple's disease. *N Engl J Med* 1995;332:390–392.
9. Rickman LS, Freeman WR, Green WR, et al. Brief report: uveitis caused by *Tropheryma whippelii* (Whipple's bacillus). *N Engl J Med* 1995;332:363–366.
10. Anderson M. Neurology of Whipple's disease. *J Neurol Neurosurg Psychiatry* 2000;68:2–5.

11. Kremer S, Besson G, Bonaz B, et al. Diffuse lesions in the CNS revealed by MR imaging in a case of Whipple disease. *Am J Neuroradiol* 2001;22:493–495.

12. Ramzan NN, Loftus E Jr, Burgart LJ, et al. Diagnosis and monitoring of Whipple disease by polymerase chain reaction. *Ann Intern Med* 1997;126:520–527.

13. Keinath RD, Merrell DE, Vlietstra R, et al. Antibiotic treatment and relapse in Whipple's disease: long-term follow-up of 88 patients. *Gastroenterology* 1985;88:1867–1873.

14. Knox DL, Bayless TM, Pittman FE. Neurologic disease in patients with treated Whipple's disease. *Medicine* 1976;55:467–476.

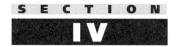

SECTION
IV

HEMATOLOGY/ MEDICAL ONCOLOGY

24

RECURRENT SPONTANEOUS HEMATOMAS IN AN ELDERLY WOMAN

SOUFIAN ALMAHAMEED
SARKIS B. BAGHDASARIAN
ELISA TSO

CASE PRESENTATION

An 85-year-old woman was transferred to our institution from a rehabilitation facility with a painful hematoma of her right thigh. The patient reported no history of trauma involving the right thigh. There was no other source of bleeding, and the review of systems was otherwise noncontributory.

Six weeks before this admission, the patient presented to another hospital with a spontaneous hematoma of her left arm. She was taking warfarin for atrial fibrillation. At the time of that admission, her INR (international normalizing ratio) was 3.3, and her hemoglobin was 6.9 g/dL. In addition to discontinuing the warfarin, she received transfusions of fresh-frozen plasma (FFP) and packed red blood cells (PRBC). Her course was complicated by compartment syndrome in her left arm, which was treated conservatively. She developed left wrist drop and was transferred from the hospital to the aforementioned rehabilitation facility.

In addition to atrial fibrillation, the patient's medical history included an 8-year history of idiopathic thrombocytopenic purpura (ITP), which had been stable on prednisone; hypertension; hypercholesterolemia; and coronary artery disease. Her surgical history included a remote cholecystectomy and umbilical hernia repair. The patient reported that she had not developed significant bleeding after either procedure. Her family history was not significant for bleeding diathesis. She did not have a history of tobacco, alcohol, or recreational drug use. Her medications on admission included prednisone 10 mg daily, furosemide, sotalol, and simvastatin.

On physical examination, the patient had a temperature of 37.5°C, heart rate of 80 beats per minute, respiratory rate of 16 breaths per minute, and blood pressure of 126/62 mm Hg. There was no icterus. Neck examination revealed a bounding carotid pulse without bruits or goiter. Her lungs were clear bilaterally. Cardiac examination revealed an irregular rhythm without murmurs. Bowel sounds were normal, and the abdomen was soft and nontender without organomegaly. Rectal examination revealed no masses and was negative for blood. There was no peripheral edema. Neurologically, she was alert and oriented. She clearly responded to questions and followed commands. Cranial nerves II to XII were intact. Strength and reflexes were normal. Skin examination did not reveal any rash, purpura, or petechiae. A large ecchymotic area covering the entire posterior aspect of the right thigh was evident and the skin overlying that area was tight and tender (Fig. 24.1).

Computed tomography of the lower extremity demonstrated a heterogeneous mass in the posterior compartment of the right thigh (Fig. 24.2). Table 24.1 summarizes initial laboratory data.

QUESTIONS/DISCUSSION

Which of the following is the least likely diagnosis?

A. von Willebrand disease (VWD)
B. Mild hemophilia A or B
C. Coagulation factor deficiency/inhibitor
D. Dysfibrinogenemia
E. ITP

The differential diagnosis of spontaneous bleeding can be divided into defects of primary or secondary hemostasis. Defects of primary hemostasis include disorders of the platelets and/or the blood vessels. Patients typically present with mucosal bleeding (epistaxis and gingival bleeding) or cutaneous bleeding (petechiae and superficial ecchymoses). Although this patient had a history of ITP, her platelet count was normal at presentation. In view of the prolonged activated partial thromboplastin time (aPTT) with a normal platelet count, VWD should be considered.

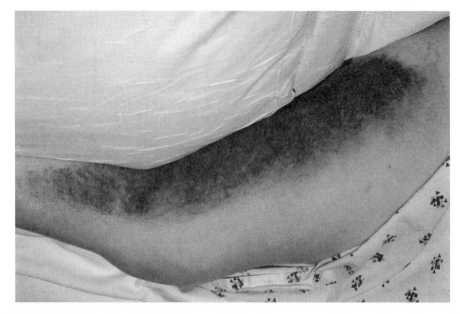

FIGURE 24.1. This patient's right thigh on admission demonstrated a large ecchymosis over the entire posterior aspect.

Defects of secondary hemostasis include disorders of the coagulation cascade, which may be caused by coagulation factor deficiencies or inhibitors of coagulation factors. The typical presentation is palpable ecchymosis extending over large areas or deep soft-tissue hematomas. Mild hemophilia A or B is associated with prolonged aPTT; most of the bleeding in these patients develops secondary to trauma or surgery (1).

In dysfibrinogenemia, the aPTT may be slightly prolonged, but almost all patients will display a prolonged thrombin time. The fibrinogen concentration is occasionally low. Patients with abnormal fibrinogen levels may have excessive bleeding, excessive thrombosis, or an absence of symptoms (2).

ITP is the least likely diagnosis in this patient.

All of the following tests are indicated in this patient except:

A. von Willebrand screen
B. Mixing studies
C. Factor IX, XI, and VIII: C (factor VIII activity) levels
D. Antiphospholipid antibody screen

The initial evaluation of patients with bleeding disorders includes a platelet count, bleeding time, prothrombin time (PT), and aPTT. Further testing depends on the results of

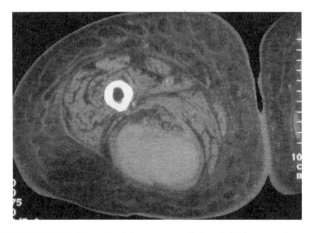

FIGURE 24.2. Computed tomogram of the right lower extremity demonstrates a large, somewhat heterogeneous, high attenuation, masslike lesion involving the posterior compartment of the right thigh. The lesion lies between the semimembranosus muscle and the long head of the biceps femoris. There is some edema within the surrounding muscles of the posterior compartment.

TABLE 24.1. ADMISSION LABORATORY DATA

	6 Weeks Prior		
	Before FFP/on Warfarin	After FFP	Presentation
Hgb	6.9 g/dL		8.3 g/dL
Platelet	151 K/μL		278 K/μL
PT	32.0 sec	14.3 sec	10.4 sec
INR	3.30	1.36	0.91
aPTT	58.9 sec	51.6 sec	59.2 sec

aPTT, activated thromboplastin time; FFP, fresh frozen plasma; INR, international normalizing ratio; PT, prothrombin time.

these tests. An abnormal platelet count or bleeding time indicates a disorder of primary hemostasis, whereas a prolonged PT, aPTT, or both indicate disorders of secondary hemostasis. A prolonged aPTT is indicative of deficiencies of the intrinsic pathway. A prolonged aPTT may be caused by heparin therapy, the presence of antiphospholipid antibodies, circulating anticoagulants, vitamin K deficiency, or liver disease. PT prolongation occurs in patients with deficiencies of extrinsic pathway coagulation factors, liver disease, vitamin K deficiency, and circulating anticoagulants. Warfarin use will predictably prolong the PT; unintentional ingestion or surreptitious use should be investigated in patients without an obvious reason for PT prolongation. During this patient's initial hospitalization, the PT normalized after fresh-frozen plasma transfusion and vitamin K administration. However, her aPTT remained elevated. The use of heparin was excluded with serum heparin assays. In this patient, VWD screening was negative, and fibrinogen level was normal.

Mixing studies are indicated in the setting of prolonged PT or aPTT of unclear etiology. Equal amounts of the patient's plasma and pooled normal plasma are mixed with subsequent measurement of aPTT and PT. Complete correction of the prolonged test indicates a coagulation factor deficiency or VWD, whereas persistent prolongation or partial correction suggests the presence of coagulation factor inhibitors. In this patient, the aPTT did not correct after mixing with normal plasma, which indicated the presence of an inhibitor to factor VIII, IX, XI, or XII.

Only factors VIII, IX, and XI were tested. Factors XI and IX were normal, whereas factor VIII—C level—was 5% (normal, 55% to 145%) (3). Factor XII was not measured because it usually causes thrombosis rather than bleeding (4).

A Bethesda assay is indicated in the setting of an abnormal mixing study to establish the presence of a coagulation factor inhibitor and measure its titer. In this assay, serial dilutions of a patient's plasma are incubated with pooled normal plasma at 37°C for 2 hours. Subsequently, coagulation factor activity is measured using a clotting assay. The reciprocal of the dilution of a patient's plasma that results in 50% factor activity is presented as Bethesda units (BU) (4). Consequently, a stronger inhibitor will result in higher Bethesda units. This patient had a measurement of 30 BU, and the diagnosis of acquired factor VIII inhibitor was made.

Antiphospholipid antibody syndrome can cause prolonged aPTT that does not correct after mixing with normal plasma; however, it is associated with thrombosis rather than bleeding. For this reason, an antiphospholipid antibody screen would not be indicated in the evaluation of this patient.

With which of the following conditions is acquired factor VIII inhibitor associated?

A. **Pregnancy**
B. **Malignancy**
C. **Rheumatoid arthritis**

D. **Systemic lupus erythematosus**
E. **All of the above**

Acquired factor VIII inhibitor is the most common acquired coagulation factor inhibitor. Its incidence is 0.2 to 1 case per 1 million individuals per year, with bimodal peaks at ages 20 to 30 years and 60 to 80 years (5). It results from immune dysregulation and emergence of a previously silent or suppressed lymphoid clone from its inhibited state. Antibodies will subsequently interact with specific epitopes on factor VIII and neutralize its procoagulant function. This disorder can cause mild to severe bleeding in patients with no previous bleeding history. It is associated with a mortality rate of 13% to 22% (6,7). Up to 50% of patients with factor VIII inhibitor have associated immune abnormalities such as lymphoproliferative disorders, pregnancy, skin diseases, drug reactions, malignancy, rheumatoid arthritis, systemic lupus erythematosus, giant cell arteritis, and inflammatory bowel disease. Our patient did not have a history or physical examination suggestive of any of these conditions.

The choice of treatment depends on the acuity and severity of bleeding and the BU titer. Since low responders (<5 BU) usually do not manifest an amnestic rise in antibody titer after reexposure to the coagulation protein, large doses of factor VIII or desmopressin acetate (DDAVP) 0.3 μg/kg may be used. DDAVP stimulates the release of factor VIII from physiologic stores (6). High responders (>10 BU) tend to mount an amnestic antibody increase after reexposure to the coagulation protein. Treatment options for high responders include bypassing agents such as prothrombin complex concentrates or recombinant factor VIIa; agents with reduced cross-reactivity such as porcine factor VIII or extracorporeal plasmapheresis with porcine factor VIII and intravenous immunoglobulin (IVIG) infusion; and immunomodulation with high-dose IVIG (6). Immunosuppression with prednisone, cyclophosphamide, or azathioprine has also been used with good results (6). Forty percent of factor VIII autoantibodies will be suppressed after 3 to 6 weeks of prednisone alone, and more than 50% of autoantibodies ultimately will be suppressed by prednisone, with or without cyclophosphamide or azathioprine (7,8).

CONCLUSION

This patient was in the high-responder group, but fortunately had very low cross-reactivity toward porcine factor VIII. Consequently, two doses of porcine factor VIII were given to the patient. She was started on cyclophosphamide 100 mg and prednisone 60 mg daily. She remained hemodynamically stable, and repeated blood tests showed stable hemoglobin, increased serum factor VIII levels, and decreased aPTT. She was transferred to a rehabilitation facility in good condition.

REFERENCES

1. Feinstein DI. Inhibitors in hemophilia. In: Hoffman R, Benz EJ Jr, Shattil SJ, et al., eds. *Hematology: basic principles and practice,* 3rd ed. Philadelphia: Churchill Livingstone, 2000:1904–1911.
2. Reitsma PH. Genetic principles underlying disorders of procoagulant and anticoagulant proteins. In: Colman RW, Hirsch J, Marder VJ, et al, eds. *Hemostasis and thrombosis: basic principles and clinical practice,* 4th ed. Philadelphia: Lippincott Williams & Wilkins, 2001:59–87.
3. Wallach J. Introduction to normal values. In: *Interpretation of diagnostic tests,* 6th ed. Boston: Little, Brown, 1996:3–30.
4. Santoro SA, Eby CS. Laboratory evaluation of hemostatic disorders. In: Hoffman R, Benz EJ Jr., Shattil SJ, et al., eds. *Hematology: basic principles and practice,* 3rd ed. Philadelphia: Churchill Livingstone, 2000:1841–1849.
5. Kessler CM. Acquired factor VIII autoantibody inhibitors: current concepts and potential therapeutic strategies for the future. *Haematologica* 2000;85(10 Suppl):57–61.
6. Kessler CM, Ludlam CA. The treatment of acquired factor VIII inhibitors: worldwide experience with porcine factor VIII concentrate. *Semin Hematol* 1993;30:22–27.
7. Green D, Lecher KA. A survey of 215 non-hemophilic patients with inhibitors to factor VIII. *Thromb Haemost* 1981;45:200–203.
8. Bossi P, Cabane J, Ninet J, et al. Acquired hemophilia due to factor VIII inhibitors in 34 patients. *Am J Med* 1998;105:400–408.

25

A 34-YEAR-OLD WOMAN WITH GROSS HEMATURIA

FIRAS Z. SIOUFI
DAVID M. CASEY

CASE PRESENTATION

A 34-year-old black woman presented to the emergency department with 1 day of gross hematuria, urinary frequency, and a sensation of incomplete voiding. She denied dysuria, fever, or chills. She had been discharged from the hospital 8 days earlier, following an upper gastrointestinal (GI) bleed, which required intensive care unit admission and blood transfusions. During her hospitalization, a Foley catheter had been placed to monitor urine output.

In addition to the recent GI bleed, the patient had a history of benign hypertension and dyspepsia. She was taking ramipril and esomeprazole, which was started following her discharge from the hospital. She denied use of over-the-counter or herbal medications. There was no family history of bleeding disorders, kidney disease, or anemia. She did not smoke and did not use alcohol or drugs.

Vital signs revealed the patient to be afebrile, with a blood pressure of 138/81 mm Hg, pulse of 84 beats per minute, respiratory rate of 16 per minute, and pulse oximetry of 97% on room air. Physical examination was essentially normal, without abdominal or flank pain, skin changes, evidence of hepatosplenomegaly, or signs of bleeding from other areas of her body.

A urine dipstick showed 3+ hemoglobin, 2+ leukocyte esterase, positive nitrite, pH 6.5, and specific gravity of 1.020. Microscopic examination showed zero to five white blood cells per high-power field and zero to three red blood cells per high-power field. Serum hemoglobin was 10 g/dL; hemoglobin was 11 g/dL upon hospital discharge 8 days earlier. Platelets were 225 K/μL, and white blood cell count was 8.8 K/μL. Coagulation parameters, serum electrolytes, and creatinine were all normal. The patient was thought to have an iatrogenic urinary tract infection (UTI) from her recent Foley catheterization, and she was discharged home on oral ciprofloxacin.

QUESTIONS/DISCUSSION

Which of the following can produce red urine without red blood cells present on microscopic examination?

A. Ingestion of beets
B. Use of rifampin
C. Myoglobinuria
D. Hemoglobinuria
E. All of the above

The initial step in evaluating a patient with gross hematuria should be a urine dipstick and examination of the urine sediment. If the dipstick is positive for blood but red blood cells are not seen in the sediment, several reasons need to be considered. The urine dipstick reacts to heme, which in the absence of red cells may represent either myoglobin or hemoglobin (1). Myoglobinuria can occur in the setting of skeletal muscle breakdown, such as trauma or rhabdomyolysis, in which case serum creatine kinase will usually be elevated. Hemoglobinuria may be caused by hemolysis, occurring in either the systemic circulation or the urinary tract itself. Red urine which is negative for blood on the dipstick can be seen in porphyria; with certain medications, including rifampin and phenazopyridine; or with ingestion of certain foods, such as beets, rhubarb, and paprika (2,3).

This patient had evidence of a UTI based on positive leukocyte esterase and nitrite, but a UTI fails to explain the presence of blood on dipstick without any red cells on microscopy. Hematuria is commonly present in UTIs; however, red cells should be seen on urine microscopy. While the recent Foley catheterization placed the patient at increased risk for developing a UTI, she may have been expected to develop symptoms sooner after discharge, rather than 8 days later. Her urine findings raise the question of whether or not she truly has a UTI. Urine dipstick has a very high negative predictive value (>90%) for UTI in the absence of leukocyte esterase and nitrite. However, the positive predictive value is only moderate (3,4). Patients with positive leukocyte esterase or nitrite on dipstick should have laboratory evaluation of the urine to confirm the diagnosis, especially when the clinical suspicion for UTI is not high.

Case Continued. One day after initial assessment in the emergency department, the patient returned, complaining of persistently bloody urine. Her vital signs at that time included blood pressure, 130/80 mm Hg; pulse, 90 beats per minute; respiratory rate, 18 per minute; and pulse oximetry, 97% on room air. Her physical examination was unchanged from the day before, except for the presence of mild icterus. Rectal examination revealed no gross or occult blood.

Laboratory studies at that time showed hemoglobin of 7.3 g/dL, mean corpuscular volume of 88 fL, platelets of 218 K/μL, white blood cell count of 7 K/μL, and reticulocyte count of 6.2%. A peripheral smear revealed normocytic anemia with slight polychromasia and no schistocytes. Additional blood work showed a bilirubin of 3.7 mg/dL, direct bilirubin of 0.3 mg/dL, lactate dehydrogenase (LDH) of 1,536 U/L, and normal coagulation studies.

What is the most likely cause of her anemia?

A. **Acute blood loss from the gastrointestinal or genitourinary tract**
B. **Hemolytic anemia**
C. **Vitamin B$_{12}$ deficiency**
D. **Bone marrow suppression**
E. **Iron deficiency**

Over 9 days, this patient suffered a drop in hemoglobin of almost 4 g/dL, and, upon this presentation, the hemoglobin dropped almost 2 g/dL in 24 hours. There was no evidence of GI bleeding on examination or by history, and the previous urinalysis did not show any red blood cells, making acute blood loss an unlikely source of her anemia. Iron deficiency anemia and anemia due to vitamin B$_{12}$ deficiency result in microcytic and macrocytic anemia, respectively, neither of which this patient had. Furthermore, anemia due to dietary deficiencies causes chronic anemia that develops gradually, not an acute anemia as seen in this patient. A process resulting in bone marrow suppression is also unlikely in this patient, as an elevated reticulocyte count, as seen in this patient, indicates that immature red cells are being released from the marrow in response to her anemia.

At this point, hemolytic anemia was thought to be the most likely cause of this patient's anemia. She had elevated indirect bilirubin and LDH, both of which are elevated in hemolysis. In addition, her chief complaint of blood in the urine can be explained by hemolysis, as she likely developed hemoglobinuria, not true hematuria. Her urine was dipstick positive for blood, yet there were no red cells on microscopic examination, which could have signified the presence of ongoing hemolysis.

Serum haptoglobin is another marker of hemolytic anemia. Haptoglobin is typically low in hemolytic anemia, as haptoglobin quickly binds free hemoglobin in the plasma. The bound complex is rapidly cleared by the mononuclear phagocyte system (5). When the binding capacity of haptoglobin is exceeded, free hemoglobin is filtered by the kidneys and reabsorbed in the proximal tubules (5). Thus, the presence of hemoglobinuria indicates that the capacity for hemoglobin retrieval by both haptoglobin and tubular reabsorption has been overcome, indicating a severe hemolytic process (5).

Which of the following is the least likely cause of this patient's hemolytic anemia?

A. **Delayed hemolytic transfusion reaction (DHTR)**
B. **Immune-mediated hemolysis secondary to medication**
C. **Non–immune-mediated hemolysis secondary to medication**
D. **Hereditary spherocytosis**

A delayed hemolytic transfusion reaction (DHTR) usually occurs 2 to 10 days after blood transfusion. This process occurs in patients who have been sensitized to red blood cell antigen during previous blood transfusions, resulting in alloantibody production at very low levels. The low levels of antibody may result in a negative alloantibody screen during the cross-matching process. During a subsequent transfusion with red blood cells bearing the particular antigen, an anamnestic response may develop, which produces delayed hemolysis. Usually, the hemolytic process is self-limited, and treatment is unnecessary. However, the hemolysis can occasionally be severe enough to require blood transfusions (6). The diagnosis is frequently made when a direct antiglobulin test (direct Coombs test) and antibody screen become positive on cross-match ordered before a subsequent transfusion. This patient could have developed a DHTR during her previous hospitalization, as she received multiple transfusions over several days.

Drug-induced hemolysis can develop by one of two mechanisms. Immune-mediated processes occur as a result of drug-induced antibody production directed against antigens on the surface of the red cell. The antibodies, which are usually IgG, are known as "warm antibodies," since they bind at body temperature (5). A direct Coombs test is almost always positive in this setting. A non–immune-mediated process can be caused by drug-induced oxidative stress. A variety of drugs that produce oxidative hemolysis through the formation of intracellular oxygen radicals have been identified. Glucose-6-phosphate dehydrogenase (G6PD) deficiency places patients at increased susceptibility to hemolysis by disrupting the hexose–monophosphate shunt pathway that normally handles oxidant stress (5). Susceptible patients are typically of African or Mediterranean descent. Culprit drugs include sulfamethoxazole, primaquine, dapsone, nitrofurantoin, methylene blue, and phenazopyridine.

Hereditary spherocytosis is a condition that can produce crises of hemolytic anemia. It may not manifest itself until adulthood. It is an autosomal dominant condition that affects red blood cell cytoskeletal proteins; a family history of anemia or splenectomy is often obtained (7,8). Patients often present with hemolytic anemia, splenomegaly, and jaundice. Spherocytes are seen on peripheral smear. However, this finding is sensitive, but not specific, as other disorders may also produce spherocytes. This patient did not have spherocytes on peripheral smear, splenomegaly, or a family history of anemia, all of which make hereditary spherocytosis unlikely.

Case Concluded

To evaluate for an antibody-mediated form of hemolytic anemia, a Coombs test was performed, which was negative. The possibility of a DHTR was also raised. To evaluate for this, samples of the patient's blood were cross-matched against aliquots from two units transfused during her admission for GI bleeding. The antibody screen was negative, making DHTR unlikely. Her hemolytic anemia was thought to be secondary to a non–immune-mediated process, which was likely due to a medication. Her only medications—ramipril, ciprofloxacin, and esomeprazole—were discontinued. Follow-up laboratory studies showed resolution of the hemolytic process, with serum LDH and bilirubin normalizing. On hospital day 3, the patient was discharged home. Follow-up hemoglobin 2 weeks later was 11.1 g/dL, which was similar to her hemoglobin upon discharge from her first hospitalization. The patient was scheduled for follow-up with a hematologist to evaluate for the presence of an enzyme deficiency that would predispose to oxidative hemolysis.

CONCLUSION

This patient presented with what initially appeared to be a UTI but was eventually diagnosed with a non–immune-mediated hemolytic anemia, likely secondary to medications. Clinicians need to recognize that what patients describe as "bloody urine" does not always represent true hematuria. A lack of red blood cells in urine with positive blood on dipstick should raise suspicion for either hemoglobinuria or myoglobinuria, both of which may indicate a severe underlying process.

REFERENCES

1. Pimstone NR. Renal degradation of hemoglobin. *Semin Hematol* 1972;9:31–42.
2. Watson WC, Luke RG, Inall JA. Beeturia: its incidence and a clue to its mechanism. *Br Med J* 1963;2:971–973.
3. Spector DA. Hematuria. In: Barker LR, Burton JR, Zieve PD, eds. *Principles of ambulatory medicine,* 5th ed. Baltimore: Williams & Wilkins, 1999: 549–553.
4. Hooton TM, Stamm WE. Diagnosis and treatment of uncomplicated urinary tract infection. *Infect Dis Clin North Am* 1997;11: 551–581.
5. Kasiske BL, Keane WF. Laboratory assessment of renal disease: clearance, urinalysis, and renal disease. In: Brenner B, ed. *Brenner & Rector's the kidney,* 6th ed. Philadelphia: WB Saunders, 2000: 1129–1170.
6. Bunn HF, Rosse W. Hemolytic anemia and acute blood loss. In: Braunwald E, Fauci AS, Kasper DL, et al., eds. *Harrison's principles of internal medicine,* 15th ed. Philadelphia: McGraw-Hill, 2001: 681–692.
7. Dzieckowski JS, Anderson KC. Transfusion biology and therapy. In: Braunwald E, Fauci AS, Kasper DL, et al., eds. *Harrison's principles of internal medicine,* 15th ed. Philadelphia: McGraw-Hill, 2001:733–739.
8. Tse WT, Lux SE. Red blood cell membrane disorders. *Br J Haematol* 1999;104:2–13.

26

A 78-YEAR-OLD MAN WITH THROMBOCYTOPENIA

ARMANDO PHILIP S. PAEZ
JAMES C. PILE

CASE PRESENTATION

A 78-year-old man with a history of coronary artery disease, gastroesophageal reflux disease, and diverticulosis presented to the emergency department with 2 days of severe lower-quadrant abdominal pain. He described the pain as constant and severe, with radiation to the back. The pain was exacerbated by eating, and associated with nausea. The patient had three episodes of melena, the last while undergoing evaluation in the emergency department. There was no hematochezia, hematemesis, or hematuria. He noted a rash on both arms but was unsure of the duration. For the preceding 2 months, the patient had been taking quinine sulfate every night for leg cramps. Additionally, he reported taking aspirin three times daily for headache. His other medications included amitriptyline, spironolactone, tamsulosin, lansoprazole, digoxin, isosorbide mononitrate, potassium chloride, and furosemide, all of which he was taking once a day.

On physical examination, the patient was afebrile with a blood pressure of 105/60 mm Hg and pulse of 70 beats per minute, without orthostatic changes. Respiratory rate was 18 per minute, with an oxygen saturation of 96% on room air. Conjunctivae were pale; oral mucosa and palate were moist with no petechiae. His neck was supple with no lymphadenopathy. Cardiovascular examination revealed regular rate and rhythm with a grade II/VI holosystolic murmur heard best at the apex. Lungs were clear to auscultation bilaterally. Abdomen was soft, with mild direct tenderness over the epigastrium and left lower quadrant on deep palpation. There was no rebound tenderness. Spleen and liver were not palpable. Bowel sounds were present. Extremities showed 2+ lower-extremity pitting edema with some venous stasis changes, with normal pedal pulses. Examination of the skin showed nonpalpable purpura over the dorsal aspect of both upper extremities. Rectal examination showed normal tone and no palpable masses. The stool was foul smelling, black in

color, and positive for occult blood. Neurologic examination was unremarkable.

Initial laboratory results showed a white blood cell count of 4.02 K/μL, hemoglobin of 10.5 g/dL, and hematocrit of 32%, with a mean corpuscular volume of 94.4 fL and a slightly elevated red cell distribution width of 15.5. Platelet count was 7,000/μL. Peripheral smear confirmed true thrombocytopenia without evidence of other abnormalities, including microangiopathic hemolytic anemia. Lactate dehydrogenase (LDH), haptoglobin, and electrolytes were within normal limits. Serum blood urea nitrogen was 33 mg/dL and serum creatinine was 1.6 mg/dL, with a known baseline of 1.3 mg/dL. Coagulation profile was normal.

QUESTIONS/DISCUSSION

What is the most likely cause of this patient's thrombocytopenia?

A. Pseudothrombocytopenia
B. Idiopathic thrombocytopenic purpura
C. Thrombotic thrombocytopenic purpura–Hemolytic uremic syndrome (TTP-HUS)
D. Drug-induced thrombocytopenia

Pseudothrombocytopenia, which is due to platelet clumping, occurs in approximately 0.1% of the population (1,2). This usually occurs in blood samples containing EDTA and is due to the binding of preformed platelet antibodies to neoepitopes exposed after EDTA exposure (3). Examination of a peripheral smear is essential in evaluating a patient with thrombocytopenia in order to rule out this artifact. This can be confirmed by peripheral smear using citrated blood. Clinically, this has not been proven to cause an increased risk of bleeding or thrombosis.

Idiopathic thrombocytopenic purpura (ITP) is essentially a diagnosis of exclusion. There are several criteria for the diagnosis of ITP, including the exclusion of the use of any medication that can cause thrombocytopenia (4). Clinically, it is difficult, if not impossible, to distinguish ITP from other causes of thrombocytopenia at the outset. This should be borne in mind, especially in cases of severe bleeding requiring immediate treatment.

This patient presented only with thrombocytopenia, without signs of hemolytic anemia. Except for mild chronic renal insufficiency, he did not have any other manifestations of hemolytic–uremic syndrome (HUS) or thrombotic thrombocytopenic purpura (TTP), such as neurologic symptoms or fever. However, quinine-induced HUS-TTP has been reported (5).

Clinically, this patient was suspected to have a drug-induced thrombocytopenia. However, as mentioned earlier, ITP could not be ruled out at this point.

Which of the following medications could have caused this patient's thrombocytopenia?

A. **Quinine**
B. **Aspirin**
C. **Amitriptyline**
D. **Digoxin**
E. **Furosemide**
F. **Spironolactone**
G. **All of the above**

All the preceding medications have been reported to cause thrombocytopenia (6–8). Apart from heparin, which is associated with both bleeding and hypercoagulability, and myelosuppressive medications, the most common causes of drug-induced thrombocytopenia are the quinine/quinidine drug group and sulfonamides (6,7).

Several criteria have been proposed to aid in the diagnosis of drug-induced thrombocytopenia (7,9–12):

- Therapy with the suspected drug should precede the thrombocytopenia, and recovery from thrombocytopenia should be complete and sustained after the drug is stopped.
- The suspected drug is the only one used before the onset of thrombocytopenia *or* there is a sustained normal platelet count after other drugs are continued or reintroduced after discontinuation of the suspected drug.
- Other causes of thrombocytopenia are excluded.
- Reexposure to the suspected drug should result in recurrent thrombocytopenia.

If a case fulfills all these criteria, then there is a definite level of causality. If three out of four criteria are met, it is probable, and if one out of four is met, it is possible. Rechallenge with the suspected offending agent is generally not appropriate after profound thrombocytopenia.

Practically, drug-induced thrombocytopenia can be diagnosed only when thrombocytopenia resolves with discontinuation of the suspected drug, as no diagnostic laboratory tests are available. When faced with a patient with isolated thrombocytopenia on multiple medications, knowing the probability of each of the drugs causing thrombocytopenia is helpful in making the decision to stop or continue individual medications.

When confronted with a suspected drug-induced thrombocytopenia, true thrombocytopenia should be established by performing a platelet count and peripheral blood smear. Coagulation tests will help rule out bleeding tendencies due to coagulation disorders. A peripheral smear is essential, as this will help identify pseudothrombocytopenia and obvious congenital platelet disorders. *In vitro* drug-specific platelet antibody testing is neither standardized nor widely available. Therefore, routine drug-specific platelet antibody testing is not recommended. Bone marrow examination may be necessary when the etiology of thrombocytopenia remains unclear.

A detailed history, a careful review of all medications, and exclusion of other causes of thrombocytopenia are crucial in evaluating these patients. A careful physical examination, paying particular attention to the oral cavity and skin, will give clues to the severity and nature of bleeding manifestations. Petechiae and purpura, mostly in the dependent areas of the body such as the ankles and feet, are nonpalpable, which helps differentiate them from vasculitic skin rashes. In contrast to isolated thrombocytopenia, coagulation disorders will likely present with deep-tissue bleeding, including hemarthroses or visceral hematomas.

Drug-induced thrombocytopenia occurs through two general mechanisms. The first is decreased platelet production, as seen with chemotherapeutic drugs and ethanol. A second mechanism is through increased platelet destruction, which may be nonimmunologic (ristocetin, protamine sulfate, bleomycin) or immunologic (quinidine/quinine, heparin, gold salts, acetaminophen, and penicillin). Most drug-induced thrombocytopenias fall into the latter category, which is idiosyncratic and antibody-mediated.

Quinine and its optical isomer, quinidine, have been well described to cause thrombocytopenia (7), as well as HUS (5,13). The platelet antibodies are drug dependent, meaning that the antibodies bind to target receptors in the presence of the drug in the blood. In most cases, glycoprotein (Gp) Ib/IX is the target for these drug-dependent antibodies; Gp IIb/IIIa has also been reported as a target (14). The binding sites on restricted sets of epitopes of quinine-dependent antibodies have been characterized (15). Immunologic drug-mediated thrombocytopenia results from the IgG Fab terminus binding to a complex comprised of the drug or its metabolite and Gp Ib/IX or Gp IIb/IIIa (Fig. 26.1) (8).

Which of the following is the most appropriate initial management of drug-induced thrombocytopenia?

A. **Platelet transfusion**
B. **Corticosteroids**

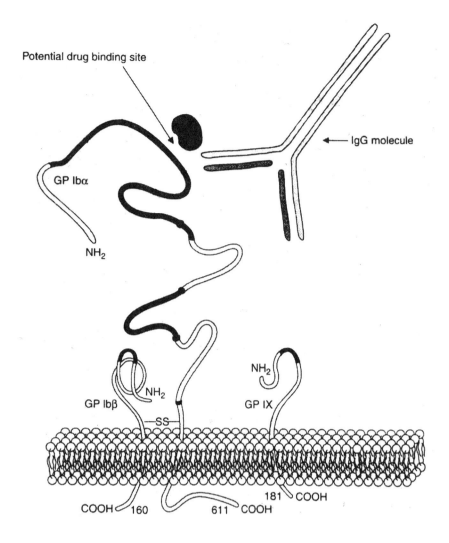

Potential drug binding site

IgG molecule

GP Ibα

NH₂

NH₂

GP Ibβ   NH₂   GP IX

SS

COOH   160   611   COOH   181   COOH

FIGURE 26.1. Proposed binding of quinine/quinidine-induced thrombocytopenia. (From Warkentin TE, Kelton JG. Thrombocytopenia due to platelet destruction and hypersplenism. In: Hoffman R, Benz E, Shattil S, et al., eds. *Hematology: basic principles and practice,* 3rd ed. New York: Churchill Livingstone, 1999:2138–2154, with permission.)

C. **Plasmapheresis**
D. **Intravenous immunoglobulin (IV IG)**
E. **Discontinuation of the suspected medication(s)**

Although there is no standard therapy for drug-induced thrombocytopenia, the first and most important step in managing drug-induced thrombocytopenia is discontinuation of the suspected drug or drugs. On admission, quinine and aspirin were stopped, while the rest of the patient's usual medications were continued. Platelets were administered in light of the severe thrombocytopenia and active bleeding. Empiric steroid treatment with prednisone 60 mg once daily was started due to an inability to completely dismiss the possibility of ITP. While no evidence exists to suggest a benefit from corticosteroids in treating drug-induced thrombocytopenia, their use is often recommended in severe cases due to the difficulty in excluding ITP (10). If drug-induced thrombocytopenia is suspected, discontinuation of the drug should result in recovery of the platelet count. With discontinuation of the drug, the platelet count may recover in 1 day, although normalization may take 2 weeks or longer. As in the case of ITP, IV IG, platelet trans-

fusions, and RhD in Rh+ individuals can be given, especially in cases of severe thrombocytopenia with active bleeding. In asymptomatic patients with platelet counts of greater than 10,000 to 20,000/μL, discontinuation of the suspected drug and careful monitoring may be sufficient. Patient education regarding the cause of thrombocytopenia is very important as well, as proper information may prevent recurrent thrombocytopenia.

Hospital Course

The patient's immediate posttransfusion platelet count was 15,000/μL. Esophagogastroduodenoscopy done immediately upon admission showed chronic gastritis. Computed tomography of the abdomen showed diverticulosis with mild inflammatory changes suggestive of diverticulitis. The platelet count rose to 26,000/μL the following day. By the second hospital day, the abdominal pain and melena had resolved. On the third day, the platelet count was 31,000/μL. Corticosteroids were stopped, and the platelet count continued to increase over the subsequent days. The patient was discharged home on the sixth hospital day with a platelet count of 87,000/μL. After 11 days off quinine and aspirin, the platelet count had normalized to 171,000/μL. Aspirin therapy was subsequently restarted in view of his significant coronary artery disease. He had no recurrence of his thrombocytopenia, pointing to quinine as the likely cause of his drug-induced thrombocytopenia.

CONCLUSION

Quinine is currently approved by the Food and Drug Administration (FDA) only for the treatment of malaria. Until 1994, it was also indicated for the treatment of nocturnal leg cramps. A metaanalysis of its efficacy showed modest efficacy in the prevention of nocturnal leg cramps in the elderly (16,17). However, its serious side effects, including thrombocytopenia in a significant number of patients, seem to outweigh the small potential benefits in the treatment of nocturnal leg cramps. On August 22, 1999, the FDA prohibited the marketing of over-the-counter quinine sulfate for leg cramps (18). Cases such as this one suggest that quinine should be used very cautiously, if at all, for this indication.

REFERENCES

1. Vicari A, Banfi G, Bonini PA. EDTA-dependent pseudothrombocytopaenia: a 12-month epidemiological study. *Scand J Clin Lab Invest* 1988;48:537–542.
2. Bartels PC, Schoorl M, Lombarts AJ. Screening for EDTA-dependent deviations in platelet counts and abnormalities in platelet distribution histograms in pseudothrombocytopenia. *Scand J Clin Lab Invest* 1997;57:629–636.
3. Fiorin F, Steffan A, Pradella P, et al. IgG platelet antibodies in EDTA-dependent pseudothrombocytopenia bind to platelet membrane glycoprotein IIb. *Am J Clin Pathol* 1998;110:178–183.
4. George JN, Woolf SH, Raskob GE, et al. Idiopathic thrombocytopenic purpura: a practice guideline developed by explicit methods for the American Society of Hematology. *Blood* 1996;88:3–40.
5. McDonald SP, Shanahan EM, Thomas AC, et al. Quinine-induced hemolytic uremic syndrome. *Clin Nephrol* 1997;47:397–400.
6. Database for Drug-induced thrombocytopenia: an update. http://moon.ouhsc.edu/jgeorge.
7. George JN, Raskob GE, Shah SR, et al. Drug-induced thrombocytopenia: a systematic review of published case reports. *Ann Intern Med* 1998;129:886–890.
8. Warkentin TE, Kelton JG. Thrombocytopenia due to platelet destruction and hypersplenism. In: Hoffman R, Benz E, Shattil S, et al., eds. *Hematology: basic principles and practice,* 3rd ed. New York: Churchill Livingstone, 1999:2138–2154.
9. Standardization of definitions and criteria of causality assessment of adverse drug reactions: drug-induced cytopenia. *Int J Clin Pharmacol Ther Toxicol* 1991;29:75–81.
10. Pedersen-Bjergaard U, Andersen M, Hansen PB. Drug-induced thrombocytopenia: clinical data on 309 cases and the effect of corticosteroid therapy. *Eur J Clin Pharmacol* 1997;52:183–189.
11. Majhail NS, Lichtin AE. What is the best way to determine if thrombocytopenia in a patient on multiple medications is drug-induced? *Cleve Clin J Med* 2002;69:259–262.
12. Rizvi MA, Kojouri K, George JN. Drug-induced thrombocytopenia: an updated systematic review. *Ann Intern Med* 2001;134:346.
13. Hou M, Horney E, Stockelberg D, et al. Multiple quinine-dependent antibodies in a patient with episodic thrombocytopenia, neutropenia, lymphopenia, and granulomatous hepatitis. *Blood* 1997;90:4806–4811.
14. Nieminen U, Kekomaki R. Quinidine-induced thrombocytopenic purpura: clinical presentation in relation to drug-dependent and drug-independent platelet antibodies. *Br J Haematol* 1992;80:77–82.
15. Chong BH, Du XP, Berndt MS, et al. Characterization of the binding domains on platelet glycoproteins Ib–IX and IIb/IIIa complexes for the quinine/quinidine dependent antibodies. *Blood* 1991;77:2190–2199.
16. Man-Son-Hing M, Wells G, Lau A. Quinine for nocturnal leg cramps: a meta-analysis including unpublished data. *J Gen Intern Med* 1998;13:600–606.
17. Man-Son-Hing M, Wells G. Meta-analysis of efficacy of quinine for treatment of nocturnal leg cramps in elderly people. *BMJ* 1995;310:13–17.
18. FDA orders stop to marketing of quinine for night leg cramps. *FDA Consumer.* July–Aug 1995.

27

A 44-YEAR-OLD WOMAN WITH SEVERE IRON-DEFICIENCY ANEMIA

JASON G. HURBANEK
SARKIS B. BAGHDASARIAN
ROBERT M. PALMER

CASE PRESENTATION

A 44-year-old black woman presented to the emergency department with 1 day of nausea and vomiting. She noted six episodes of emesis of yellowish gastric secretions but denied hematemesis. The vomiting was associated with periumbilical pain that did not radiate. The patient denied diarrhea and reported regular bowel movements without melena or hematochezia. She denied any previous history of similar symptoms. On review of systems, she noted weakness and fatigue for 1 year. Her fatigue was worse on exertion, but she was able to perform her desk job without difficulty. She denied fever, chills, arthralgias, skin rash, shortness of breath, chest pain, or weight loss. Gynecologic history revealed regular 28-day cycles with menses of approximately 7 days that required four soaked pads per day. Upon presentation, the patient was on the last day of her menses. The patient had never been pregnant and denied contraceptive use.

The patient denied any significant past medical history, including diabetes mellitus, coronary artery disease, hypertension, hyperlipidemia, thyroid disease, gallstones, or anemia. She also denied any previous surgeries. She was not taking any medications. The patient smoked two packs of cigarettes per week and denied any alcohol or drug use. Family history was negative for any significant disease.

Physical examination revealed an uncomfortable patient. Vital signs showed a temperature of 37.9°C, heart rate of 108 beats per minute, and blood pressure of 152/79 mm Hg supine and 125/68 mm Hg sitting. Her mucous membranes were dry. Examination of the neck revealed a bounding carotid pulse without bruits or goiter. Her lungs were clear bilaterally. Cardiac examination revealed tachycardia with normal first and second heart sounds and a grade III/VI systolic ejection murmur heard best at the left lower sternal border. Her bowel sounds were normal, and her abdomen was soft but tender in the suprapubic area. Rectal examination revealed no masses and was negative for blood. She had an enlarged uterus consistent with 14- to 16-week gestational size and vaginal blood clots on pelvic exam. There was no peripheral edema. Neurologic examination was nonfocal.

QUESTIONS/DISCUSSION

Which of the following is the least likely diagnosis?

A. **Gastroenteritis**
B. **Uterine fibroids**
C. **Pregnancy**
D. **Colon cancer**

Vomiting is a nonspecific complaint that can be due to a myriad of medical conditions. Patients with gastroenteritis can present with abdominal pain and vomiting. These patients often do not have diarrhea; therefore, this diagnosis should be considered in this patient. The enlarged uterus on bimanual exam and menorrhagia are consistent with uterine leiomyomas (fibroids). However, it is essential to rule out pregnancy in a woman of childbearing age with this presentation. Colon cancer is the least likely diagnosis, given her history and physical examination.

Initial laboratory data revealed normal electrolytes and renal function. Complete blood count revealed a white blood count of 7.15 K/μL, hemoglobin of 3.1 g/dL, hematocrit of 12.4%, and platelets of 160 K/μL. Repeat hemoglobin and hematocrit were 2.9 g/dL and 11.5%, respectively. Urine pregnancy test was negative.

Which of the following is the appropriate first step in the evaluation of this patient?

A. **Pelvic ultrasound**
B. **O-negative blood transfusion**
C. **Hydration with normal saline**

D. Anemia studies with peripheral blood smear

Although all the preceding should be considered, the first step in caring for this patient, given her signs of volume depletion, is hydration with normal saline while preparing typed and cross-matched blood for transfusion. Without a clear source of rapid blood loss and her relative hemodynamic stability, immediate transfusion with O-negative blood is not indicated. Pelvic ultrasound and anemia studies are indicated in this setting but should be done after the patient has been adequately volume resuscitated.

Further evaluation of this patient's anemia revealed a mean corpuscular volume of 62 fL, mean corpuscular hemoglobin concentration of 25 g/dL, and red cell distribution width of 21.6. Other studies included iron of 18 μg/dL, total iron-binding capacity of 483 μg/dL, ferritin of 2 ng/mL, transferrin saturation of 4%, and reticulocyte count of 2%. A peripheral blood smear was consistent with hypochromic, microcytic anemia (Fig. 27.1).

Which of the following statements regarding laboratory studies for iron-deficiency anemia is true?

A. Total iron-binding capacity (TIBC) is the most specific test for iron-deficiency anemia.

B. TIBC is unaffected by pregnancy and oral contraceptives.

C. Inflammation has no effect on serum ferritin levels.

D. Ferritin levels less than 10 to 15 ng/mL are highly specific for iron-deficiency anemia.

E. Hypochromic, microcytic indices are pathognomonic of iron deficiency.

There is no clinical situation other than iron deficiency in which extremely low serum ferritin levels are seen (1,2). Ferritin concentrations of less than 10 to 15 ng/mL are 59% sensitive and 99% specific for iron-deficiency anemia (3). Ferritin is an acute phase reactant that can be elevated in liver disease, infection, inflammation, and malignancy. Therefore, clinicians need to realize that a patient with iron-deficiency anemia and any of these diagnoses may have a normal or high ferritin level.

An increased TIBC is the second most accurate test for predicting iron-deficiency anemia. An elevated TIBC results in decreased transferrin saturation. One study demonstrated that a transferrin saturation of less than 15% was 80% sensitive and 50% to 65% specific for iron-deficiency anemia (4). The specificity of the test is diminished because TIBC is decreased in certain circumstances in which plasma transferrin concentration increases, including pregnancy and oral contraceptive use (5).

Hypochromic microcytic anemia is also seen with anemia of chronic disease and thalassemia. Therefore, it is important to rule out these disorders before beginning iron supplementation. Anemia of chronic disease is often normocytic, and in contrast to iron-deficiency anemia, the ferritin level is usually normal or high.

In adults, iron-deficiency anemia develops and progresses based on the balance between iron absorption and loss. For example, iron stores in premenopausal women are generally decreased due to menstrual losses that average an extra 1 mg loss of iron per day (6). The Third National Health and Nutrition Examination Survey reported that iron-deficiency anemia was present in 1%

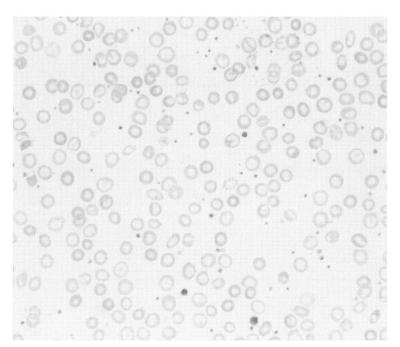

FIGURE 27.1. This patient's peripheral blood smear demonstrated hypochromic, microcytic anemia. Hypochromic, microcytic anemia can be seen with iron-deficiency anemia, anemia of chronic disease, and thalassemia (original magnification, ×40). (Courtesy of Jeffrey Fine, M.D., Cleveland Clinic Foundation Department of Pathology.)

to 2% of adults in the United States (7). Although the most common complaints of iron-deficiency anemia include weakness, headache, fatigue, and irritability, some patients may complain of glossal pain, reduced salivary secretions, and atrophy of the tongue papillae. Pagophagia, or chewing on ice, is considered quite specific for iron deficiency (8,9).

This patient tolerated transfusion with four units of packed red blood cells. Pelvic ultrasound showed uterine fibroids with total obscuration of the endometrial echo complex.

All of the following statements regarding uterine leiomyomas are true except:

A. **The differential diagnosis includes pregnancy, adenomyosis, polyps, endometrial hyperplasia, endometrial carcinoma, and congenital anomalies.**
B. **Black women have a lower incidence of leiomyomas than other women.**
C. **Diagnosis is made by bimanual examination and confirmed with a pelvic ultrasound.**
D. **Treatment options include hysterectomy, uterine artery embolization, myomectomy, gonadotropin-releasing hormone (GnRH) agonist therapy, androgenic agents (danazol), or progestins.**
E. **Leiomyomas are associated with recurrent miscarriage, infertility, premature labor, and complications of labor.**

Leiomyomas are the most common solid pelvic tumors in women. They are clinically apparent in 20% to 25% of women during reproductive years (10,11). Black women carry a two- to threefold increased risk of leiomyomas (12). On examination, the uterus is enlarged, is mobile, and may be palpated above the symphysis. Although ultrasound confirms the diagnosis, other modalities are helpful in diagnosis. Magnetic resonance imaging can distinguish leiomyomas, adenomyomas, and leiomyosarcomas. Hysterosalpingogram, sonohysterogram, or hysteroscopy are other useful diagnostic modalities.

Surgery is the primary therapy for patients with large or symptomatic leiomyomas. Although hysterectomy provides a definitive cure for leiomyomas, myomectomy and uterine artery embolization are options for women wishing to preserve childbearing potential. Medical treatments take advantage of the fact that leiomyomas need estrogen for growth. One study demonstrated that a 3-month treatment regimen with GnRH agonists decreased uterine volume by 40% to 60% (13). Other medical treatments, including androgenic agents and progestins, can control menorrhagia associated with leiomyomas.

Case Conclusion

Following transfusion, the patient's hemoglobin and hematocrit increased to 7.0 g/dL and 22.9%, respectively, and remained stable over the next 2 days. After 3 days in the hospital, the patient was discharged on oral ferrous sulfate. Long-term treatment options for the patient's fibroids were discussed and follow-up with gynecology was arranged.

CONCLUSION

Uterine fibroids are not typically considered a cause for severe anemia. However, this case demonstrates that previously undiagnosed fibroids can produce massive blood loss. This patient had atypical symptoms related to her fibroids, presenting with periumbilical pain and vomiting. Clinicians need to consider the diagnosis of fibroids in women with iron-deficiency anemia and abdominal complaints. Patients should be reassured that effective long-term treatment options are available for uterine fibroids.

REFERENCES

1. Fairbanks VF. Laboratory testing for iron status. *Hosp Pract* 1991;26(Suppl 3):17–24.
2. McMahon LF Jr, Ryan MJ, Larson D, et al. Occult gastrointestinal blood loss in marathon runners. *Ann Intern Med* 1984;100: 846–847.
3. Tran TN, Eubanks SK, Schaffer KJ, et al. Secretion of ferritin by rat hepatoma cells and its regulation by inflammatory cytokines and iron. *Blood* 1997;90:4979–4986.
4. Hansen TM, Hansen NE. Serum ferritin as indicator of iron responsive anaemia in patients with rheumatoid arthritis. *Ann Rheum Dis* 1986;45:596–602.
5. Eschbach JW, Cook JD, Scribner BH, et al. Iron balance in hemodialysis patients. *Ann Intern Med* 1977;87:710–713.
6. Brittenham GM. Disorders of iron metabolism: iron deficiency and overload. In: Hoffman R, Benz EJ Jr., Shattil SJ, et al., eds. *Hematology: basic principles and practice*, 3rd ed. New York: Churchill Livingstone, 2000:397–428.
7. Looker AC, Dallman PR, Carroll MD, et al. Prevalence of iron deficiency in the United States. *JAMA* 1997;277:973–976.
8. Osaki T, Ueta E, Arisawa K, et al. The pathophysiology of glossal pain in patients with iron deficiency and anemia. *Am J Med Sci* 1999;318:324–329.
9. Reynolds RD, Binder HJ, Miller MB, et al. Pagophagia and iron-deficiency anemia. *Ann Intern Med* 1968;69:435–440.
10. Buttram VC Jr, Reiter RC. Uterine leiomyomata: etiology, symptomatology, and management. *Fertil Steril* 1981;36:433–445.
11. Cramer SF, Patel A. The frequency of uterine leiomyomas. *Am J Clin Pathol* 1990;94:435–438.
12. Marshall LM, Spiegelman D, Barbieri RL, et al. Variation in the incidence of uterine leiomyoma among premenopausal women by age and race. *Obstet Gynecol* 1997;90:967–973.
13. Stewart EA, Friedman AJ. Steroidal treatment of myomas: preoperative and long-term medical therapy. *Semin Reprod Endocrinol* 1992;10:344–357.

28

A 71-YEAR-OLD WOMAN WITH PERSISTENT LYMPHADENOPATHY

BRIDGET P. SINNOTT
RODERICK ADAMS

CASE PRESENTATION

A 71-year-old woman presented for evaluation of persistent lymphadenopathy (LAN) and eosinophilia. The patient reported that she was healthy until 5 years before admission, at which time she developed jaundice. She was diagnosed with coombs positive autoimmune hemolytic anemia (AIHA), for which she was treated with prednisone. Her work-up at that time included computed tomography (CT) of the abdomen and pelvis, which revealed diffuse intraabdominal and pelvic lymphadenopathy. Serial CT scans of her chest, abdomen, and pelvis revealed progression of the LAN from the pelvic and inguinal chains into the axillary, mediastinal, and periaortic areas. Multiple bone marrow biopsies and lymph node biopsies of inguinal, cervical, and axillary nodes were negative for malignancy. Two courses of corticosteroids did not significantly improve the lymphadenopathy.

One year before this presentation, the patient was asymptomatic except for mild fatigue. Over the 4 months before presentation, she developed drenching night sweats, lip ulceration, and diffuse swelling. She also gained 35 pounds. Several weeks before presentation, she developed dyspnea on minimal exertion, decreased appetite, and pruritus. Review of systems was otherwise remarkable for early satiety, dry cough, minimal arthralgias, and urinary frequency.

About 4 months before presentation, the patient underwent a left axillary lymph node biopsy that showed atypical lymphoid hyperplasia without evidence of lymphoma. One month later, the patient underwent a bone marrow biopsy that showed a normocellular marrow without evidence of lymphoma.

Her past medical history was remarkable for type 2 diabetes mellitus, hypothyroidism, and childhood asthma. Surgical history included a hysterectomy and cholecystectomy. She had a history of exposure to tuberculosis, but had been found to be PPD (Purified Protein Derivative skin test for tuberculosis) negative. Her medications on admission were glyburide and levothyroxine. She denied alcohol or tobacco use. She resided in rural Pennsylvania. She was retired, having worked in a bank, hardware store, and bakery. She did not have any pets or any history of animal or insect bites. She had no history of foreign travel. Her family history was negative for hematologic malignancies.

QUESTIONS/DISCUSSION

Lymph nodes should be assessed for all of the following characteristics except:

A. **Location**
B. **Size**
C. **Consistency**
D. **Mobility**
E. **Thrills**

Lymph nodes should be examined for all of the preceding except for thrills.

- *Location:* Localized LAN suggests a local process and prompts a search for pathology in the area of nodal drainage. Enlarged supraclavicular and scalene nodes are always abnormal (1). Virchow node is an enlarged left supraclavicular node that is associated with metastatic gastrointestinal cancer (1). Generalized LAN is more suggestive of systemic pathology.
- *Size:* The size of individual lymph nodes and their rate of enlargement is important. Abnormal nodes are generally greater than 1 cm in diameter (1). Rapidly enlarging LAN is suggestive of an infectious etiology. In contrast, slowly enlarging LAN is more suggestive of malignancy or other noninfectious etiologies.
- *Consistency:* Lymph nodes that develop in response to infection and inflammation tend to feel soft. Firm, rubbery nodes are more typically found in lymphoma and chronic leukemia. Hard lymph nodes are found in

metastatic cancer and postinflammatory fibrotic lymphadenopathy.

- *Mobility:* It is important to assess the mobility of lymph nodes in relation to surrounding structures and overlying skin. Normal lymph nodes are freely mobile. Matted lymph nodes suggest malignancy or inflammation in the surrounding tissues.
- *Tenderness:* Tenderness on lymph node examination is suggestive of rapid enlargement, which typically occurs with inflammatory processes (2). Occasionally, tenderness may result from hemorrhage or malignancy.

It is also important to assess for the presence of organomegaly. The combination of splenomegaly and generalized lymphadenopathy favors certain diagnoses, most notably lymphoproliferative disorders, including lymphoma and leukemia (2).

Physical examination on admission revealed a temperature of 37.4°C, blood pressure of 134/59 mm Hg, pulse of 111 beats per minute, and respiratory rate of 24 per minute. In general, the patient was mildly dyspneic at rest, with evidence of anasarca. Head and neck examination did not reveal any oral ulcers. There were multiple, firm, hard, nontender cervical lymph nodes bilaterally, ranging from 1 to 5 cm in diameter. There were multiple, bilateral, firm, hard, nontender axillary lymph nodes. Chest examination revealed left basilar crackles. She had left breast edema, without evidence of cellulitis. Her cardiovascular examination was normal except for tachycardia. Her abdomen was soft, with evidence of diffuse mild tenderness, hepatomegaly to 2 cm below the costal margin, and a palpable splenic tip. She had 4+ pitting edema to her hips and lymphedema in her left arm; there was no synovitis. Neurologic examination was nonfocal. Examination of the skin revealed multiple excoriations.

Which of the following conditions could have produced generalized lymphadenopathy in this patient?

A. **Lymphoma**
B. **Tuberculosis**
C. **Sarcoidosis**
D. **Angioimmunoblastic lymphadenopathy**
E. **All of the above**

All the preceding are potential etiologies for this patient's generalized lymphadenopathy. Lymphadenopathy (LAN) can be a primary or secondary manifestation of numerous disorders. A history of symptoms suggestive of malignancy or infection, such as fever, night sweats, fatigue, and weight loss, should be sought. A history of exposure to tuberculosis, pets, travel, risk factors for human immunodeficiency virus (HIV), and medication use should be sought. Distinguishing localized and generalized LAN can help in the formulation of a differential diagnosis. Localized LAN involves only one lymph node region, such as the inguinal region,

whereas generalized LAN involves multiple lymph node groups. This patient's history and physical examination was consistent with a picture of generalized lymphadenopathy, which has a broad differential diagnosis (Table 28.1).

Generalized LAN with night sweats and pruritus are consistent with lymphoma in a 71-year-old lady. Although the duration of her generalized LAN and associated weight gain are not typical features of lymphoma, these features do not rule out a diagnosis of lymphoma. Lymphadenopathy associated with neoplastic processes is typically painless and frequently develops at a more indolent rate than lymphadenopathy associated with infection.

LAN secondary to disseminated tuberculosis is a possibility, despite the patient's prior negative PPD. She had night sweats, which are common with tuberculosis. However, a patient with disseminated tuberculosis would likely develop more systemic symptoms, such as fever, weight loss, and productive cough.

Sarcoidosis frequently presents with hilar and mediastinal LAN, but it can occasionally present with generalized LAN (1). Although this patient's prior lymph node biopsies did not show caseating granulomas, several features of her presentation are potentially consistent with sarcoidosis, including arthralgias and dyspnea.

Angioimmunoblastic lymphadenopathy is a rare cause of indolent generalized LAN. It is associated with eosinophilia, autoimmune hemolytic anemia, generalized edema, and hepatosplenomegaly (3). Many features of this patient's history are consistent with angioimmunoblastic lymphadenopathy.

Laboratory work-up on admission included a white blood cell count of 12.78 K/μL, with a differential of 67% neutrophils, 13% lymphocytes, 12% eosinophils, and 5% monocytes. Hemoglobin was 8.9 g/dL, with a mean corpuscular volume of 87 fL, and platelets were 348 K/μL. Peripheral blood smear revealed mild eosinophilia, normocytic anemia with slight polychromasia, and neutrophilic

TABLE 28.1. DIFFERENTIAL DIAGNOSIS OF GENERALIZED LYMPHADENOPATHY

Viral infection: Epstein–Barr virus, cytomegalovirus, human immunodeficiency virus, rubella, hepatitis B
Bacterial infection: Tuberculosis, syphilis, brucellosis, leptospirosis, Lyme disease
Parasitic infection: Toxoplasmosis, malaria
Fungal infection: Histoplasmosis, coccidioidomycosis, paracoccidioidomycosis
Hematologic: Hodgkin disease, non-Hodgkin lymphoma, acute lymphoblastic leukemia, chronic lymphocytic leukemia, angioimmunoblastic lymphadenopathy
Medications: Phenytoin, hydralazine, allopurinol
Miscellaneous: Sarcoidosis, systemic lupus erythematosus, rheumatoid arthritis, hyperthyroidism, chronic granulomatous disorders

leukocytosis without left shift. Electrolytes, blood urea nitrogen, creatinine, and thyroid stimulating hormone were all normal. Hepatic function panel was normal except for an alkaline phosphatase of 133 U/L and albumin of 3.0 g/dL. Lactate dehydrogenase was elevated at 303 U/L, and both the erythrocyte sedimentation rate (72 mm/hr) and C-reactive protein (2.6 mg/dL) were elevated. Urinalysis was normal except for three to five red blood cells per high-power field.

Blood cultures and serologies for toxoplasmosis, rubella, herpes simplex virus, HIV, and *Strongyloides* were negative. Fungal serologies for *Aspergillus, Blastomyces, Coccidioides,* and *Histoplasma* were negative. A repeat PPD with anergy panel was nonreactive.

Which of the following radiographic studies is least appropriate for the evaluation of this patient's symptoms?

A. **Chest x-ray**
B. **Abdominal ultrasound**
C. **Computed tomography (CT scan) of the chest/ abdomen/pelvis**
D. **Lymphangiogram**

Radiographic studies can define the size and extent of lymphadenopathy more precisely than clinical examination. All the preceding studies are appropriate except for a lymphangiogram. A chest x-ray is important to rule out hilar lymphadenopathy or a pulmonary infiltrate, which may be secondary to lymphoma, tuberculosis, sarcoidosis, fungal infection, or lung cancer. Abdominal ultrasound is useful as a rapid and noninvasive method of confirming the extent of organomegaly. CT scanning can clarify the extent and location of adenopathy not evident on physical examination. The description of the lymph nodes on CT may also help in narrowing the differential diagnosis. CT can also guide radiologists in selecting the most appropriate lymph nodes for sampling. CT scanning has replaced lymphangiography as the most appropriate tool to assess lymphadenopathy.

In this patient, chest x-ray revealed pulmonary venous congestion with bilateral pleural effusions. Abdominal ultrasound demonstrated hepatomegaly. CT of the chest revealed extensive axillary and mediastinal adenopathy, and CT of the abdomen revealed intraabdominal and retroperitoneal adenopathy with splenomegaly (Figs. 28.1 and 28.2). These findings were considered suggestive of a lymphoproliferative process. Review of prior abdominal/pelvic CT scans revealed pelvic, inguinal, periaortic, and retroperitoneal lymphadenopathy. Hepatomegaly and splenomegaly were also noted.

At this stage, which of the following tests is most appropriate to establish a diagnosis?

A. **Excisional lymph node biopsy**

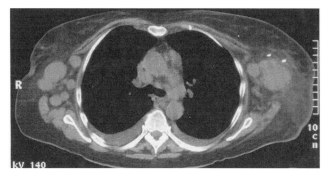

FIGURE 28.1. Computed tomography of the chest demonstrating extensive axillary and mediastinal adenopathy.

B. **Fine-needle aspiration (FNA)**
C. **Bone marrow biopsy**
D. **Exploratory laparotomy**

Although this patient had undergone multiple unrevealing biopsies, excisional lymph node biopsy is the most appropriate test at this stage, since it allows histologic examination of an intact core of tissue, which provides information about nodal architecture and the presence of abnormal cells or microorganisms. FNA of a lymph node is less sensitive than excisional biopsy due to sampling errors and difficulty in recognizing well-differentiated lymphoma. Bone marrow biopsy is appropriate in patients with an unrevealing excisional lymph node biopsy in whom lymphoma or lymphoproliferative disease is suspected. Exploratory laparotomy is not typically needed to obtain a tissue diagnosis and would not be appropriate at this point in the evaluation.

A repeat lymph node biopsy revealed evidence of a peripheral T-cell lymphoma with features of angioimmunoblastic lymphadenopathy.

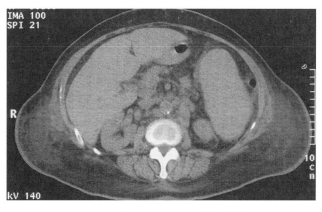

FIGURE 28.2. Computed tomography of the abdomen demonstrating intraabdominal and retroperitoneal adenopathy, hepatomegaly, and splenomegaly.

CONCLUSION

Angioimmunoblastic lymphadenopathy (AILD) is a rare lymphoproliferative disorder that usually affects older adults. Diffuse lymphadenopathy, hepatosplenomegaly, autoimmune hemolytic anemia, rash, and hypergammaglobulinemia are common features of AILD. AILD is considered a disease of T-cell origin; about 18% of cases transform into immunoblastic or large-cell lymphoma (3). The etiology remains unclear, although several reports describe an association with Epstein–Barr virus (4). Generally, symptoms develop over several weeks. However, as in this case, the onset can be insidious, occurring over years (3).

Immunologic abnormalities associated with AILD include polyclonal hypergammaglobulinemia and coombs positive AIHA (4,5). Monoclonal gammopathy, especially late in the course of the disease, has also been described (6). Normocytic anemia is a common finding, and eosinophilia has also been associated with this disorder (5). In addition to lymphadenopathy, generalized or localized edema and pleural effusions are notable clinical findings in AILD (7).

Combined chemotherapeutic regimens are used to treat AILD, with 25% of patients developing complete and sustained remission (4). Stage and tumor bulk do not appear to correlate with disease activity or prognosis in AILD (4). Overwhelming infections rather than lymphoma itself account for the majority of deaths in AILD (5).

Lymphadenopathy is a common problem in clinical practice. A thorough history and physical examination are imperative in crafting a differential diagnosis. It is important to characterize lymphadenopathy as acute or chronic and localized or generalized. The overall presentation of the patient should guide further investigations. In this case, the presentation was somewhat atypical and required an extensive work-up to determine the etiology of her chronic generalized lymphadenopathy.

REFERENCES

1. Henry PH, Longo DL. Enlargement of the lymph nodes and spleen. In: Braunwald E, Fauci AS, Kasper DL, et al., eds. *Harrison's principles of internal medicine,* 15th ed. New York: McGraw-Hill, 2001:360–365.
2. Talley NJ, O'Connor S. The haematological system. In: *Clinical examination,* 3rd ed. Oxford: Blackwell Science Ltd, 1996: 223–246.
3. Pangalis GA, Moran EM, Nathwani BN, et al. Angioimmunoblastic lymphadenopathy: long-term follow-up study. *Cancer* 1983;52:318–321.
4. Sallah S, Gagnon GA. Angioimmunoblastic lymphadenopathy with dysproteinemia: emphasis on pathogenesis and treatment. *Acta Haematol* 1998; 99:57–64.
5. Knecht H. Angioimmunoblastic lymphadenopathy: ten years' experience and state of current knowledge. *Semin Hematol* 1989; 26:208–215.
6. Offit K, Macris NT, Finkbeiner JA. Monoclonal hypergammaglobulinemia without malignant transformation in angioimmunoblastic lymphadenopathy with dysproteinemia. *Am J Med* 1986; 80:292–294.
7. Ganesan TS, Dhaliwal HS, Dorreen MS, et al. Angioimmunoblastic lymphadenopathy: a clinical, immunological and molecular study. *Br J Cancer* 1987;55:437–442.

29

A 54-YEAR-OLD WOMAN WITH BACK PAIN

MICHAEL J. LEE
ROBERT J. PELLEY

CASE PRESENTATION

A 54-year-old woman was admitted from the office of an orthopedic surgeon for disabling back pain and compression fractures. The patient noted progressive midthoracic back pain for 7 months. Associated with this, she had right midthigh pain that was exacerbated with activity and weight bearing. The pain was not completely relieved with rest. Over the preceding few weeks, her back and thigh pain rapidly progressed to the point where she became wheelchair bound. At presentation, the pain was 8 out of 10 in intensity and radiated in a bandlike pattern from her midback toward her chest. The patient also reported generalized fatigue, anorexia, and weight loss.

Her review of systems was significant for intermittent chills and fevers. She also noted increasing abdominal girth. She reported occasional nausea and nonbilious, nonbloody emesis, which she did not relate to meals or any other stimulus. She noted dyspnea on exertion with a flight of stairs. She denied any loss of bowel or bladder function, hemoptysis, hematemesis, hematuria, melena, hematochezia, dysuria, or change in bowel habits.

The patient's past medical history was significant for coronary artery disease with a previous myocardial infarction, hypertension, gastroesophageal reflux disease, and choledocholithiasis. Her surgical history was significant for two cesarean sections, an ovarian cystectomy 29 years prior, laparoscopic cholecystectomy three years prior, and a total abdominal hysterectomy with bilateral salpingo-oophorectomy for bleeding uterine leiomyomas. The patient denied any tobacco, drug, or alcohol abuse. Her last Pap smear was 3 years before presentation, and her last mammogram was 9 months before presentation. Both of these tests were normal.

For her symptoms, the patient had seen her primary care physician, who prescribed various muscle relaxants and pain medications, which provided no improvement. Because of the lack of improvement, her physician referred her to our

institution for further evaluation and management. A skeletal survey revealed bony destruction of the inferior ramus of the right hip and sclerosis of the proximal portion of the right femur (Fig. 29.1). The skeletal survey also showed compression fractures of the sixth through tenth thoracic vertebrae and generalized lytic and blastic disease of the ribs.

Physical Examination

The patient had a temperature of 36.9°C, respiratory rate of 12 per minute, pulse of 91 beats per minute, and blood pressure of 176/91 mm Hg. In general, she was alert and oriented to person, place, and time, and in no apparent distress. The examination revealed no neck masses or cervical,

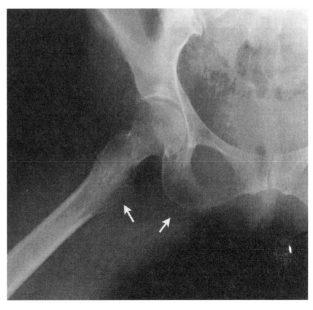

FIGURE 29.1. X-ray of the right hip and femur. The *arrows* demonstrate lytic disease in the inferior ramus and sclerosis of the proximal femur.

submandibular, supraclavicular, epitrochlear, or inguinal adenopathy. Examination of the left breast revealed tenderness at the 2 o'clock position extending toward the tail of the breast with a small, palpable mass. Pulmonary and cardiac examinations were normal. The abdomen was soft and nontender with normal bowel sounds. No masses were palpable. Rectal examination revealed occult-negative brown stool; no masses were present. The patient was diffusely tender along her mid and lower thoracic spine. The patient had a normal cranial nerve examination. She had normal strength in her upper extremities and left lower extremity but had 3 out of 5 strength in the right lower extremity, with the examination greatly limited due to pain. Muscle tone was normal. Upper-extremity reflexes were normal. Patellar reflexes were diminished bilaterally, and Achilles reflexes were absent. Babinski sign was negative bilaterally. Sensation was grossly intact.

QUESTIONS/DISCUSSION

What is the most likely cause of the patient's constellation of signs and symptoms?

A. **Neoplasm**
B. **Vertebral osteomyelitis**
C. **Osteoporosis**
D. **Paget disease**

Metastatic disease of unknown primary comprises approximately 10% to 15% of all malignancies. With a prevalence of 13.8 per 100,000 patients, it is the eighth most common malignancy. It has a higher frequency than ovarian cancer, rectal cancer, and non-Hodgkin lymphoma (1,2). Unknown primary tumor portends a poor prognosis. The mortality is 75% in the first year, and the average life expectancy from the date of diagnosis is approximately 6 months (2). A clinical presentation suggestive of a cancer of unknown primary consists of four general features (1):

- A short time course of symptoms
- Localized symptoms, such as pain, swelling, or cough
- Constitutional symptoms, including anorexia, fever, fatigue, and weight loss
- Obvious abnormalities on physical examination, such as palpable masses at a single site or multiple sites

In this case the patient had constitutional symptoms and rapidly progressive pain localized primarily to her skeletal system. She also had findings on examination localizing to her left breast and axilla, as well as pain over her thoracic spine. These findings suggested an unknown primary tumor. The results of the skeletal survey also increased the suspicion for metastatic disease of unknown primary.

Vertebral osteomyelitis is part of the differential diagnosis of back pain with constitutional symptoms. However, vertebral osteomyelitis is more common in men and

involves the lumbar spine (50% of cases) more frequently than the thoracic spine (35% of cases) (3). Sources of bacteremia such as a catheter-related infection, urosepsis, endocarditis, or soft-tissue infection are usually obvious. Most patients experience slowly progressive, dull pain over several months, rather than the acute acceleration of pain this patient experienced. The presence of multiple compression fractures is also not a feature of vertebral osteomyelitis. Furthermore, localizing signs such as breast tenderness with an axillary mass are uncommon in vertebral osteomyelitis. The usual focal finding on examination is pain over the involved vertebrae and paraspinous structures. Radiographically, osteomyelitis appears as irregular erosions of contiguous vertebral bodies with narrowing of the interposing disk space. Other diseases of the spine, such as malignancy, rarely involve the disk space (3).

Osteoporosis can also lead to compression fractures. Only 25% to 30% of patients experience acute onset of pain with vertebral compression fractures secondary to osteoporosis (4). The pelvis and long bones are also affected. However, constitutional symptoms and localizing symptoms are not present. The severe pain of the initial fracture usually subsides in 6 to 10 weeks (4). Chronic pain is usually due to strain on adjacent soft tissue structures, including muscles, ligaments, and tendons. Severe unremitting back pain must raise the thought of malignancy. Radiographically, diffuse osteopenia is seen without the lytic or blastic involvement.

Paget disease is another potential cause of vertebral compression fractures. As with osteoporosis, constitutional symptoms are not part of the clinical presentation. Many patients are asymptomatic. Headache, facial pain, increasing hat size, and lumbar back pain are common presenting symptoms. Hip pain similar to degenerative joint disease may be due to Paget or secondary osteoarthritis (5). Radiographically, Paget disease involves the pelvis, femur, skull, tibia, lumbosacral spine, clavicles, and ribs (5). Depending on the phase of the disease, radiographs may reveal lytic disease and/or sclerosis.

Which of the following is not a routine part of the evaluation of a cancer of unknown primary?

A. **Computed tomography (CT scan) of the abdomen and pelvis**
B. **Rectal examination**
C. **Carcinoembryonic antigen (CEA), CA 15-3, CA 19-9**
D. **Thorough history and physical**
E. **Prostate-specific antigen (PSA) in men**

The evaluation of a cancer of unknown primary should be detailed and systematic. If a primary cancer is not found upon initial evaluation, it is unlikely that a more extensive assessment will provide a diagnosis. In up to 30% of patients with cancer of unknown primary, the site of origin is not found at autopsy (2). Necroscopy studies have shown that the most likely site of primary disease for patients with symptoms above the diaphragm is the lung and for patients with symptoms below the diaphragm is the pancreas. A thorough, yet focused, evaluation is appropriate in the evaluation of these patients.

A complete history should include questions about exposures to carcinogens, such as solvents, radiation, and tobacco (6). Clinicians should inquire as to whether or not patients are current on age and gender-appropriate cancer screening. A thorough review of systems is important. For instance, a history of urinary hesitancy in a man would raise the question of prostate cancer, hematuria would suggest a genitourinary malignancy, and gastrointestinal (GI) bleeding would raise suspicion for a GI source. A personal history of malignancy as well as any family history of malignancy should be elicited. A complete physical examination, including breast, pelvic, rectal, and prostate examinations, should be performed (1,2,6,7). A basic laboratory evaluation, including a complete blood count, liver function tests, a serum chemistry profile, and a urinalysis checking for occult blood, is necessary (2). If myeloma is suspected, serum and urine protein electrophoresis can be diagnostic.

A chest x-ray and CT scan of the abdomen and pelvis are required radiographic studies as per European Society of Medical Oncology (ESMO) guidelines and some of the literature (2,7). There is still controversy over the utility of computed tomography of the abdomen and pelvis. Even though 20% to 30% of these scans may show a primary tumor, principally in the pancreas, a mortality benefit has not been demonstrated (1). The diagnosis of a breast or ovarian primary can confer a survival advantage to patients. Therefore, mammography and imaging of the pelvis in female patients, either by CT or pelvic ultrasound, should be performed (1). The signs and symptoms of the patient should guide the performance of further radiographic studies and other tests, such as colonoscopy or upper endoscopy.

The most accurate tumor-specific markers are α-fetoprotein (AFP), β-human chorionic gonadotropin (β-HCG), and prostate specific antigen (PSA). In a young male with primarily midline disease, AFP and β-HCG can help to exclude a germ cell tumor. PSA can also be used to exclude prostate cancer in men (2,7). The specificities of CEA, CA 15-3, and CA 19-9 are too low to identify a primary site; their utility has been established only for monitoring disease activity in known primary sites (1,6). For instance, CEA may be elevated in hepatitis, pancreatitis, or renal failure, without a malignancy present. About 35% to 75% of patients with thyroid, lung, breast, ovarian, endometrial, lung, biliary, gastric, colon, or pancreatic cancer can have elevated CEA levels (6).

Which of the following tumors metastasize to bone?

A. **Lung**
B. **Breast**

C. **Hodgkin disease**
D. **Multiple myeloma**
E. **All of the above**

The most common malignancy of bone is metastatic disease. It is the third most common site of metastatic disease, behind only lung and liver. The tumors that most commonly metastasize to bone are breast, lung, prostate, renal, and thyroid malignancies. The frequency of bone metastases for breast and prostate cancers is highest (6). Metastases to the spinal cord are frequently due to malignancies of the breast, lung, prostate, myeloma, and lymphoma. Lung cancer tends to metastasize to the cervical and thoracic spine; lymphoma, to the thoracic and lumbar spine; and prostate cancer, to the lumbar spine (2). Knowing which tumors metastasize to specific locations can help to focus further evaluation, although any tumor can metastasize to any area. Table 29.1 shows the common sites of metastasis of primary cancers (2).

Laboratory and Radiographic Data

The patient's calcium was 10.0 mg/dL, with an elevated alkaline phosphatase of 618 U/L. The remainder of her blood work was within normal limits. Chest x-ray revealed atelectasis and bony disease as noted on the skeletal survey. A brain CT did not show intracranial disease. CT scans of the chest, abdomen, and pelvis (Fig. 29.2) showed minimal left axillary lymphadenopathy, a small mass in the lateral portion of the left breast, extensive lytic lesions in the thoracic spine, and small hepatic lesions in the left lobe of the liver that were suspicious for metastatic disease.

Hospital Course: Given the patient's extensive spinal disease, right-lower-extremity weakness, and hyporeflexia, she was started on dexamethasone to reduce spinal cord swelling in the event of cord compromise. Emergent mag-

TABLE 29.1. COMMON SITES OF METASTATIC CANCER

Site of Metastasis	Primary Cancer Type
Bone PQRST	Breast, lung, Hodgkin disease, multiple myeloma, prostate, thyroid, kidney
Brain "4 ps"	Breast, lung, melanoma, pancreas, prostate
Liver	Breast, lung, pancreas, gastrointestinal
Lung	Breast, lung, melanoma, gastrointestinal, pancreas, sarcoma
Peritoneum/ascites	Gastrointestinal, ovary, pancreas
Pleural effusions	Breast, lung, ovary, pancreas
Skin	Breast, kidney, lung, lymphoma, melanoma
Spinal cord	Breast, lung, lymphoma, prostate

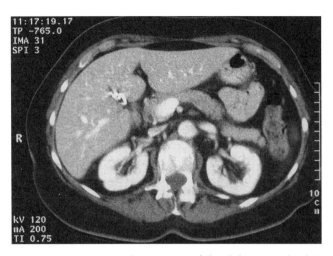

FIGURE 29.2. Computed tomogram of the abdomen and pelvis showing spinal metastases and possible metastases in the left lobe of the liver.

netic resonance imaging (MRI) of the cervical, thoracic, and lumbar spines was performed to rule out spinal cord compression. The MRI revealed mild pathologic compression deformities at the third, fourth, sixth, seventh, eighth, tenth, and eleventh thoracic vertebrae. There was mild retropulsion of the dorsal cortex at T10, with mild impingement on the anterior aspect of the lower thoracic cord (Fig. 29.3). A spine specialist evaluated the patient and felt that there was no immediate cord compromise. An elec-

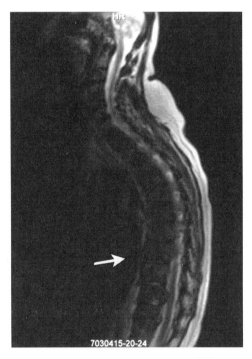

FIGURE 29.3. Magnetic resonance imaging of the spine showing diffuse compression fractures, with the *arrow* showing retropulsion at T10.

tive reduction of the T10 compression fracture with kyphoplasty and a bone biopsy were performed for tissue diagnosis. An ultrasound-guided breast biopsy was also performed.

What is the most common histopathologic type causing cancer of unknown primary?

A. Adenocarcinoma
B. Squamous cell carcinoma
C. Poorly differentiated carcinoma
D. Undifferentiated neoplasm

Adenocarcinoma comprises approximately 60% of cancers of unknown primary (8). Squamous cell carcinoma comprises 5% to 8%; poorly differentiated neoplasm, 2% to 5%; and poorly differentiated adenocarcinomas, 30% to 40% of cancers of unknown primary (1,8). Obtaining a pathologic diagnosis is important because it suggests a possible primary site and potential treatment. In this case, both biopsies demonstrated adenocarcinoma (Fig. 29.4). Immunohistochemical studies confirmed the diagnosis of infiltrating lobular carcinoma of the breast, consistent with the clinical picture. Specific tests for estrogen/progesterone receptors and HER-2/NEU receptors were negative. These tests predict tumor responsiveness to hormonal therapy. The importance of the status of specific receptors also applies for male patients with histologic evidence of prostate or testicular cancer.

The overall prognosis for cancer of unknown primary is poor, but there are treatable subgroups. For most patients, treatment should strive for improved quality of life rather than a cure. Hypercalcemia should be treated medically, and radiation therapy should be used to limit pain and other complications of bony metastases (4). Paracentesis and thoracentesis for symptomatic malignant ascites and pleural effusions, respectively, should be performed. Recurrent malignant pleural effusions may require sclerosis or decortication. Surgery may be indicated for bleeding or obstruction (2). Palliative low-toxicity chemotherapy or supportive care is recommended for patients with adenocarcinoma metastatic to liver or bone (7). Patients with poorly differentiated carcinoma/adenocarcinoma involving predominantly lymph nodes should undergo cisplatin-based combination chemotherapy (1,7). Adenocarcinomas with peritoneal carcinomatosis should be treated as FIGO (International Federation of Gynecology and Obstetrics) stage III ovarian cancer (7). Women with isolated axillary lymph nodes should be treated as having breast cancer of a similar stage (1,2,7). Squamous cell carcinoma with cervical lymph nodes is likely due to an underlying head and neck cancer. In the setting of squamous cell carcinoma involving inguinal lymph nodes, investigation for a primary tumor should include the anorectal and perineal areas. Both of these groups are treated with aggressive local therapy with surgery and/or radiation, with or without chemotherapy (1,2). Lastly, hormonal therapy is used in women with

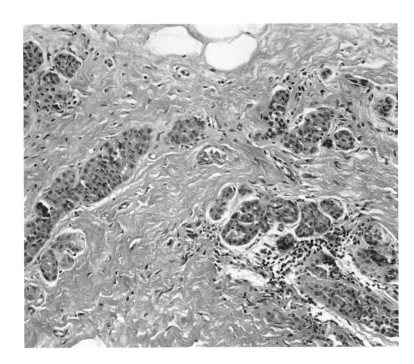

FIGURE 29.4. This patient's breast biopsy demonstrated infiltrating lobular carcinoma of the breast. The lobules are expanded and are filled by epithelial cells. Malignant cells are seen infiltrating the stroma in rows called Indian files.

receptor-positive breast tumors and men with PSA-positive staining tumors, as discussed earlier.

Follow-up

The initial abdominal CT scan was done with contrast, which can obscure breast cancer metastases. A noncontrast CT scan might have helped the radiologist determine if the lesions in the left lobe of the liver were metastases. However, follow-up studies did reveal that the lesions were metastases, as initially suspected. The patient was treated with radiation therapy for her bony disease and with adriamycin and cyclophosphamide for receptor-negative metastatic breast cancer. Four months after the initial diagnosis, the patient was still alive.

CONCLUSION

Clinicians need to consider metastatic carcinoma of an unknown primary in the appropriate setting. In evaluating these patients, a detailed history and physical examination may provide crucial information leading to the diagnosis of the primary when radiographic and other screening tests may fail. The overall prognosis for a cancer of unknown primary is poor; however, a histopathologic diagnosis is essential because some patients may have curable or treatable disease.

REFERENCES

1. Hillen HF. Unknown primary tumours. *Postgrad Med J* 2000;76: 690–693.
2. Markman M. The dilemma of evaluating and treating cancer of unknown primary site. *Cleve Clin J Med* 1997;64:73–75.
3. Maguire JH. Osteomyelitis. In: Braunwald E, Fauci AS, Kasper DL, et al., eds. *Harrison's principles of internal medicine,* 15th ed. New York: McGraw-Hill, 2001:825–829.
4. Lindsay R, Cosman F. Osteoporosis. In: Braunwald E, Fauci AS, Kasper DL, et al., eds. *Harrison's principles of internal medicine,* 15th ed. New York: McGraw-Hill, 2001:2226–2237.
5. Krane SM, Schiller AL. Paget's disease and other dysplasias of bone. In: Braunwald E, Fauci AS, Kasper DL, et al., eds. *Harrison's principles of internal medicine,* 15th ed. New York: McGraw-Hill, 2001:2237–2245.
6. Hage WD, Aboulafia AJ, Aboulafia DM. Incidence, location, and diagnostic evaluation of metastatic bone disease. *Orthop Clin North Am* 2000;31:515–528.
7. ESMO minimum clinical recommendations for diagnosis, treatment and follow-up of cancers of unknown primary site (CUP). *Ann Oncol* 2001;12:1057–1058.
8. Hammar SP. Metastatic adenocarcinoma of unknown primary origin. *Hum Pathol* 1998;29:1393–1402.

30

LOW BACK PAIN IN A 78-YEAR-OLD MAN

SNEHAL G. THAKKAR
CHELIF JUNOR
GORDAN SRKALOVIC

CASE PRESENTATION

A 78-year-old black man presented to the emergency department with a 6-week history of daily, intermittent, sharp low-back pain. The patient reported that the symptoms began after moving a refrigerator. He also described progressive lower-extremity weakness, as noted by his decreased functional ability at home. He denied any numbness or tingling of the lower extremities, as well as any urinary or bowel incontinence. Nonsteroidal antiinflammatory drugs (NSAIDs) and rest did not provide any relief of his symptoms. He also reported a 10- to 15-pound weight loss over the previous 6 months.

His past medical history was significant for prostate cancer diagnosed 4 years earlier. He underwent a transurethral resection of the prostate (TURP) and was being treated with monthly leuprolide injections. Recent prostate-specific antigen (PSA) levels were within normal limits. There was no history of prior exposure to tuberculosis, and the patient denied any indwelling catheters, recent back surgery, or infections.

Vital signs showed a temperature of 38.1°C, blood pressure of 142/78 mm Hg, pulse of 94 beats per minute, and a respiratory rate of 17 per minute. The patient was in no apparent distress. Physical examination revealed fine bibasilar rales and point tenderness along the entire length of the lumbar spine. No palpable deformities of the spinous processes were appreciated. Neurologic examination was significant only for 4 out of 5 strength in the proximal lower extremities. Straight-leg raise did not reproduce his symptoms, and his lower-extremity reflexes were normal. The patient did not have any sensory deficits, and rectal tone was normal.

APPROACH TO THE PATIENT WITH REFRACTORY LOW BACK PAIN

At some point in their lives, more than 80% of the adult population experience low back pain. Ninety percent of these patients recover with conservative management within 4 weeks (1). Given the many causes of low back pain, the 10% of patients who do not respond to conservative therapy during those initial 4 weeks pose a diagnostic challenge (1).

QUESTIONS/DISCUSSION

Based on this patient's presenting symptoms and prior medical history, which of the following is the least likely cause of this patient's low back pain?

A. Neoplasm
B. Osteomyelitis
C. Disc herniation
D. Ankylosing spondylitis

Neoplasm: Neoplastic disease of the spine results from either primary or metastatic disease. Primary tumors include those involving the marrow, bone, or cartilage of the spine. Multiple myeloma is the most common primary malignancy of bone in adults. Back pain is the presenting symptom in 35% of cases of multiple myeloma (2,3). Metastatic spinal disease is 25 times more common than primary neoplastic processes, due mostly to the large volume of blood that flows slowly through bidirectional venous channels (Batson plexus) in the epidural space around the spine. There is direct communication between the blood spaces and the vertebral marrow (4). Tumors that commonly metastasize to the spine include those of the prostate, lung, breast, kidney, and gastrointestinal tract (5).

Osteomyelitis: The patient's presentation of fever and localized back pain should raise concern for an infectious etiology. Most patients with osteomyelitis have fever, leukocytosis, an elevated erythrocyte sedimentation rate (ESR), and focal back pain worsened by percussion. Many patients do not have obvious risk factors for osteomyelitis (6). It is reasonable to consider osteomyelitis as a possible etiology for this patient's pain.

Disc herniation: The patient indicated that his symptoms developed after he moved a refrigerator. He demonstrated some proximal muscle weakness but did not have other physical findings suggestive of a radiculopathy. The presence of sciatica is only 80% sensitive and 40% specific for a herniated disc (7). Even though true sciatica was not established in our patient, this should not entirely exclude the diagnosis of a herniated disc.

Ankylosing spondylitis: The patient's presenting symptoms make this diagnosis the least likely. Classically, ankylosing spondylitis presents insidiously in adults less than 40 years of age. Pain is often worse in the morning upon rising or after inactivity. The pain usually improves with movement. This patient demonstrated good range of motion throughout his cervical, thoracic, and lumbar spine. Moreover, the symptoms did not improve throughout the day with increased activity.

Which of the following diagnostic tests are appropriate to evaluate this patient's back pain?

A. **Complete blood count (CBC)**
B. **Plain radiographs of the spine**
C. **Magnetic resonance imaging (MRI) of the spine**
D. **Computed tomography (CT scan) of the spine**
E. **All of the above**

This patient presented with findings that would be considered "red flag" signs and symptoms, including age greater than 60 years, history of cancer, unexplained weight loss, unremitting back pain despite conservative measures for longer than 4 to 6 weeks (1). Although an elevated white blood cell count in the setting of high ESR is not specific, it may suggest an infectious process. Anemia may represent a manifestation of chronic disease or infiltrative disease of the bone marrow. Therefore, a CBC would be appropriate in the initial evaluation of this patient.

Patients who present with low back pain typically do not require plain x-rays, as the diagnostic yield is very low. Retrospective studies have shown that x-rays were normal or demonstrated changes of equivocal clinical significance in greater than 75% of patients with low back pain (8). However, anyone presenting with "red flags" should undergo anteroposterior and lateral views to assess for fracture, tumor, or infection (1). Oblique views of the spine are useful in less than 3% of patients and are not usually indicated (9).

TABLE 30.1. SERUM PROTEIN ELECTROPHORESIS

	Patient Values (mg/dL)	Normal Values (mg/dL)
Albumin	2.44	4.0–5.4
α_1-globulin	0.25	0.08–0.22
α_2-globulin	0.65	0.5–0.9
β-globulin	0.54	0.5–1.0
γ-globulin	6.92	0.6–1.35

TABLE 30.2 SERUM MONOCLONAL PROTEIN ANALYSIS

	Patient's Values (mg/dL)	Normal Values (mg/dL)
IgG	6,950	717–1,411
IgA	17	78–391
IgM	11	53–334
κ	8,100	534–1,267
λ	51	253–653

Although MRI is expensive, it is widely used for several reasons. It is a noninvasive test that does not expose patients to radiation. MRI can evaluate a large area of the spine and can assess changes in the disc and vertebral body (10). MRI offers the best resolution of the spinal canal and spinal cord. In comparison to MRI, CT scan provides better evaluation of skeletal anatomy. CT is considered superior to MRI for spinal trauma and vertebral fractures. Clinicians also need to recognize that both MRI and CT scan may show evidence of pathology in asymptomatic patients. Studies have suggested that 30% to 70% of asymptomatic subjects may have disk protrusion or abnormal nonspecific disk changes (11).

All the preceding tests are appropriate in this patient.

Case Continued: Initial laboratory studies revealed a white blood cell count of 7.2 K/μL, hemoglobin of 7.8 g/dL (baseline hemoglobin, 11 to 12 g/dL), and a platelet count of 103 K/μL. ESR was normal. Urinalysis was negative for blood, protein, or leukocytes.

Additional blood work revealed a creatinine of 1.6 g/dL and an elevated total protein of 11.0 g/dL. Because of the elevated total protein, a serum protein electrophoresis (SPEP) was sent, the results of which are shown in Table 30.1. The elevated γ-globulin fraction prompted a monoclonal protein analysis, which is shown in Table 30.2.

Since the monoclonal gammopathy was suspicious for multiple myeloma, a bone marrow biopsy was performed. This revealed 87% plasma cells and established the diagnosis of multiple myeloma. Initial plain films of the spine showed evidence of compression fractures at L3 and T12 and widespread osteopenia. MRI confirmed the presence of compression fractures and did not show any evidence of spinal cord compression.

Which of the following clinical manifestations occurs least often among patients presenting with multiple myeloma?

A. **Skeletal destruction**
B. **Anemia**
C. **Hypercalcemia**
D. **Renal insufficiency**
E. **Hyperviscosity syndrome**

Skeletal destruction: Bone pain, especially involving the chest and back, is present in two-thirds of patients presenting with multiple myeloma. The pain is constant and is worse with movement, as opposed to the pain of metastatic disease, which is worse at night. Skeletal destruction results from the proliferation of plasma cells within the bone marrow and the resultant increase in the amount of osteoclast-activating factors (12–15). Cytokines such as interleukin-1, lymphotoxin, and tumor necrosis factor mediate this process. Bone scans are not helpful to assess these patients because multiple myeloma is rarely associated with osteoblastic bone formation (16). Osteolytic lesions, osteopenia, and fractures are common. All these processes may result in other clinical manifestations, such as hypercalcemia.

Anemia: The anemia associated with multiple myeloma is most often normochromic, normocytic; however, patients may rarely present with megaloblastic and macrocytic anemias (17,18). Several factors contribute to anemia in patients with multiple myeloma, including decreased red cell production secondary to marrow infiltration, diminished erythropoietin production due to renal dysfunction, and the direct effect of cytokines on erythropoiesis (16).

Hypercalcemia: Similar to the mechanism producing skeletal abnormalities, hypercalcemia occurs due to an imbalance between osteoclastic and osteoblastic activity within the bony microenvironment (12–15). Approximately 25% of myeloma patients develop this complication at some stage of the disease. Hypercalcemia is also the most common cause of renal failure in myeloma patients (16). Hypercalcemia and the resultant hypercalciuria lead to osmotic diuresis and volume depletion, which contributes to prerenal azotemia. Hypercalcemic patients usually require aggressive treatment with intravenous fluids and bisphosphonates.

Renal insufficiency: Although the most common cause of renal insufficiency in multiple myeloma patients is hypercalcemia, amyloid deposition, recurrent infections, and infiltration of the kidney by myeloma cells may also play a role. The so-called myeloma kidney, which may accentuate the anemia, occurs due to the deposition of light-chain tubular casts, which produces interstitial nephritis. Renal pathology is noted in approximately 25% of myeloma patients (16). Other factors potentially contributing to worsening renal function include the use of NSAIDs for pain control, contrast dye, and nephrotoxic chemotherapeutic agents.

Hyperviscosity: Although potentially destructive, hyperviscosity is a relatively uncommon complication. Among the choices listed, it is the least common manifestation of multiple myeloma. The M components in myeloma can lead to problems when the immunoglobulin levels exceed a certain level (16,19,20). Despite the infrequency with which hyperviscosity occurs, a high level of suspicion

should be maintained, as prompt plasmapheresis may alleviate potential organ damage.

Other clinical manifestations seen in multiple myeloma include neurologic symptoms, infections, and coagulopathies.

DIAGNOSIS OF MULTIPLE MYELOMA

Multiple myeloma accounts for about 1% of all malignancies and approximately 10% of all hematologic malignancies. The prevalence is slightly higher in men than in women, and the incidence is almost twice that for blacks as it is for whites. The median age at diagnosis is 65, with only 3% diagnosed below 40 years of age (16).

The diagnosis of multiple myeloma is often delayed because of the variety and obscurity of presenting symptoms. An older patient may have subtle findings such as unexplained back pain, recurrent infection, anemia, or renal insufficiency. Findings such as hyperproteinemia, proteinuria, anemia, and hypoalbuminemia should warrant an evaluation for multiple myeloma. Initial evaluation for multiple myeloma includes a complete blood count, complete skeletal survey, SPEP, urine protein electrophoresis (UPEP) with immunofixation, quantitative immunoglobulin levels, a 24-hour urine protein measurement, and bone marrow biopsy.

The diagnostic criteria for multiple myeloma follow (21).

The major criteria are:

 I. Plasmacytoma on tissue biopsy
 II. Bone marrow plasmacytosis with greater than 30% plasma cells
III. Monoclonal globulin spike on SPEP exceeding 3.5 g/dL for IgG or 2.0 g/dL for IgA; greater than or equal to 1 g/day of κ or γ light-chain excretion on UPEP in the presence of amyloidosis

The minor criteria are:

  I. Bone marrow plasmacytosis, 10% to 30%
 II. Monoclonal globulin spike present, but less than the level required to fulfill major criterion III
III. Lytic bone lesions
IV. Suppressed uninvolved immunoglobulins: IgM less than 50 mg/dL, IgA less than 100 mg/dL, or IgG less than 600 mg/dL

The diagnosis is established if one major and one minor criterion are met, or if three minor criteria are met, including both minor criteria I and II. A staging system (Durie–Salmon system) is in place to quantify the extent of the disease. Once the diagnosis of multiple myeloma is made and the disease is staged, the next step is to implement a treatment strategy.

Which of the following treatment options would be palliative, rather than curative for multiple myeloma?

A. Oral prednisone and melphalan
B. Bone marrow transplantation
C. Thalidomide
D. Radiation therapy

Oral prednisone/melphalan: The treatment protocol of oral prednisone and melphalan was introduced almost 30 years ago and continues to be standard therapy. Various other alkylating agent-based combinations have been introduced, but their response rates continue to be only comparable to the combination of melphalan and prednisone.

Bone marrow transplantation: Bone marrow transplantation is an area of controversy. Although the French Myeloma Group has continued to show improved 5-year survival rates when comparing the combination of autologous bone marrow transplant and chemotherapy to chemotherapy alone, the results seem applicable to only a certain subset of myeloma patients (21). Allogeneic bone marrow transplant has also been evaluated; however, 90% of patients with myeloma are ineligible for allogeneic bone marrow transplant because of their age, lack of a human leukocyte antigen (HLA)–matched sibling donor, or inadequate renal, pulmonary, or cardiac function (21).

Thalidomide: The results from recent clinical trials involving thalidomide combined with dexamethasone in patients with refractory or relapsed myeloma have been encouraging. Although ongoing trials are helping to develop treatment protocols, the preliminary results suggest a significant role for thalidomide (22).

Radiation therapy: This essentially plays a palliative role in the treatment of multiple myeloma. Once a mainstay of treatment, its use has been supplanted by the introduction of chemotherapeutic options. Despite its limited role, it remains the treatment of choice for cases involving impending pathologic fractures, spinal cord compression, and meningeal myelomatosis (20).

CONCLUSION

Following discharge, the patient was started on systemic chemotherapy with melphalan and prednisone for 4 days at a time on a monthly basis. His back pain persisted despite medical and surgical treatments, and he was referred to an outpatient chronic pain management clinic.

REFERENCES

1. Agency for Health Care Policy and Research. *Acute low back problems in adults: assessment and treatment. Quick reference guide.* Rockville, MD: U.S. Public Health Service, 1994, AHCPR publication 95-0643.
2. Hewell GM, Alexanian R. Multiple myeloma in young persons. *Ann Intern Med* 1976;84:441–443.
3. Kyle RA. Multiple myeloma: review of 869 cases. *Mayo Clin Proc* 1975;50:29–40.
4. Posner JB. Back pain and epidural spinal cord compression. *Med Clin North Am* 1987;71:185–205.
5. Gilbert RW, Kim JH, Posner JB. Epidural spinal cord compression from metastatic tumor: diagnosis and treatment. *Ann Neurol* 1978;3:40–51.
6. Kapeller P, Fazekas F, Krametter D, et al. Pyogenic infectious spondylitis: clinical, laboratory and MRI features. *Eur Neurol* 1997;38:94–98.
7. Deyo RA, Rainville J, Kent DL. What can the history and physical examination tell us about low back pain? *JAMA* 1992;268:760–765.
8. Scavone JG, Latshaw RF, Rohrer GV. Use of lumbar spine films: statistical evaluation at a university teaching hospital. *JAMA* 1981;246:1105–1108.
9. Scavone JG, Latshaw RF, Weidner WA. Anteroposterior and lateral radiographs: an adequate lumbar spine examination. *Am J Roentgenol* 1981;136:715–717.
10. Arce D, Sass P, Abul-Khoudoud H. Recognizing spinal cord emergencies. *Am Fam Physician* 2001;64:631–638.
11. Boden SD, Davis DO, Dina TS, et al. Abnormal magnetic-resonance scans of the lumbar spine in asymptomatic subjects: a prospective investigation. *J Bone Joint Surg Am* 1990;72:403–408.
12. Michigami T, Shimizu N, Williams PJ, et al. Cell–cell contact between marrow stromal cells and myeloma cells via VCAM-1 and alpha(4)beta(1)-integrin enhances production of osteoclast-stimulating activity. *Blood* 2000;96:1953–1960.
13. Hjertner O, Torgersen ML, Seidel C, et al. Hepatocyte growth factor (HCF) induces interleukin-11 secretion from osteoblasts: a possible role for HGF in myeloma-associated osteolytic bone disease. *Blood* 1999;94:3883–3888.
14. Pruzanski W, Watt JG. Serum viscosity and hyperviscosity syndrome in IgG multiple myeloma: report on 10 patients and a review of the literature. *Ann Intern Med* 1972;77:853–860.
15. Preston FE, Cooke KB, Foster ME, et al. Myelomatosis and the hyperviscosity syndrome. *Br J Haematol* 1978;38:517–530.
16. Munshi NC, Tricot G, Barlogie B. Plasma cell neoplasms. In: DeVita VT Jr, Hellman S, Rosenberg SA, eds. *Cancer: principles and practice of oncology,* 6th ed. Philadelphia: Lippincott Williams & Wilkins, 2001:2465–2499.
17. Gomez AR, Harley JB. Multiple myeloma and pernicious anemia. *W V Med J* 1970;66:38–41.
18. Miramon Lopez J, Ruiz Cantero A, Morales Jimenez J, et al. [A new case of association of multiple myeloma and megaloblastic anemia]. *An Med Interna* 1999;16:654–655.
19. Chandy KG, Stockley RA, Leonard RC, et al. Relationship between serum viscosity and intravascular IgA polymer concentrations in IgA myeloma. *Clin Exp Immunol* 1981;46:653–661.
20. Hussein MA, Juturi JV, Lieberman I. Multiple myeloma: present and future. *Curr Opin Oncol* 2002;14:31–35.
21. Attal M, Harousseau JL, Stoppa AM, et al. A prospective, randomized trial of autologous bone marrow transplantation and chemotherapy in multiple myeloma. Intergroupe Français du Myélome. *N Engl J Med* 1996;335:91–97.
22. Weber DM, Rankin K, Gavino M, et al. Thalidomide with dexamethasone for resistant multiple myeloma. *Blood* 2000;96:167a.

31

A 62-YEAR-OLD MAN WITH EDEMA AND HEPATOSPLENOMEGALY

EYAD AL-HATTAB
BINDU SANGANI

CASE PRESENTATION

A 62-year-old man with no significant past medical history presented to the emergency department with a 2-week history of bilateral lower-extremity swelling and scrotal swelling. The patient initially noticed ankle and foot swelling in addition to difficulty ambulating, which he attributed to a "heaviness" in his lower extremities. The edema subsequently extended to the upper thighs and groin. The patient denied any erythema or warmth of the lower extremities but did notice bilateral calf pain.

The patient also noted shortness of breath when walking up hills and a decreased energy level for 1 year before admission. He denied chest pain, paroxysmal nocturnal dyspnea, orthopnea, palpitations, abdominal distension, pain, or change in bowel or urinary habits. He did not describe any weight loss or early satiety; in fact, he had noted an unspecified weight gain over the 2 weeks before admission.

Although the patient had an episode of bronchitis several months before admission, he denied any cough, fever, chills or sputum production. He also recalled an episode of shingles approximately 10 years earlier but had not seen a physician regularly over the 34 years before admission. His only medication on admission was a daily aspirin. The patient did not have a history of tobacco or alcohol abuse.

Physical examination revealed a pale, middle-aged man in no acute distress. His temperature was 37.2°C, blood pressure 128/65 mm Hg, pulse 100 beats per minute, and respiratory rate 12 per minute. The jugular venous pressure was elevated to 8 cm at 30 degrees. Lungs were clear to auscultation. Cardiac examination revealed a hyperdynamic precordium, with normal heart sounds. Abdominal examination revealed a distended abdomen, with the liver span extending 4 cm below the costal margin and a palpable spleen tip in the right lower quadrant. Bowel sounds were normal. There was no evidence of ascites or distended umbilical veins. There was 3+ pitting edema of both lower extremities up to the inguinal region and sacrum; multiple varicosities were noted in both lower extremities. There was no cervical, axillary, or inguinal adenopathy.

QUESTIONS / DISCUSSION

Which of the following is the least likely to cause this patient's bilateral leg edema?

A. **Congestive heart failure**
B. **Deep venous thrombosis**
C. **Cirrhosis of the liver**
D. **Nephrotic syndrome**

Clinicians need to consider if there is a history of any disorder, such as coronary artery disease, hypertension, or alcohol abuse, that would predispose to the development of edema or if there is a history of use of medications that can cause cardiac, hepatic, or renal disease. On examination, the location and distribution of the edema, as well as an estimation of the central venous pressure, may provide important clues in determining the etiology of the edema (1,2).

Congestive heart failure (CHF) typically causes edema in the dependent parts of the body. Pressures in the right atrium and central venous system are elevated. Increased right-sided filling pressures can be estimated by measuring the jugular venous pressure or directly measuring with a central venous catheter. CHF needs to be considered in this patient presenting with bilateral leg swelling and dyspnea when climbing hills.

Cirrhosis of the liver can produce edema of the lower extremities and ascites as a result of hepatic venous outflow blockade causing portal hypertension. Venous pressures in structures distal to the hepatic vein, including the right atrium, are usually reduced or normal. Signs of portal hypertension, such as distended abdominal wall veins or splenomegaly, are suggestive of, but not diagnostic of, primary hepatic disease. Although this patient has no known history of liver disease or any known risk factors, cirrhosis cannot be ruled out, given his presentation.

Patients with nephrotic syndrome frequently present with periorbital and peripheral edema. Two factors contribute to the fluid retention in this condition: primary sodium retention due to the underlying renal disease and a diminished transcapillary oncotic pressure gradient, which occurs most often in cases of severe hypoalbuminemia (3).

Deep venous thrombosis (DVT) causes lower-extremity edema but is the least likely cause of this patient's edema. DVT usually causes acute, unilateral leg swelling.

Laboratory testing revealed white blood cell count of 2.31 K/μL, hemoglobin of 5.6 g/dL, and platelet count of 97 K/μL. The mean corpuscular volume was 90 fL. Electrolytes were normal. Blood urea nitrogen was 25 mg/dL, and creatinine was 1.2 mg/dL. Transaminases, alkaline phosphatase, and bilirubin were normal; however, albumin was mildly decreased at 3.4 g/dL. Urinalysis did not reveal any proteinuria. An electrocardiogram revealed sinus tachycardia, left atrial enlargement, and nonspecific ST–T wave abnormalities. A chest x-ray revealed a normal cardiac silhouette and blunting of the right costophrenic angle, thought to be consistent with basilar atelectasis and/or effusion. No focal infiltrates were noted.

Which of the following can cause pancytopenia?

A. Leukemia
B. Parvovirus B19 infection
C. Vitamin B$_{12}$ deficiency
D. Nonsteroidal antiinflammatory drugs (NSAIDs)
E. All of the above

All the preceding entities can cause pancytopenia, a condition that typically represents bone marrow failure. When evaluating patients with pancytopenia, clinicians need to consider the various mechanisms by which pancytopenia develops. Aplastic anemia is a condition in which pancytopenia develops due to a hypocellular bone marrow. Aplastic anemia can be congenital, as in Fanconi anemia, or acquired. Common causes of acquired aplastic anemia include radiation, chemotherapeutic drugs, other medications (including nonsteroidal antiinflammatory drugs and sulfonamides), viral infections [including parvovirus B19 and human immunodeficiency virus (HIV)-1], and immune disorders (including systemic lupus erythematosus). Marrow infiltration, as seen in leukemia, lymphoma, metastatic tumor, and myelofibrosis, can also result in pancytopenia. Patients with vitamin B$_{12}$ or folate deficiency and myelodysplasia can also develop pancytopenia as a result of ineffective hematopoiesis (4).

Which of the following tests is most likely to determine the etiology of this patient's pancytopenia?

A. Reticulocyte count
B. Peripheral blood smear
C. Vitamin B$_{12}$ level

D. Bone marrow biopsy
E. None of the above

To evaluate a pancytopenic patient, the functional state of the bone marrow must be assessed. The reticulocyte count and the corrected reticulocyte count can estimate bone marrow function. Both a peripheral blood smear and vitamin B$_{12}$ level can be helpful, but ultimately are not diagnostic. A low serum B$_{12}$ level does not provide definitive proof that B$_{12}$ deficiency is the cause of pancytopenia.

The best means of determining bone marrow function and evaluating for underlying pathology is a bone marrow biopsy and aspirate. Pathologists can examine the bone marrow for its architecture, its cellularity, evidence of dysplastic changes (both nuclear and cytoplasmic), fibrosis, iron stores, and evidence of granulomas (5–7). Cytogenetic studies can also be performed, which can help determine prognosis and guide the choice of therapy (8).

Case Continued. In this patient, B$_{12}$ level was 1,595 pg/mL (normal, 221 to 700 pg/mL). The reticulocyte count was 2.7%, with an absolute reticulocyte count of 62, which was considered inappropriately low for the severity of this patient's anemia. The peripheral smear showed leukoerythroblasts (immature granulocytes and nucleated red cells) and teardrop-shaped red blood cells, features consistent with myelophthisis. Myelophthisis may occur in many disorders, including primary myelofibrosis, chronic myeloid leukemia, metastatic cancer, lymphoma, plasma cell dyscrasias, and infections (8).

Following these tests, this patient underwent a bone marrow aspirate and biopsy. The bone marrow was not easily aspirated (a "dry" tap). The histology showed marrow fibrosis associated with an increased number of atypical megakaryocytes, thought to be consistent with a diagnosis of myelofibrosis.

Myelofibrosis with Myeloid Metaplasia

Myelofibrosis with myeloid metaplasia (MMM) is classified as a chronic myeloproliferative disease, a category that also includes essential thrombocytosis and polycythemia vera. These disorders result from a clonal stem cell disorder, which leads to the production of abnormal hematopoietic cells (9). These abnormal cells inappropriately release fibrogenic cytokines and/or growth factors in the bone marrow, invade the bloodstream, and colonize extramedullary sites. This process results in ineffective erythropoiesis. In idiopathic myelofibrosis, the ineffective erythropoiesis, dysplastic megakaryocyte hyperplasia, and increased number of immature granulocytes are accompanied by reactive bone marrow fibrosis (myelofibrosis) (8). Bone marrow fibrosis in MMM results from the release of stimulatory factors from the myeloproliferative clonal cell population, which produces a prominent infiltrate of fibroblasts and coarse bundles of extracellular matrix in the bone marrow (9).

The incidence of myelofibrosis with myeloid metaplasia is estimated to be 0.73 per 100,000 persons per year in males and 0.40 per 100,000 persons per year in females. Median age at diagnosis ranges from 54 to 62 years, with approximately 20% of patients younger than 55 years of age at presentation (9). Myelofibrosis can occur in a variety of benign and malignant disorders (Table 31.1), some of which are treatable (10).

Which of the following are complications of myelofibrosis?

A. Infection
B. Extramedullary hematopoiesis
C. Congestive heart failure
D. Hemorrhage
E. All of the above

Many of the complications of myelofibrosis occur due to the deficiencies in the cell lines. Patients who are leukopenic are prone to overwhelming infections and sepsis. Extramedullary hematopoiesis often occurs as a compensatory mechanism in response to marrow fibrosis and can lead to various complications, including hepatomegaly and splenomegaly, which can develop so rapidly that it can cause splenic infarction. Extramedullary hematopoiesis can also involve the lymph nodes, resulting in lymphadenopathy; serosal surfaces, leading to pleural effusions, pericardial tamponade, and ascites; the lungs, causing a pneumonia-like process; the genitourinary system, causing ureteral obstruction; and the paraspinal or epidural spaces, leading to compression of the spinal cord and nerve roots (8,9). The main causes of mortality in patients with myelofibrosis and myeloid metaplasia are infection, hemorrhagic events, and heart failure. Up to 20% of patients who live 10 years after the diagnosis of the disease develop an aggressive form of leukemia. MMM carries the worst prognosis of the chronic myeloproliferative disorders, with a median survival of 3.5 to 5.5 years. Several well-defined indicators portend a poorer prognosis, including age greater than 56, hemoglobin less than 10 g/dL, platelet count less than 100,000/mm^3, leukopenia, leukocytosis, circulating blasts, and karyotype abnormalities (8,9).

Which of the following treatment(s) is/are currently used to treat myelofibrosis?

A. Supportive measures
B. **Androgens and/or corticosteroids**
C. **Hydroxyurea**
D. **Splenectomy**
E. **All of the above**

Currently, supportive measures remain the cornerstone of treatment in myelofibrosis with myeloid metaplasia. Typical supportive measures include red cell and platelet transfusions and appropriate treatment of infections. Although many medications have been used in myelofibrosis, none have shown a proven survival benefit. Androgen preparations and corticosteroids may alleviate the associated anemia; however, less than one-third of patients respond, a response that is frequently transient. This anemia also typically fails to respond to erythropoietin.

Up to 28% of patients with myelofibrosis, especially in the early stages, may develop leukocytosis or thrombocytosis, rather than leukopenia or thrombocytopenia (9). Hydroxyurea remains the drug of choice to control the leukocytosis, thrombocytosis, or organomegaly in these patients.

Splenectomy is indicated for patients with evidence of hypersplenism and for patients with splenomegaly resulting in gastric obstruction. Given the potential for perioperative complications, patients taken for splenectomy need to be carefully selected. Other treatment modalities for which the efficacy remains unclear include splenic irradiation, allogeneic and autologous stem cell transplantation, and antifibrotic and antiangiogenic therapies.

Follow-up

The patient's symptoms on presentation were most likely exacerbated by the cardiac condition discovered coincidentally with his myelofibrosis. An echocardiogram showed moderately severe mitral stenosis with moderate mitral regurgitation, moderate tricuspid regurgitation, and severe right ventricular dysfunction. His valvular dysfunction was thought to be due to rheumatic heart disease. The patient was supported with blood transfusions and appropriate management for heart failure. He was discharged home with follow-up with an oncologist and a cardiologist.

As an outpatient, he required frequent blood transfusions. Five months later, he expired in the intensive care unit after presenting to the emergency department with neutropenic sepsis.

CONCLUSION

An evaluation of pancytopenia should focus on the various causes of bone marrow failure. The best way to evaluate any bone marrow process is with a bone marrow biopsy, which can provide a diagnosis, predict prognosis, and help guide treatment. Myelofibrosis, as seen in this patient, needs to be included in the differential diagnosis of pancytopenia. It causes bone marrow failure as a result of bone marrow

TABLE 31.1. CAUSES OF MYELOFIBROSIS

Carcinoma metastatic to the marrow	Chronic myelogenous leukemia
Infection	Polycythemia vera
Lymphoma	Idiopathic myelofibrosis
Hodgkin disease	Systemic mastocytosis
Acute leukemia	Thorium dioxide exposure
Hairy cell leukemia	Systemic lupus erythematosus
Multiple myeloma	Renal osteodystrophy

fibrosis. Patients with myelofibrosis develop extramedullary hematopoiesis, which can result in a multitude of complications.

REFERENCES

1. Rose BD. Approach to the patient with edema. UpToDate Online 10.1, 2002. December 20, 2002, *www.uptodate.com.*
2. Yale SH, Mazza JJ. Approach to diagnosing lower extremity edema. *Compr Ther* 2001;27:242–252.
3. Humphreys MH. Mechanisms and management of nephrotic edema. *Kidney Int* 1994;45:266–281.
4. Dallman PR, Mentzer WC. Anemia. In: Rudolph AM, Hoffman JIE, Rudolph CD, eds. *Rudolph's pediatrics,* 20th ed. Stamford, CT: Appleton & Lange, 1996:1172–1221.
5. Bain BJ. Bone marrow aspiration. *J Clin Pathol* 2001;54: 657–663.
6. Bain BJ. Bone marrow trephine biopsy. *J Clin Pathol* 2001;54: 737–742.
7. Young NS. Aplastic anemia, myelodysplasia, and related bone marrow failure syndromes. In: Braunwald E, Fauci AS, Kasper DL, et al., eds. *Harrison's principles of internal medicine,* 15th ed. New York: McGraw-Hill, 2001:692–701.
8. Tefferi A. Myelofibrosis with myeloid metaplasia. *N Engl J Med* 2000;342:1255–1265.
9. Barosi G. Myelofibrosis with myeloid metaplasia: diagnostic definition and prognostic classification for clinical studies and treatment guidelines. *J Clin Oncol* 1999;17:2954–2970.
10. Spivak JL. Polycythemia vera and other myeloproliferative diseases. In: Braunwald E, Fauci AS, Kasper DL, et al., eds. *Harrison's principles of internal medicine,* 15th ed. New York: McGraw-Hill, 2001:701–706.

32

PELVIC PAIN IN A 58-YEAR-OLD WOMAN

TONI CHOUEIRI
RONY M. ABOU-JAWDE
ROBERT J. PELLEY

CASE PRESENTATION

A 58-year-old woman presented with sharp pelvic pain for 6 days. The patient described intermittent pain located low in the pelvic area that radiated to the lower back and lower extremities. Defecation and urination exacerbated the pain, and analgesics relieved it. She had never experienced similar pain. The patient denied any nausea, vomiting, or fever; there was no change in bowel habits, hematochezia, or melena. She denied any urinary urgency, frequency, incontinence, or hematuria. The patient had not experienced any vaginal bleeding or weight loss.

Two months before presentation, she was diagnosed with an extranodal marginal zone B cell lymphoma of the lung by thoracoscopic wedge resection of a mass discovered on a chest x-ray done to evaluate dyspnea. Extensive metastatic work-up at that time was negative, including:

- Complete blood count and differential
- Bone marrow aspirate and biopsy 1 week before this presentation
- Esophagogastroduodenoscopy radiolabelled urea breath test to rule out concomitant gastric lymphoma

Past surgical history included total abdominal hysterectomy with bilateral salpingo-oophorectomy for endometriosis. Her family history included hypertension and diabetes mellitus. The patient did not have a history of tobacco or alcohol abuse.

Physical examination revealed a woman in moderate distress with temperature of 36.7°C, pulse of 88 beats per minute, blood pressure of 98/48 mm Hg, respiratory rate of 18 per minute, and oxygen saturation of 90% on room air. Abdominal examination revealed tenderness on deep palpation of the left lower quadrant. There was no distension, and bowel sounds were normal. Musculoskeletal examination revealed severe tenderness of the thoracic and left lumbar regions. Neurologic examination was nonfocal. The remainder of her physical examination was normal.

QUESTIONS/DISCUSSION

Given this patient's back pain and history of non-Hodgkin lymphoma, the most important condition to rule out initially is:

A. **Spinal cord compression**
B. **Abdominal lymphoma**
C. **Nephrolithiasis**
D. **Bowel obstruction**

Spinal cord compression is a common complication of malignancy that causes back pain and, at times, irreversible loss of neurologic function. Metastatic tumor from any primary site can produce cord compression (1). Prostate, breast, and lung cancer each account for 15% to 20% of cases; renal cell carcinoma, non-Hodgkin lymphoma, and multiple myeloma each account for 5% to 10% of cases (2). Pain is typically the first symptom of cord compression, occurring in 83% to 95% of patients (3); pain often precedes neurologic symptoms by several weeks. Since the outcome depends most upon the patient's neurologic status at the initiation of treatment, the goal must be to diagnose patients before the development of neurologic symptoms, such as lower-extremity weakness, numbness, paresthesias, or loss of bladder and bowel function. Once these late symptoms develop, the spinal cord damage is generally irreversible. Although all the preceding conditions are potential explanations for this patient's pain, spinal cord compression is the one condition that must be diagnosed immediately.

Magnetic resonance imaging (MRI) of the spine did not reveal any cord compression. Laboratory findings showed normal electrolytes and creatinine. Complete blood count revealed a white blood cell count of 16,000/μL, hemoglobin of 11.3 g/dL, and platelet count of 267,000/μL. The hemoglobin had been 14.8 g/dL 2 months earlier.

Renal ultrasound did not show hydronephrosis or calculi, making a diagnosis of nephrolithiasis far less likely. Acute abdominal series showed no obstruction.

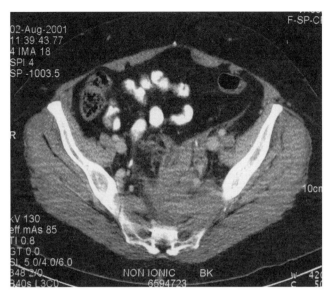

FIGURE 32.1. Computed tomogram of the abdomen and pelvis showing a soft-tissue density abutting the external and internal iliac vessels, with extension into the presacral space and deep pelvis.

Computed tomography (CT) of the abdomen and the pelvis (Fig. 32.1) showed a soft-tissue density abutting the internal and external iliac vessels, with extension into the presacral space and deep pelvis. There was no evidence of bony erosion.

Which of the following is now the most likely diagnosis?

A. **Extension of non-Hodgkin lymphoma (NHL)**
B. **Retroperitoneal hematoma**
C. **Retroperitoneal sarcoma**
D. **None of the above**

Extension of NHL: The patient underwent resection of an extranodal marginal zone B cell lymphoma of the lung, also called low-grade B cell lymphoma of mucosa-associated lymphoid tissue (MALT). MALT comprises about 5% of all non-Hodgkin lymphoma and almost 50% of all gastric lymphomas (4). A coexistence of lung and gastrointestinal MALT tumors has been described. This type of lymphoma is usually indolent and remains localized for a prolonged period (5,6). However, patients with tumors outside the gastrointestinal (GI) tract seem to progress more often than those with GI tumors. CT findings include mesenteric and retroperitoneal lymphadenopathy, rather than a soft-tissue mass (7).

Retroperitoneal hematoma: A retroperitoneal hematoma is common. It has been described with trauma, cardiac catheterization, ruptured tubal pregnancy, anticoagulants such as heparin, pheochromocytoma of the adrenal gland, and inherited or acquired bleeding disorders (8–13). CT findings include the presence of a soft-tissue mass, some-

times with a high-attenuation component if there is still active bleeding. The pain is typically transient and improves after a few days. The mass usually resolves within several weeks (14). The CT findings in this case are compatible with a retroperitoneal hematoma.

Retroperitoneal sarcoma: Most patients who develop a retroperitoneal sarcoma present with an asymptomatic abdominal mass. Less commonly, neurologic or musculoskeletal symptoms involving the lower extremities may result from local invasion or compression of retroperitoneal neurovascular structures (15). Sarcomas of the retroperitoneal tissues have a poorer prognosis than other soft-tissue sarcomas (16). Common CT findings include the presence of an extensive mass with necrotic, cystic, and heterogeneous areas (17). The CT findings in this case are not typical of a retroperitoneal sarcoma.

The patient's symptoms were improving on small doses of analgesics.

Which of the following options is most appropriate to evaluate this patient further?

A. **Observation**
B. **Chemotherapy**
C. **CT-guided biopsy of the mass**
D. **Surgery and radiation therapy**

In this case, a CT-guided biopsy could establish the etiology of the mass. In a retrospective review of CT-guided biopsies of the retroperitoneum, aspiration accurately suggested the correct diagnosis in 100% of cases of metastatic disease, 93% of cases of lymphoma, and 100% of cases of unusual benign disorders. It was also possible to diagnose the specific type of lymphoma in 93% of cases. Complications associated with the procedure were rare (18). In a prospective analysis of 1,000 procedures at the Mayo Clinic, with 722 performed in the area of the liver, retroperitoneum, pancreas, pelvis, and adrenal glands, CT-guided biopsy was 91.8% sensitive and 98.9% specific for the diagnosis of lymphoma. Eleven patients developed complications, including seven hematomas, three pneumothoraces, and one case of hematuria. Only one patient required surgery (19).

Observation is not appropriate at this time since a tissue diagnosis is warranted, given the known history of lymphoma and the potential for curative treatment.

Starting chemotherapy for lymphoma or radiotherapy and surgery for a potential retroperitoneal sarcoma without having a tissue diagnosis is also not appropriate.

A CT-guided biopsy was performed successfully and showed granulation tissue and spindle cell proliferation, suggesting fibrosis. Meanwhile, the patient steadily improved, so that she could ambulate without difficulty.

Given that the symptoms started 1 day after the bone marrow biopsy, coinciding with a 25% drop in hematocrit, a retroperitoneal hematoma seemed very likely. The results

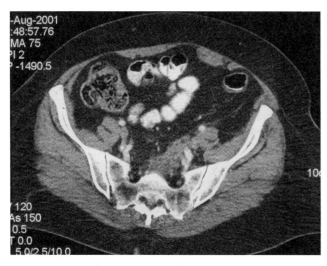

FIGURE 32.2. Follow-up computed tomogram of the abdomen and pelvis showing 80% resolution of the soft-tissue density.

of the CT-guided biopsy further strengthened the likelihood of a retroperitoneal hematoma. The patient was discharged home on tapering doses of analgesics, and a follow-up abdominal CT showed 80% resolution of the soft-tissue mass (Fig. 32.2).

Bone marrow biopsy has traditionally been considered a safe procedure, even when coagulopathy or thrombocytopenia is present (20). However, injury to the retroperitoneal vessels of the posterior iliac crest, although very rare, can be a serious complication of bone marrow biopsy. Such injuries have occurred in Paget disease, multiple myeloma, and osteoporosis (21–23).

CONCLUSION

Clinicians need to remember retroperitoneal bleeding as a potential complication of bone marrow biopsy, even if the conditions mentioned earlier are not present. In this case, it was feared that the patient had an extension of her lymphoma. If the lymphoma had indeed progressed, her prognosis would have been worse, with chemotherapy the likely treatment. The CT scan findings in this patient help to establish the diagnosis of a retroperitoneal bleed. A high-attenuation signal suggests active bleeding. That was not present in this patient, who probably bled only shortly after the biopsy. CT-guided biopsy is a useful tool in determining the etiology of a retroperitoneal mass and helping to guide subsequent treatment.

REFERENCES

1. Bach F, Larsen BH, Rohde K, et al. Metastatic spinal cord compression: occurrence, symptoms, clinical presentations and prognosis in 398 patients with spinal cord compression. *Acta Neurochir (Wien)* 1990;107:37–43.
2. Constans JP, de Divitiis E, Donzelli R, et al. Spinal metastases with neurological manifestations. Review of 600 cases. *J Neurosurg* 1983;59:111–118.
3. Loblaw DA, Laperriere NJ. Emergency treatment of malignant extradural spinal cord compression: an evidence-based guideline. *J Clin Oncol* 1998;16:1613–1624.
4. Tsang RW, Gospodarowicz, MK, Pintilie M, et al. Stage I and II MALT lymphoma: results of treatment with radiotherapy. *Int J Radiat Oncol Biol Phys* 2001;50:1258–1264.
5. Thieblemont C, Berger F, Dumontet C, et al. Mucosa-associated lymphoid tissue lymphoma is a disseminated disease in one third of 158 patients analyzed. *Blood* 2000;95:802–806.
6. Thieblemont C, Bastion Y, Berger F, et al. Mucosa-associated lymphoid tissue gastrointestinal and nongastrointestinal lymphoma behavior: analysis of 108 patients. *J Clin Oncol* 1997;15:1624–1630.
7. Balthazar EJ, Noordhoorn M, Megibow AJ, et al. CT of small-bowel lymphoma in immunocompetent patients and patients with AIDS: comparison of findings. *Am J Roentgenol* 1997;168:675–680.
8. Feliciano DV. Management of traumatic retroperitoneal hematoma. *Ann Surg* 1990;211:109–123.
9. Kalinowski EA, Trerotola SO. Postcatheterization retroperitoneal hematoma due to spontaneous lumbar arterial hemorrhage. *Cardiovasc Intervent Radiol* 1998;21:337–339.
10. Lev-Gur M, Adachi A, Greston WM, et al. Retroperitoneal hematoma from a ruptured tubal pregnancy as an unusual cause of pelvic mass. A case report. *J Reprod Med* 1986;31:271–273.
11. Dabney A, Bastani B. Enoxaparin-associated severe retroperitoneal bleeding and abdominal compartment syndrome: a report of two cases. *Intensive Care Med* 2001;27:1954–1957.
12. Gulla N, Patriti A, Capitanucci L. A case of "silent" pheochromocytoma presenting as spontaneous retroperitoneal hematoma. *Ann Ital Chir* 2000;71:735–737.
13. Kondo E, Utsumi M, Hattori M, et al. Acquired factor VIII-specific antibody disorder accompanied by a life-threatening retroperitoneal hematoma. *Intern Med* 1995;34:901–903.
14. Kastan DJ, Burke TH. Images in clinical medicine: retroperitoneal hemorrhage. *N Engl J Med* 2000;342:702.
15. Lawrence W Jr, Donegan WL, Natarajan N, et al. Adult soft tissue sarcomas: a pattern of care survey of the American College of Surgeons. *Ann Surg* 1987;205:349–359.
16. Linehan DC, Lewis JJ, Leung D, et al. Influence of biologic factors and anatomic site in completely resected liposarcoma. *J Clin Oncol* 2000;18:1637–1643.
17. Dai JR. Computed tomography of retroperitoneal neoplasms. *Zhonghua Zhong Liu Za Zhi* 1992;14:455–457. Chinese.
18. Knelson M, Haaga J, Lazarus H, et al. Computed tomography-guided retroperitoneal biopsies. *J Clin Oncol* 1989;7:1168–1173.
19. Welch TJ, Sheedy PF 2nd, Johnson CD, et al. CT-guided biopsy: prospective analysis of 1,000 procedures. *Radiology* 1989;171:493–496.
20. Bird AR, Jacobs P. Trephine biopsy of the bone marrow. *S Afr Med J* 1983;64:271–276.
21. Ben-Chetrit E, Flusser D, Assaf Y. Severe bleeding complicating percutaneous bone marrow biopsy. *Arch Intern Med* 1984;144:2284.
22. Gupta S, Meyers ML, Trambert J, et al. Massive intra-abdominal bleeding complicating bone marrow aspiration and biopsy in multiple myeloma. *Postgrad Med J* 1992;68:770.
23. McNutt DR, Fudenberg HH. Bone marrow biopsy and osteoporosis. *N Engl J Med* 1972;286:46.

33

A 41-YEAR-OLD WOMAN WITH ANEMIA AND THROMBOCYTOPENIA

AHMED A. ABSI
MOHAMMED S. GHANAMAH

CASE PRESENTATION

A 41-year-old woman presented to the outpatient clinic with a 2-day history of right-lower-quadrant abdominal pain and gross hematuria. The patient denied any visual disturbances, focal weakness, numbness, nausea, vomiting, fever, or chills. She reported a past medical history of nephrolithiasis, β-thalassemia minor, uterine fibroids, and fibromyalgia. Her medications included an oral contraceptive agent and acetaminophen.

On physical examination, her temperature was 37.8°C, her pulse was 100 beats per minute, and her blood pressure was 125/75 mm Hg. Her conjunctivae were pale, and several ecchymoses were noted over the anterior tibial region. Lungs were clear to auscultation, and cardiac examination revealed normal first and second heart sounds without murmurs. The abdomen was flat, with active bowel sounds and no tenderness. The liver and the spleen were not enlarged.

Laboratory studies revealed a hemoglobin of 8.2 g/dL, mean corpuscular volume of 65.8 fL, platelets of 12 K/μL, and white blood cell count of 9.93 K/μL. Blood urea nitrogen was 20 mg/dL, and creatinine was 0.9 mg/dL. Red blood cells were present in the urine.

QUESTIONS/DISCUSSION

In assessing this patient's anemia and thrombocytopenia, which of the following is the best next test?

A. **Serum lactate dehydrogenase (LDH)**
B. **Peripheral blood smear**
C. **Bone marrow biopsy**
D. **Coagulation studies [activated partial thromboplastin time (aPTT), international normalized ratio (INR)]**
E. **Repeat complete blood count (CBC) with sodium citrate**

Any laboratory evaluation of thrombocytopenia should start with a CBC and examination of the peripheral blood smear. Examination of the peripheral blood smear is important to rule out thrombotic thrombocytopenic purpura–hemolytic uremic syndrome (TTP–HUS) and acute leukemia, both of which require prompt treatment to prevent serious morbidity and mortality. The peripheral blood smear can help to identify abnormal platelet morphology, which may be an indicator of an inherited disorder. Reviewing the peripheral smear can also facilitate diagnosing disorders that are characterized by decreased platelet production, such as leukoerythroblastic syndromes and myelodysplastic states.

Repeating a blood count using sodium citrate or heparin as the anticoagulant is helpful in ruling out ethylenediaminetetraacetic acid (EDTA)–induced platelet clumping, which can cause pseudothrombocytopenia. Almost 0.1% of normal subjects have EDTA-dependent agglutinins, which can lead to platelet clumping and erroneous platelet counts (1). Repeat blood sampling with the use of an alternate anticoagulant can help diagnose pseudothrombocytopenia.

Bone marrow aspiration and biopsy are indicated in those cases of severe thrombocytopenia for which the etiology is not clear by history, physical examination, or laboratory evaluation. The bone marrow biopsy may help to confirm a diagnosis that has been suggested by the laboratory evaluation. The presence of normal to increased numbers of megakaryocytes in the marrow indicates that the thrombocytopenia is due, at least in part, to increased peripheral destruction. The absence of megakaryocytes or a decreased number of megakaryocytes in the bone marrow is consistent with decreased bone marrow production. A bone marrow biopsy may also help in diagnosing myelodysplastic disorders or invasive marrow disorders.

A serum lactate dehydrogenase (LDH) level is important in the evaluation of hemolytic anemia. LDH may be elevated due to red blood cell destruction as well as systemic tissue ischemia. Coagulation studies are important in differentiating disseminated intravascular coagulation (DIC) from TTP–HUS. Patients with DIC will typically have prolonged prothrombin (PT) and partial thromboplastin times (PTT), whereas the coagulation studies in TTP–HUS should be relatively normal.

Case Continued: A peripheral blood smear showed red blood cell (RBC) fragments, polychromasia, and occasional target cells. Additional testing showed a reticulocyte count of 7.1%, LDH of 880 U/L, total bilirubin of 2.1 mg/dL (conjugated 0.2 mg/dL), PT of 11.2 seconds, PTT 23.2 of seconds, and INR of 0.98. Urine human chorionic gonadotropin was negative. Coombs test was also negative.

The patient was admitted to the hospital, and within four hours she became confused and experienced a generalized clonic seizure. One hour after the seizure, the patient was easily arousable and followed commands. She was oriented to self and place only. Cranial nerves were intact. Motor examination revealed normal strength bilaterally. Reflexes, as well as sensory and cerebellar examinations, were normal.

What is the most likely diagnosis?

A. TTP–HUS
B. Disseminated intravascular coagulation
C. Sepsis
D. Evans syndrome

The proper approach to any medical problem starts with appropriately defining the problem. This woman's anemia is characterized by an elevated reticulocyte count, elevated LDH, elevated indirect bilirubin, and evidence of RBC fragments on peripheral smear. These findings point to a destructive process as the cause of her anemia, which could be classified as "microangiopathic hemolytic anemia."

TTP and HUS are multisystem disorders characterized by thrombocytopenia, microangiopathic hemolytic anemia, and ischemic manifestations, which result from platelet agglutination in the arterial microvasculature. HUS is a disorder that overlaps with TTP; the final manifestation of both disorders is the formation of platelet microthrombi in the setting of a microangiopathic hemolytic anemia. HUS differs from TTP in that the predominant effect seen in HUS is in the kidneys, with deposition of platelet microthrombi in the glomeruli. Many still consider TTP and HUS to be essentially the same disorder, but with different initiating events, especially in children, where HUS is associated with verotoxin-producing *Escherichia coli* (2).

Sepsis with DIC must be excluded in acutely ill patients who present with fever, thrombocytopenia, multiorgan dysfunction, and microangiopathic hemolysis. Appropriate antimicrobial and supportive therapy should be initiated as soon as appropriate cultures have been obtained. PT, PTT, and fibrin degradation products are elevated in DIC, and fibrinogen is usually decreased. Sepsis was an unlikely diag-

nosis in this patient, as she remained hemodynamically stable with normal blood pressure and temperature and did not have an obvious source of infection on presentation. DIC was excluded based on normal coagulation parameters.

Patients with Evans syndrome have concomitant autoimmune hemolytic anemia and immune thrombocytopenic purpura. Evans syndrome can be diagnosed on the basis of a positive direct Coombs test, a lack of RBC fragments on peripheral blood smear, and a lack of involvement of other organ systems.

At this point, TTP was considered the most likely diagnosis, as the patient had a combination of microangiopathic hemolytic anemia, thrombocytopenia, and neurologic manifestations. TTP classically consists of the pentad of microangiopathic hemolytic anemia, thrombocytopenia, fever, renal dysfunction, and neurologic manifestations. Neurologic symptoms include confusion, focal neurologic deficits, sensorimotor deficits, aphasia, seizures, and coma. Not all five components of the pentad are required to make the diagnosis. HUS is usually not associated with fever or neurologic manifestations, as the primary effects are seen in the kidney. TTP–HUS may be associated with various disease states, such as breast cancer and gastric adenocarcinoma. Certain infections, including human immunodeficiency virus (HIV)-1 and *E. coli* 0157:H7, have also been associated with TTP–HUS. Medications may also predispose to the development of TTP–HUS. Medications most often implicated include quinine, ticlopidine, clopidogrel, tacrolimus, cyclosporine, and mitomycin (3).

A number of pathophysiologic mechanisms have been considered to account for TTP–HUS. The most widely accepted theory is that the presence of an inhibiting autoantibody to the von Willebrand factor (vWF)–cleaving protease or an inherited deficiency of this enzyme results in the presence of unusually large multimeric forms of vWF that form occlusive hyaline thrombi with platelets (3). In *E. coli* 0157:H7-associated HUS, the pathogenesis is believed to be related to the elaboration of verotoxins that preferentially bind to specific glycolipid receptors on vascular endothelial cells, leading to endothelial injury and localized intravascular thrombosis. The renal vascular endothelium is particularly susceptible to this type of injury (3).

Laboratory studies in TTP routinely show severe hemolytic anemia, which is characterized by an elevated reticulocyte count, elevated indirect bilirubin, and very low serum haptoglobin. The peripheral smear demonstrates schistocytes (RBC fragments) and confirms true thrombocytopenia. The serum creatinine is variably elevated and typically higher in HUS than in TTP. LDH levels are often dramatically elevated.

Which of the following is the appropriate treatment for this patient?

A. Plasma exchange therapy
B. Corticosteroids and intravenous immunoglobulin

C. Anticoagulation with heparin
D. Splenectomy
E. Platelet transfusion

The mortality rate for TTP approaches 100% without treatment. However, some patients have improved after transfusion of blood or plasma, which led to the realization that plasma-based therapy may be an effective treatment for TTP. Plasma exchange reverses the platelet consumption that causes the thrombus formation and symptoms that are characteristic of TTP. Plasma transfusion presumably supplies the missing enzyme, while plasma exchange can remove the acquired autoantibody and the von Willebrand factor multimers (3). As soon as hemolytic microangiopathic anemia with thrombocytopenia is identified and TTP is suspected, therapy should commence. Plasma exchange should be performed on a daily basis until neurologic symptoms, if present, have resolved, and normal LDH levels and platelet counts are maintained for at least 3 days (3). Serial observations indicate that neurologic symptoms and serum LDH tend to improve within the first 3 days, whereas the platelet count may take a few more days to recover (4). In patients with renal dysfunction, recovery of function is unpredictable and often incomplete. If instituted in a timely manner, plasma exchange results in a greater than 90% survival rate (5).

In patients who do not respond or have an incomplete response, the most important principle is to increase the dose of plasma exchange. Other potentially helpful modalities include corticosteroids, vincristine, and infusion of intravenous immunoglobulin; however, these medications are not an alternative to continuing plasma exchange (5).

Splenectomy has been tried in refractory patients with variable results. Splenectomy is usually reserved for patients who do not respond to exchange with fresh-frozen plasma or cryosupernatant. Since splenectomy can enhance the response to plasma exchange, patients who undergo splenectomy should continue to receive plasma exchange postoperatively until remission is achieved (3).

Heparin is not indicated in the treatment of TTP–HUS. Platelet transfusion is also not indicated and may worsen neurologic symptoms and renal dysfunction. Platelet transfusion can lead to the generation of new or expanding thrombi, as the infused platelets are consumed (6).

This patient was started on plasma exchange therapy. She received six sessions for the first 7 days, in combination with prednisone at a dose of 1 mg/kg/day. By the seventh day, her platelet count was 110 K/µL, and the LDH level was normal. Her neurologic complications resolved completely.

The patient was discharged home and observed closely as an outpatient. Three months later, she presented to her hematologist with right-lower-quadrant abdominal pain, a platelet count of 22 K/µL, and an LDH level of 735 U/L.

CONCLUSION

Relapses, defined as recurrence of TTP 30 or more days after the completion of successful therapy, are common in patients who respond to the initial course of therapy. Relapses should be distinguished from exacerbations, which occur when daily plasma exchange is tapered or discontinued. Relapses usually occur within the first year, but occasionally are seen as late as 10 years after initial presentation. Patients who responded initially to plasma exchange treatment will likely respond again (3). Splenectomy during remission may reduce the incidence of TTP relapses, which occur in up to 30% of patients (7).

This patient relapsed three times within a 6-month period. With each relapse, she responded completely to plasmapheresis and corticosteroids. The patient underwent a splenectomy after her third relapse. She has been in remission since then.

REFERENCES

1. Vicari A, Banfi G, Bonini PA. EDTA-dependent pseudothrombocytopaenia: a 12-month epidemiological study. *Scand J Clin Lab Invest* 1988;48:537–542.
2. Karmali MA, Petric M, Lim C, et al. The association between idiopathic hemolytic uremic syndrome and infection by verotoxin-producing *Escherichia coli. J Infect Dis* 1985;151:775–782.
3. Elliott MA, Nichols WL. Thrombotic thrombocytopenic purpura and hemolytic uremic syndrome. *Mayo Clin Proc* 2001;76: 1154–1162.
4. Thompson CE, Damon LE, Ries CA, et al. Thrombotic microangiopathies in the 1980s: clinical features, response to treatment, and the impact of the human immunodeficiency virus epidemic. *Blood* 1992;80:1890–1895.
5. Bunn HF, Rosse W. Hemolytic anemias and acute blood loss. In: Braunwald E, Fauci AS, Kasper DL, et al., eds. *Harrison's principles of internal medicine,* 15th ed. Philadelphia: McGraw-Hill, 2001: 681–692.
6. Lind SE. Thrombocytopenic purpura and platelet transfusion. *Ann Intern Med* 1987;106:478.
7. Crowther MA, Heddle N, Hayward CP, et al. Splenectomy done during hematologic remission to prevent relapse in patients with thrombotic thrombocytopenic purpura. *Ann Intern Med* 1996; 125:294–296.

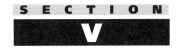

SECTION V

INFECTIOUS DISEASES

34

A PATIENT WITH HUMAN IMMUNODEFICIENCY VIRUS INFECTION WITH FEVER AND SHORTNESS OF BREATH

JOSE RAFAEL ROMERO
SARKIS B. BAGHDASARIAN
OLYMPIA A. TACHOPOULOU
THOMAS F. KEYS

CASE PRESENTATION

A 45-year-old man with human immunodeficiency virus (HIV) infection was admitted to the hospital with fever, shortness of breath, and vomiting. Three weeks before admission, the patient noted increased abdominal girth. One week later, he developed low-grade fevers, persistent shortness of breath, and intermittent vomiting. These symptoms intensified over the following week, and the patient was brought to the emergency department. On review of systems, the patient denied chest pain, other gastrointestinal complaints, neurologic symptoms, or urinary symptoms.

The patient had been diagnosed with HIV-1 infection 12 years earlier. At the time of diagnosis, he presented with neurosyphilis, complicated by multiple strokes related to meningovascular involvement. He developed neurologic deficits, including moderate expressive aphasia, dysphagia, paraplegia, and left-upper-extremity paralysis, resulting in nursing home placement.

His past medical history was significant for aspiration pneumonia 6 years earlier, complicated by empyema; esophageal strictures requiring multiple dilatations; percutaneous gastrostomy (PEG) tube placement; seizure disorder; deep venous thrombosis of the right lower extremity 2 years earlier; and presumed *Pneumocystis carinii* pneumonia (PCP) 6 months before admission.

Six months before this presentation, the patient was started on antiretroviral therapy with lamivudine and zidovudine. A recent CD4 count was 196 cells/mm^3, and a viral load was 2,144 copies/mL. His admission medications were amitriptyline, phenobarbital, hydroxyzine, metoclopramide, sucralfate, lamivudine, zidovudine, and trimethoprim–sulfamethoxazole (TMP–SMX).

Vital signs included a blood pressure of 130/72 mm Hg, heart rate of 129 beats per minute, temperature of 38.6°C, and respiratory rate of 24 per minute. Pulse oximetry was 93% on 5 L nasal O$_2$. Chest examination revealed rales in the right upper lobe and normal heart sounds. The abdomen was mildly distended, soft, and nontender, with normal bowel sounds. The extremities had 1+ pitting edema. Neurologic examination was unchanged from previous examinations. The remainder of the examination was normal.

QUESTIONS/DISCUSSION

Which infectious processes should be considered in the initial evaluation of this patient?

A. Community-acquired pneumonia
B. Aspiration pneumonia
C. Tuberculosis
D. Opportunistic infections
E. All of the above

In patients with HIV presenting with respiratory symptoms and fever, infection is the primary initial consideration. Infection is the major cause of fever in HIV-infected patients, accounting for 90% of cases in one series (1). Table 34.1 lists infectious agents that can cause fever and respiratory symptoms in HIV patients.

Susceptibility to diverse infectious agents varies according to the degree of immunosuppression. With a relatively intact immune system, HIV patients develop infections due to the same microorganisms that infect the general population. As the disease progresses, opportunistic infections play

TABLE 34.1. ETIOLOGY OF FEVER AND RESPIRATORY SYMPTOMS IN HUMAN IMMUNODEFICIENCY VIRUS PATIENTS

Infectious Agents

Bacterial	*Streptococcus pneumoniae, Haemophilus influenzae, Staphylococcus aureus, Mycobacterium tuberculosis, Mycobacterium avium* complex, *Mycoplasma pneumoniae, Chlamydia, Legionella*
Fungal	Cryptococcosis, histoplasmosis, coccidioidomycosis, candidiasis, blastomycosis, sporotrichosis
Parasitic	*Pneumocystis carinii, Strongyloides stercoralis, Cryptosporidium, Microsporidia,* toxoplasmosis
Viral	Cytomegalovirus, HSV, VZV, adenovirus, influenza, parainfluenza

Noninfectious Causes

Neoplastic	Kaposi sarcoma, lymphoma (non-Hodgkin and Hodgkin), lymphoid interstitial pneumonitis, bronchogenic carcinoma
Drugs	Thyroid hormone, amphetamines, phencyclidine, cocaine, monoamine oxidase inhibitors, tricyclic antidepressants, antipsychotics, lithium, halothane, succinylcholine, salicylates, phenothiazines, ethanol, sulfonamides
Metabolic	Hyperthyroidism, adrenal insufficiency
Other	Collagen vascular disease
	Granulomatous diseases (sarcoidosis)
	Idiosyncratic reactions (malignant hyperthermia, transfusion reaction)
	Pulmonary embolism
	Pulmonary hypertension
	Acute myocardial infarction

HSV, herpes simplex virus; VZV, varicella zoster virus.

a more important role. The patient's travel and medical history, geographic location, and socioeconomic status may affect the likelihood of certain opportunistic infections.

Community-acquired pneumonia is the most frequent pulmonary infection in HIV patients (2). Nosocomial pneumonia is also common and should be considered in any patient who has been hospitalized recently or resides in a nursing home. Aspiration is a major concern in this patient, who has a history of vomiting and severe neurologic impairment.

A recent CD4 count was 196 cells/mm^3, which makes certain opportunistic infections less likely. PCP occurs more frequently with a CD4 count below 200 cells/mm^3. *Mycobacterium avium intracellulare* (MAI) most often attacks individuals with advanced HIV disease, usually when CD4 counts are less than 50 cells/mm^3. Tuberculosis should be strongly considered if there is a history of exposure, or if a 5TU PPD produces 5 mm or more of induration. Neither was present in this patient. Viruses such as cytomegalovirus, herpes virus, and varicella-zoster are rare causes of fever and pulmonary symptoms in HIV-infected patients. Fungi, especially *Cryptococcus neoformans* and *Histoplasma capsulatum*, should also be considered. Intestinal parasites such as *Strongyloides stercoralis* may cause pulmonary symptoms in immunocompromised hosts, but this is very rare.

A number of noninfectious causes might explain this patient's presentation. They should also be considered in the initial differential diagnosis (Table 34.1).

After obtaining appropriate cultures, the patient was started empirically on antibiotics for suspected aspiration/nosocomial pneumonia. TMP–SMX was continued and antiretroviral therapy was stopped.

Initial laboratory results included white blood cell count of 14.5 K/µL with 73% neutrophils and 22% lymphocytes. A metabolic profile revealed the following: sodium, 137 mmol/L; potassium, 3.7 mmol/L; chloride, 99 mmol/L; bicarbonate, 14 mmol/L; glucose, 87 mg/dL; aspartate aminotransferase, 104 U/L, alanine aminotransferase, 73 U/L; alkaline phosphatase, 152 U/L; and total bilirubin, 1.0 mg/dL. Amylase and lipase were normal.

An arterial blood gas on 3 L/min of oxygen revealed pH of 7.39, P_{CO_2} of 23 mm Hg, P_{O_2} of 73 mm Hg, and bicarbonate of 14 mmol/L. Urinalysis was remarkable for 3+ ketones and 30 mg/dL of protein. A plain film of the abdomen did not reveal any evidence of obstruction. A portable chest x-ray revealed hypoinflated lungs with apparent widening of the superior mediastinum. Elevation of the right hemidiaphragm was described. There was no focal consolidation.

What is this patient's acid–base disorder?

A. **Anion gap metabolic acidosis**
B. **Non–anion gap metabolic acidosis**
C. **Respiratory alkalosis**
D. **Mixed anion gap metabolic acidosis/non–anion gap acidosis**
E. **Mixed anion gap metabolic acidosis/respiratory alkalosis**

This patient has a mixed acid–base disorder consisting of a wide anion gap (AG) metabolic acidosis with respiratory alkalosis. The increase in AG equals the decrease in serum bicarbonate (HCO_3), findings that would not be consistent with a coexisting normal AG metabolic acidosis. Furthermore, a P_{CO_2} of 23 mm Hg is lower than expected by a compensatory mechanism (should be 29; P_{CO_2} should equal $[(1.5 \times HCO_3) + 8]$). The lower than expected P_{CO_2} suggests respiratory alkalosis. In this patient, potential causes of respiratory alkalosis include central nervous system infection, psychogenic hyperventilation, pneumonia, atelectasis, and pulmonary embolism.

The differential diagnosis of an anion gap metabolic acidosis should include diabetic ketoacidosis, lactic acidosis, renal failure, rhabdomyolysis, and toxic ingestion. A blood lactic acid level in this patient was 7.5 mmol/L. Ketones were noted in the urine; this could be due to decreased feeding, as well as vomiting, which had been present for the 2 weeks preceding admission. Lactic acid overproduction and/or underutilization may cause lactic acidosis. Under normal circumstances, most of the lactate produced in the body is cleared in the liver, so liver dysfunction may result in lactate accumulation (3).

Computerized tomography (CT) of the abdomen and chest were performed (Figs. 34.1 and 34.2). Pulmonary embolism (PE) was considered a possible diagnosis in this patient. PE can cause hypoxia, tachypnea, tachycardia, fever, and lactic acidosis. A spiral CT scan of the chest was negative for PE. A duplex ultrasound of the lower extremities only showed a remote deep venous thrombosis in the right external iliac and common femoral veins. Acute myocardial infarction was ruled out by normal serial cardiac enzymes. There was no evidence of congestive heart failure on examination or chest x-ray.

The abnormal transaminases and alkaline phosphatase could be caused by a viral hepatotrophic virus (such as cytomegalovirus, Epstein–Barr virus, hepatitis B virus, or hepatitis C virus), disseminated fungal infection, or mycobacterial infection. Screening studies for these infections were negative.

Lymphoproliferative disease, including lymphoma, may produce fever; respiratory symptoms, including hyperventilation; and thereby lactic acidosis. However, lymphoproliferative disease is unlikely in this patient with negative CT

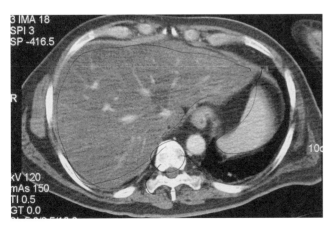

FIGURE 34.1. Computed tomogram of the abdomen and pelvis demonstrating fatty infiltration of the liver. The pancreas was normal, and there was no evidence of neoplasia.

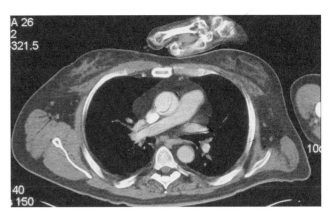

FIGURE 34.2. Computed tomogram of the chest demonstrating normal vascular structures, absence of neoplasia, and fatty infiltration of mediastinum (lipomatosis).

scans of the chest and the abdomen for lymphadenopathy. Medication toxicity may also cause these findings.

The most likely cause for lactic acidosis in this patient is:

A. **Antiretroviral therapy**
B. **Sepsis**
C. **Nonalcoholic steatohepatitis (NASH) with resultant liver dysfunction**
D. **Muscle breakdown due to lipodystrophy**

This patient was recently started on antiretroviral therapy with lamivudine and zidovudine. Antiretroviral agents have been associated with severe side effects, such as lipodystrophy syndrome, hypertriglyceridemia, fat redistribution, hepatic steatosis, and lactic acidosis syndrome (4).

Lactic acidosis syndrome may occur 5 to 13 months after the onset of antiretroviral treatment (5). Multiple agents have been implicated as causes of the syndrome, including zidovudine, didanosine, stavudine, zidovudine/zalcitabine, and combinations of lamivudine with the other nucleoside reverse transcriptase inhibitors (NRTIs) (6–8). An incidence of 20.9 cases per 1,000 person-years has been reported (9).

Presenting symptoms are usually nonspecific and include nausea, vomiting, abdominal pain, fatigue, dyspnea, and fever (10). The diagnosis is confirmed by demonstrating elevated lactic acid, moderately to severely decreased bicarbonate, and an associated anion gap of 20 to 40 mmol/L (4). Mild to moderate elevation of liver function tests has also been described (9).

The syndrome varies in severity but may result in death, with a reported mortality as high as 60% (11). Death usually results from cardiovascular complications or progressive liver or multi-organ failure (12). Hepatomegaly and diffuse fatty infiltration of the liver are often demonstrated in imaging studies or at autopsy. Histologic examination of the liver demonstrates microvesicular, macrovesicular, or mixed steatosis (13).

Although the mechanism by which NRTIs produce toxicity is unclear, inhibition of the mitochondrial DNA polymerase gamma, an enzyme required for mitochondrial replication, has been postulated (14). NRTI-related lactic acidosis shares several clinical features with inherited mitochondrial disorders, including lipomatosis, neuropathy, and hepatic steatosis.

Unfortunately, no specific treatment is available for this syndrome. Once the diagnosis is suspected, NRTIs must be stopped, and additional antiretroviral agents should be held to avoid the development of viral resistance. However, in many reported cases, acidosis has been progressive even after discontinuation of these drugs (15,16). Recent reports have described success with empiric use of agents such as coenzyme Q (10), riboflavin (6), thiamine (17), and L-carnitine (18). The exact mechanism by which these agents work is unknown. Treatment with mechanical ventilation and bicarbonate infusions has not changed the course of disease in several cases (19,20).

Although no recommendations are available for screening for lactic acidosis–steatosis, the syndrome should be suspected in patients receiving NRTIs who present with fatigue, nausea, nonspecific abdominal pain, or dyspnea without pulmonary findings, as well as in those patients with unexplained anion gap acidosis and elevated transaminases. New techniques, such as the measurement of mitochondrial DNA to nuclear DNA ratio, may be used as tools for screening (21). Reinstitution of NRTI therapy is not recommended, and an alternative antiretroviral regimen should be selected (22).

CONCLUSION

The patient's clinical picture remained unchanged for 3 days with persistent fever to 38.5°C. Because of the high suspicion for NRTI-associated lactic acidosis syndrome, empiric antibiotic therapy was discontinued. Supportive measures, including treatment with coenzyme Q, L-carnitine, thiamine, riboflavin, and vitamin E, were begun. By hospital day 5, the patient's fever had resolved. Vital signs returned to normal, and his pulmonary symptoms improved. Transaminase levels decreased but remained mildly elevated. Serum lactate levels returned to normal, and the acidosis resolved. The patient was discharged to the nursing home on hospital day 10 in improved condition. His family subsequently decided against aggressive management and the patient expired 2 months later.

REFERENCES

1. Masci JR. Symptom-oriented evaluation and management. In: *Outpatient management of HIV infection,* 3rd ed. Boca Raton, FL: CRC Press, 2001:109–130.
2. Zimmerli W. Pneumonia in patients with HIV infection. *Ther Umsch* 2001;58:620–624.
3. Kreisberg RA. Lactate homeostasis and lactic acidosis. *Ann Intern Med* 1980;92:227–237.
4. Stenzel MS, Carpenter CC. The management of the clinical complications of antiretroviral therapy. *Infect Dis Clin North Am* 2000;14:851–878.
5. Sundar K, Suarez M, Banogon PE, et al. Zidovudine-induced fatal lactic acidosis and hepatic failure in patients with acquired immunodeficiency syndrome: report of two patients and review of the literature. *Crit Care Med* 1997;25:1425–1430.
6. Kakuda TN. Pharmacology of nucleoside and nucleotide reverse transcriptase inhibitor-induced mitochondrial toxicity. *Clin Ther* 2000;22:685–708.
7. Dalton SD, Rahimi AR. Emerging role of riboflavin in the treatment of nucleoside analogue-induced type B lactic acidosis. *AIDS Patient Care STDS* 2001;15:611–614.
8. Mokrzycki MH, Harris C, May H, et al. Lactic acidosis associated with stavudine administration: a report of five cases. *Clin Infect Dis* 2000;30:198–200.
9. Lonergan JT, Behling C, Pfander H, et al. Hyperlactatemia and hepatic abnormalities in 10 human immunodeficiency virus-infected patients receiving nucleoside analogue combination regimens. *Clin Infect Dis* 2000;31:162–166.
10. Brinkman K. Editorial response: hyperlactatemia and hepatic steatosis as features of mitochondrial toxicity of nucleoside analogue reverse transcriptase inhibitors. *Clin Infect Dis* 2000;31:167–169.
11. Falco V, Rodriguez D, Ribera E, et al. Severe nucleoside-associated lactic acidosis in human immunodeficiency virus-infected patients: report of 12 cases and review of the literature. *Clin Infect Dis* 2002;34:838–846.
12. Coghlan ME, Sommadossi JP, Jhala NC, et al. Symptomatic lactic acidosis in hospitalized antiretroviral-treated patients with human immunodeficiency virus infection: a report of 12 cases. *Clin Infect Dis* 2001;33:1914–1921.
13. Goldfarb-Rumyantzev AS, Jeyakumar A, Gumpeni R, et al. Lactic acidosis associated with nucleoside analog therapy in an HIV-positive patient. *AIDS Patient Care STDS* 2000;14:339–342.
14. Brinkman K, ter Hofstede HJ, Burger DM, et al. Adverse effects of reverse transcriptase inhibitors: mitochondrial toxicity as common pathway. *AIDS* 1998;12:1735–1744.
15. Megarbane B, Goldgran-Toledano D, Guerin JM, et al. Fatal lactic acidosis in a patient infected by HIV and treated with stavudine and didanosine. *Pathol Biol* 2000;48:505–507.
16. Chariot P, Drogou I, de Lacroix-Szmania I, et al. Zidovudine-induced mitochondrial disorder with massive liver steatosis, myopathy, lactic acidosis, and mitochondrial DNA depletion. *J Hepatol* 1999;30:156–160.
17. Arici C, Tebaldi A, Quinzan GP, et al. Severe lactic acidosis and thiamine administration in an HIV-infected patient on HAART. *Int J STD AIDS* 2001;12:407–409.
18. Claessens YE, Cariou A, Chiche JD, et al. L-Carnitine as a treatment of life-threatening lactic acidosis induced by nucleoside analogues. *AIDS* 2000;14:472–473.
19. Lasso M, Perez J, Noriega LM, et al. Fatal lactic acidosis in a patient with acquired immunodeficiency syndrome treated with highly active antiretroviral therapy: report of a case. *Rev Med Chil* 2000;128:1139–1143.
20. Bissuel F, Bruneel F, Habersetzer F, et al. Fulminant hepatitis with severe lactate acidosis in HIV-infected patients on didanosine therapy. *J Intern Med* 1994;235:367–371.
21. Cote HC, Brumme ZL, Craib KJ, et al. Changes in mitochondrial DNA as a marker of nucleoside toxicity in HIV-infected patients. *N Engl J Med* 2002;346:811–820.
22. Khouri S, Cushing H. Lactic acidosis secondary to nucleoside analogue antiretroviral therapy. *AIDS Read* 2000;10:602–606.

35

A 22-YEAR-OLD WOMAN WITH SYSTEMIC LUPUS ERYTHEMATOSUS AND BRAIN LESIONS

SHADI N. DAOUD
OLYMPIA A. TACHOPOULOU
SUSAN J. REHM

CASE PRESENTATION

A 22-year-old woman was transferred to our institution for further management of systemic lupus erythematosus (SLE). A month prior to transfer, the patient presented to her primary care physician with arthralgias, lip swelling, oral ulcers, epistaxis, cough, pleuritic chest pain, and a malar rash. She was admitted to a hospital and diagnosed with SLE. Treatment included high-dose corticosteroids and hydroxychloroquine. During the hospitalization, she developed renal and hepatic dysfunction, deep venous thromboses, mental status changes, and *Staphylococcus aureus* bacteremia. The patient was transferred to our institution for further evaluation and therapy.

The patient was previously healthy except for psoriatic arthritis. She had not traveled outside the United States and denied any exposure to tuberculosis. She did not own any pets, but did grow up on a farm with many animals.

A week after admission to our institution, the patient developed a seizure and respiratory distress. Upon examination, her temperature was 37.0°C; blood pressure, 110/82 mm Hg; pulse, 92 beats per minute; and respiratory rate, 18 per minute. She was lethargic and appeared unwell. Scaling consistent with psoriasis was present over the extensor surfaces of her legs. She had a malar rash, oral ulcer, and mild swelling of her lips. Breath sounds were diminished in both bases, left greater than right, and there were scattered rhonchi on the left. Cardiac examination did not reveal any murmurs or gallops. There was no lymphadenopathy. She had no meningeal signs. Her neurologic examination revealed subtle left-lower-extremity weakness that had been present since admission. The rest of the physical examination was unremarkable.

Laboratory results were significant for a platelet count of 20,000/μL, hemoglobin of 8.6 g/dL, and white cell count of 5.11 K/μL. Her blood urea nitrogen was 56 mg/dL, and

creatinine was 1.2 mg/dL. Blood cultures again revealed methicillin-susceptible *Staphylococcus aureus*. Chest x-ray revealed small bilateral pleural effusions, which had been present previously, and new left perihilar and right basilar nodular lesions. Computed tomography (CT) of the brain revealed low-attenuation lesions in multiple vascular distributions (Fig. 35.1). Magnetic resonance imaging (MRI) of

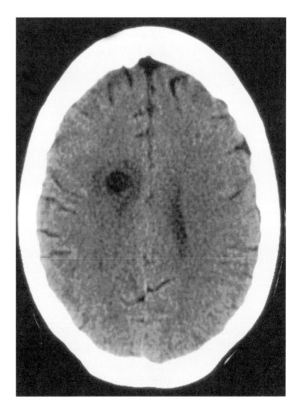

FIGURE 35.1. Computed tomography scan of the brain performed as part of the initial evaluation of this patient's seizure revealed low-attenuation lesions in multiple vascular distributions.

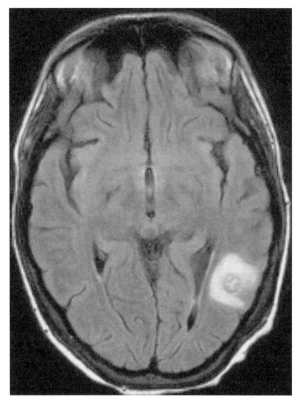

FIGURE 35.2. Magnetic resonance imaging of the brain confirmed the presence of the multiple intracranial lesions seen on computed tomography.

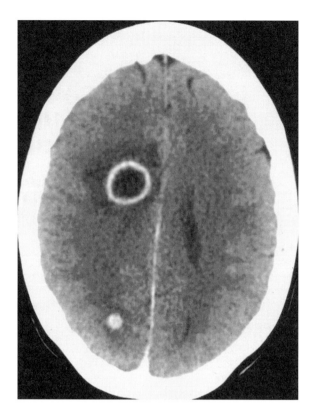

FIGURE 35.3. Follow-up computed tomography scan of the brain after 1 month of treatment with vancomycin revealed new intracranial lesions.

the brain performed the same day confirmed the presence of multiple intraaxial masses (Fig. 35.2). The findings on both CT and MRI were thought to be consistent with brain abscesses.

The patient responded to broad-spectrum antibiotic therapy for presumed pneumonia and staphylococcal brain abscesses. Due to the development of a rash while on piperacillin/tazobactam, vancomycin was used for longer-term therapy for the brain abscesses. Follow-up imaging of the brain did not show any new lesions, and the patient was discharged home. A repeat CT scan performed 1 month later showed new lesions (Fig. 35.3).

QUESTIONS/DISCUSSION

Which of the following is the least likely cause of the new lesions seen on CT?

A. **Vasculitis**
B. **Primary central nervous system (CNS) lymphoma**
C. **Intracranial hemorrhage**
D. **Infection with an opportunistic pathogen**
E. **Abscess due to vancomycin intermediately susceptible *Staphylococcus aureus* (VISA)**

The aim of immunosuppressive treatment is to reduce the host inflammatory response in order to control the symptoms and manifestations of conditions such as SLE. However, immunosuppression also reduces cell-mediated and humoral immunity, which increases the risk of infection. The approach to a patient with a suspected CNS infection depends on the presentation. Patients with mass lesions can present with a focal neurologic deficit, stroke, or seizure. Patients with meningeal infections often present with fever and nuchal rigidity, although these signs may not be present in certain opportunistic infections. Patients often have a clear sensorium. In contrast, patients with encephalitis have an altered level of consciousness. A mass lesion (brain abscess) is the most common manifestation of CNS infection in the compromised host (1). Suppression of the inflammatory response to infection can alter the typical symptoms of CNS infections; therefore, immunosuppressed patients often present with only headache or fever without any focal neurologic deficits (2).

Noninfectious causes, which can closely mimic CNS infections, should also be considered. SLE can involve any region of the brain and meninges; CNS events, including vasculitis, may occur when SLE is active in other organ systems. Patients who have thrombocytopenia as a result of either chemotherapy or their underlying illness can present with a CNS bleed that can mimic a brain abscess (1).

Immunosuppressed patients, especially those with underlying human immunodeficiency virus (HIV) infection, are at increased risk of developing malignancies that can either originate in the CNS or metastasize to the CNS. Infections due to vancomycin intermediately susceptible *Staphylococcus aureus* are extraordinarily rare; approximately a dozen cases have been reported worldwide through the end of 2001 (3). A VISA abscess is the least likely diagnosis.

Which of the following is the next appropriate diagnostic test?

A. **Stereotactic brain biopsy**
B. **Lumbar puncture for CSF analysis and cultures**
C. **Electroencephalogram (EEG)**
D. **Blood cultures**

Routine studies of blood and urine are rarely helpful, and blood cultures are only occasionally positive in patients with brain abscesses (4). Although the cerebrospinal fluid (CSF) is often abnormal in patients with brain abscess, the findings are often nonspecific. Moreover, lumbar puncture is often contraindicated in the presence of an intracranial mass because of the risk of cerebral herniation (4). EEG is rarely helpful for diagnostic purposes unless there is high clinical suspicion for certain neurologic disorders. In Creutzfeldt–Jacob disease, periodic complexes are seen; focal or lateralized periodic slow-wave complexes in an acutely encephalopathic patient may suggest the diagnosis of herpes simplex encephalitis (5).

The introduction of CT and MRI has revolutionized the diagnostic and therapeutic approach to brain abscesses. A brain abscess typically appears on a contrast-enhanced CT as a hypodense lesion surrounded by an underlying enhancing ring. A variable hypodense area of edema extends beyond the ring. Unfortunately, this CT appearance is not specific, and other processes, including neoplasm, granuloma, and a resolving hematoma, may have the same appearance. MRI permits multiplanar imaging, better distinguishes gray and white matter, and is less influenced by bony artifacts. MRI also has higher sensitivity for the detection of brain abscesses than CT scan. For patients with intracranial mass lesions, every effort must be made to make a specific diagnosis, which usually requires a tissue specimen for microbiologic and histopathologic evaluation (4). Therefore, a stereotactic brain biopsy is the most appropriate test at this point in the evaluation.

A stereotactic brain biopsy was performed. Histopathologic examination of the tissue revealed hyaline septate hyphae with acute angle branching.

The histologic appearance is most consistent with which of the following infections?

A. **Toxoplasmosis**
B. **Aspergillosis**
C. **Cryptococcosis**
D. **Cytomegalovirus**
E. **Nocardiosis**

The histologic picture is consistent with aspergillosis. Cultures grew *Aspergillus fumigatus.* Brain abscess due to *Aspergillus* species is uncommon, occurring primarily in the setting of immunosuppression. Neutropenia and therapy with corticosteroids are the most common predisposing factors (1,6). In SLE, CNS aspergillosis occurs most frequently in the setting of disseminated infection (7,8). It is difficult to diagnose invasive aspergillosis serologically, and investigational DNA diagnostic methods have not yet proven to be clinically useful (9). Thus the diagnosis of *Aspergillus* brain abscess depends on the combination of clinical judgment and demonstration of the fungus in a tissue specimen obtained from the presumed site of infection. *Aspergillus* is a rapidly growing fungus and is often cultured in one to three days. However, longer periods may be required to see growth if the inoculum is very small (10,11).

Toxoplasma gondii is an intracellular protozoan parasite. Toxoplasmosis is the most common cause of secondary CNS infection in acquired immunodeficiency syndrome (AIDS) patients, representing 50% to 60% of mass lesions in this group. Common presenting symptoms include fever, unilateral or bilateral headache, and mental status changes. Toxoplasmosis usually appears as a solitary or multiple ring-enhancing lesions in the basal ganglia, deep white matter, or gray–white junction. Definitive diagnosis requires the demonstration of trophozoites on brain biopsy. However, the combination of a compatible radiographic picture and clinical improvement after 10 to 14 days of antibiotic therapy can allow clinicians to reach a presumptive diagnosis (12).

Cryptococcosis is caused by the yeast *Cryptococcus neoformans.* It usually manifests as disseminated disease in individuals with deficiencies of cell-mediated immunity. Cryptococcal meningitis has been reported to occur in up to 7% of patients with AIDS (13). In patients with cryptococcal meningitis, cryptococcal antigen is detected in 99% of serum samples and 91% of CSF samples (14). Titers are typically significantly higher in HIV-infected patients with cryptococcal meningitis than in HIV-negative patients with the disease (15,16). Cryptococci can sometimes be demonstrated in CSF with an India ink stain, which shows large encapsulated yeast cells. In contrast to HIV-negative patients, there are often minimal CSF abnormalities in HIV-positive patients with cryptococcal meningitis (17–19). CT of the brain may demonstrate meningeal enhancement and, occasionally, an enhancing lesion known as a cryptococcoma, but the scan is often normal (12).

Cytomegalovirus (CMV) is the most important viral pathogen affecting solid organ transplant patients. Up to 50% of allograft recipients develop symptomatic CMV infection, usually 1 to 4 months after transplantation. Central nervous system disease due to CMV is rare; presenting features may include mental status changes, psychomotor slowing, cranial nerve palsies, or retinitis. CT shows nodular, enhancing ventriculoencephalitis. Polymerase chain reaction (PCR) for CMV in the CSF is sensitive and specific, but clinical correlation is important in establishing a diagnosis (12). Central nervous system CMV infection is very rare in patients with SLE. PCR for CMV was negative in this patient.

Nocardiosis is an opportunistic infection that has been described in association with SLE (20,21). *Nocardia* is a Gram-positive, partially acid-fast staining filamentous organism that has a beaded, branching appearance on microscopic examination. Nocardiosis may present as lung nodules (sometimes with cavitation), CNS abscess, or meningitis (22). Prophylaxis with co-trimoxazole is recommended for patients receiving more than 20 mg/day of prednisone for more than 1 month. Treatment of active nocardial infection depends on antimicrobial susceptibility, as some *Nocardia* species are resistant to multiple antibiotics.

Which of the following is the most appropriate treatment for this patient?

A. **Pyrimethamine/sulfadiazine**
B. **Fluconazole**
C. **Amphotericin B**
D. **Itraconazole**

Amphotericin B is the major antifungal agent for the treatment of invasive aspergillosis and is appropriate treatment for this patient. The most extensive clinical experience has been with conventional amphotericin B. Even at a daily dose of 1 to 1.5 mg/kg, mortality remains high in seriously ill patients. In the past few years, lipid-based formulations of amphotericin B have been developed in an attempt to reduce nephrotoxicity associated with long-term, high-dose therapy (23). The efficacy of lipid-based formulations for the treatment of CNS aspergillosis appears to be similar to standard amphotericin B preparations. Itraconazole is active against *Aspergillus* species, but its use is not recommended in serious or life-threatening infections such as brain abscesses.

Fluconazole is useful for the treatment of oropharyngeal and esophageal candidiasis, and it is an effective initial and maintenance treatment for cryptococcal meningitis in patients with AIDS. However, fluconazole is not active against *Aspergillus* species. Pyrimethamine in combination with sulfadiazine is the treatment of choice for toxoplasmosis (24).

This patient was started on a long-term course of amphotericin B at a dose of 1 mg/kg. Clinically, she was asymptomatic, and follow-up imaging showed regression of her brain lesions.

CONCLUSION

Immunocompromised hosts are susceptible to a wide variety of complications and opportunistic infections, in addition to the regular infections seen in immunocompetent hosts. Therefore, a high index of suspicion must be maintained in these patients, and every effort should be made to obtain a tissue diagnosis in order to start appropriate and potentially life-saving therapy.

REFERENCES

1. Cunha BA. Central nervous system infections in the compromised host: a diagnostic approach. *Infect Dis Clin North Am* 2001;15:567–590.
2. Simon DM, Levin S. Infectious complications of solid organ transplantations. *Infect Dis Clin North Am* 2001;15:521–549.
3. Fridkin SK. Vancomycin-intermediate and -resistant *Staphylococcus aureus:* What the infectious disease specialist needs to know. *Clin Infect Dis* 2001;32:108–115.
4. Roos KL, Tyler KL. Bacterial meningitis and other suppurative infections. In: Braunwald E, Fauci AS, Kasper DL, et al., eds. *Harrison's principles of internal medicine,* 15th ed. New York: McGraw-Hill, 2001:2462–2471.
5. Aminoff M. Electrophysiologic studies of the central and peripheral nervous systems. In: Braunwald E, Fauci AS, Kasper DL, et al., eds. *Harrison's principles of internal medicine,* 15th ed. New York: McGraw-Hill, 2001:2331–2336.
6. Andriole VT. Aspergillus infections: problems in diagnosis and treatment. *Infect Agents Dis* 1996;5:47–54.
7. Gonzalez-Crespo MR, Gomez-Reino JJ. Invasive aspergillosis in systemic lupus erythematosus. *Semin Arthritis Rheum* 1995;24:304–314.
8. Katz A, Ehrenfeld M, Livneh A, et al. Aspergillosis in systemic lupus erythematosus. *Semin Arthritis Rheum* 1996;26:635–640.
9. Castagnola E, Bucci B, Montinaro E, et al. Fungal infections in patients undergoing bone marrow transplantation: an approach to a rational management protocol. *Bone Marrow Transplant* 1996;18(Suppl 2):97–106.
10. Denning DW. Diagnosis and management of invasive aspergillosis. *Curr Clin Top Infect Dis* 1996;16:277–299.
11. Latge JP. Tools and trends in the detection of *Aspergillus fumigatus. Curr Top Med Mycol* 1995;6:245–281.
12. Zunt JR. Central nervous system infection during immunosuppression. *Neurol Clin* 2002;20:1–22.
13. Currie BP, Casadevall A. Estimation of the prevalence of cryptococcal infection among patients infected with the human immunodeficiency virus in New York City. *Clin Infect Dis* 1994;19:1029–1033.
14. Chuck SL, Sande MA. Infections with *Cryptococcus neoformans* in the acquired immunodeficiency syndrome. *N Engl J Med* 1989;321:794–799.
15. Zuger A, Louie E, Holzman RS, et al. Cryptococcal disease in patients with the acquired immunodeficiency syndrome: diagnostic features and outcome of treatment. *Ann Intern Med* 1986;104:234–240.
16. Pappas, PG, Perfect JR, Cloud GA. et al. Cryptococcosis in human immunodeficiency virus-negative patients in the era of effective azole therapy. *Clin Infect Dis* 2001;33:690–699.
17. Kovacs JA, Kovacs AA, Polis M, et al. Cryptococcosis in the acquired immunodeficiency syndrome. *Ann Intern Med* 1985;103:533–538.
18. Kaplan MH, Rosen PP, Armstrong D. Cryptococcosis in a can-

cer hospital: clinical and pathological correlates in forty-six patients. *Cancer* 1977;39:2265–2274.

19. Dismukes WE. Cryptococcal meningitis in patients with AIDS. *J Infect Dis* 1988;157:624–628.

20. Mok CC, Yuen KY, Lau CS. Nocardiosis in systemic lupus erythematosus. *Semin Arthritis Rheum* 1997;26:675–683.

21. Leong KP, Tee NW, Yap WM, et al. Nocardiosis in patients with systemic lupus erythematosus. *J Rheumatol* 2000;27:1306–1312.

22. Bouza E, Moya JG, Munoz P. Infections in systemic lupus erythematosus and rheumatoid arthritis. *Infect Dis Clin North Am* 2001;15:335–361.

23. Hiemenz JW, Walsh TJ. Lipid formulations of amphotericin B: Recent progress and future directions. *Clin Infect Dis* 1996;22 (Suppl 2):S133–S144.

24. Bennett JE. Diagnosis and treatment of fungal infections. In: Braunwald E, Fauci AS, Kasper DL, et al., eds. *Harrison's principles of internal medicine,* 15th ed. New York: McGraw-Hill, 2001: 1168–1171.

36

A 59-YEAR-OLD DIABETIC MAN WITH A PAINFUL HAND ULCER

KHALID TABBARAH
TONI CHOUEIRI
OLYMPIA A. TACHOPOULOU
STEVEN P. LAROSA

CASE PRESENTATION

A 59-year-old diabetic man was seen in the outpatient clinic for a painful right hand ulcer. The patient had injured the tip of his right fifth finger 4 days earlier. The lesion progressed to an ulcer with foul-smelling discharge over the next 2 days. Oral ciprofloxacin over the previous 3 days did not produce an improvement. The patient did not have fevers or chills but complained of excruciating pain.

The patient had been treated for insulin-requiring diabetes mellitus since age 35. He had also been diagnosed with congestive heart failure (left ventricular ejection fraction, 20%), atrial fibrillation, and peripheral arterial disease. He had required hemodialysis for the preceding 2 years for end-stage renal disease due to diabetic nephropathy and received thrice-weekly hemodialysis through a left brachiocephalic fistula. He had undergone a right below-knee amputation for osteomyelitis 10 years earlier. His medications included calcium acetate and aspirin. The patient was allergic to penicillin.

Physical examination revealed a morbidly obese, middle-aged white man. He was afebrile at 37°C and weighed approximately 135 kg. His pulse was 84 beats per minute. The stump of his right below-knee amputation was healed, but his left leg showed chronic venous stasis changes, hyperpigmentation, cyanosis, and onycholysis involving the first and second toes. A patent brachiocephalic fistula was seen in his left arm. His left hand had changes consistent with dry gangrene of the second distal phalanx and black discoloration of the nail bed of the third finger. His right hand had an ulcer on the dorsum of the distal phalanx of the fifth digit, with foul-smelling discharge (Fig. 36.1). The area was

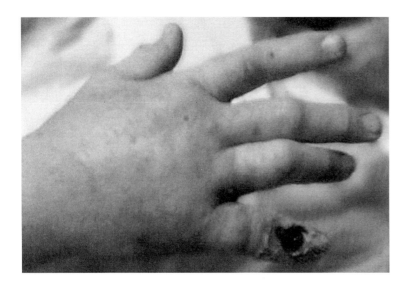

FIGURE 36.1. Ulcer involving the dorsum of the distal phalanx of this patient's right fifth digit.

swollen and markedly tender. Pulses were decreased in both upper extremities. On palpation, crepitus was felt along the dorsum of the hand. The remainder of the physical examination was unremarkable. White blood cell count was 27.33 K/μL with 86% neutrophils, and creatine kinase was elevated at 611 U/mL.

QUESTIONS/DISCUSSION

Which of the following is the appropriate next course of action?

A. **Discharge home with conservative measures and close follow-up**
B. **Discharge home on oral antibiotics with close follow-up**
C. **Admit to the hospital for intravenous antibiotics**
D. **Admit to the hospital for surgical debridement and intravenous antibiotics**
E. **None of the above**

Crepitation is the clinical sign of the presence of gas in the tissues. This is indicative of tissue hypoxia and incomplete oxidation by facultative and anaerobic bacteria. The hypoxia must be reversed to stop the progression of the infection (1). The involved area must be aggressively debrided (2). In certain cases, however, edema may obscure the presence of crepitus (3). Plain films, computed tomography, or magnetic resonance imaging may be useful in this setting. Radiographic imaging is necessary in patients with rapidly progressive disease or with evidence of the systemic inflammatory response syndrome (4). Broad-spectrum antibiotics covering Gram-positive, Gram-negative, and anaerobic bacteria should be started. Appropriate antibiotic regimens include piperacillin/tazobactam, the combination of ampicillin, gentamicin, and clindamycin, or ticarcillin/clavulanic acid. Wound cultures for aerobes, anaerobes, and fungi should be sent. Repeated debridement may be needed if the patient does not improve rapidly. If the vascular supply is inadequate or if the limb is nonfunctional, then amputation is recommended. Debridement and amputation wounds should be packed open and frequently inspected (5).

The above clinical presentation is pathognomonic for clostridial infection.

A. **True**
B. **False**

In the past, the presence of gas in the tissues was often considered indicative of the presence of clostridial gas gangrene. However, gas-forming infections in surgical patients can be due to *Clostridium* sp., *Peptostreptococcus* sp., *Bacteroides* sp., or one of the aerobic coliforms (6).

Which of the following diagnoses is consistent with this patient's presentation?

A. **Clostridial cellulitis**
B. **Nonclostridial crepitant cellulitis**
C. **Clostridial myonecrosis**
D. **Synergistic necrotizing cellulitis**
E. **Necrotizing fasciitis**
F. **All of the above**

Clostridial cellulitis often follows surgery or local trauma, especially in the presence of tissue devitalization or wound contamination. The muscle is spared in this type of infection. There is serous or purulent drainage, and tissue gas may be present. However, pain and systemic toxicity are minimal.

Nonclostridial crepitant cellulitis is an infection similar to clostridial cellulitis but is caused by other microorganisms, including *Peptostreptococcus, Bacteroides* sp., Enterobacteriaceae, and *Staphylococcus aureus.* Bacteria other than *Clostridia* cause crepitant cellulitis more frequently in diabetic patients (1).

Clostridial myonecrosis (gas gangrene) has a fulminant course, is extremely painful, and commonly involves systemic toxicity. Crepitus can occasionally be detected, and gas in the tissues may be seen on plain radiographs. In advanced cases, the skin can appear bronze-brown to darker in color, edematous, and mottled, with multiple bullae with profuse serosanguinous drainage (7). A foul odor, if present, is indicative of co-infection with other anaerobes rather than a pure clostridial infection (1). The diagnosis is confirmed when surgical exploration reveals muscle necrosis. Gas is sometimes released on entering the muscle compartment, and cultures grow *Clostridium* spp. (7).

Necrotizing fasciitis involves the superficial fascia and subcutaneous tissue. The diagnosis is made during surgery, when tissue necrosis and the undermining of surrounding structures are demonstrated. Necrotizing fasciitis can be caused by group A *Streptococcus* (Type 2) or non–group A streptococci with anaerobes or facultative anaerobes (Type 1) (8). Necrotizing fasciitis is typically painful and may be associated with a foul-smelling exudate and tissue gas (in mixed infections with anaerobes). It is rapidly progressive across fascial planes and has severe systemic toxicity. Variable skin changes due to thrombosis, ranging from normal-appearing skin to edema and erythema, to blister formation, and to cyanosis and gangrene, develop. Tissue anesthesia develops secondary to necrosis that involves the skin, superficial fascia, and subcutaneous tissues. The muscle is usually spared (1).

Synergistic necrotizing cellulitis, a form of necrotizing fasciitis, is characterized by severe pain and tenderness at the affected skin site (9). Crepitus can be found in 25% of

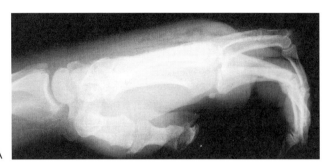
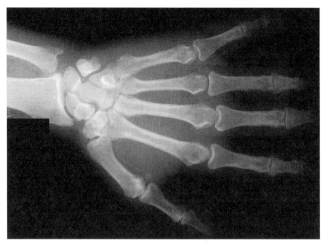

A   B

FIGURE 36.2. Radiographs of the right hand demonstrating the presence of subcutaneous gas.

cases, and exudates are usually foul-smelling, frequently described as "brown dishwater pus." Synergistic necrotizing cellulitis is also rapidly progressive and can be accompanied by marked systemic toxicity. It is characterized by extensive fascial and muscle necrosis, and secondary necrosis of the skin and subcutaneous tissues develops. The presence of muscle involvement differentiates it from necrotizing fasciitis. It typically occurs in obese diabetics with cardiac or renal disease (10).

The patient was admitted to the hospital. A radiograph of the right hand and forearm revealed subcutaneous gas (Fig. 36.2). Intravenous ciprofloxacin and clindamycin were begun. The patient underwent ray amputation of the right fourth and fifth digits that night. The wound was left to heal by secondary intention (Fig. 36.3). Wound cultures revealed a polymicrobial infection with anaerobes, including *Bacteroides fragilis.* Neither *Clostridium perfringens* nor aerobes were isolated. Histopathologic examination showed necrosis involving the soft tissues, including muscle, and extending into the underlying bone.

CONCLUSION

The patient was diagnosed with synergistic necrotizing cellulitis. He had a complicated hospital course. Despite appropriate antibiotic treatment, his hand did not heal, and he lost function of his remaining fingers. A below-elbow amputation of his right arm was subsequently required. Histopathologic examination revealed gangrenous necrosis of the skin and soft tissues. He was discharged soon afterward in stable condition.

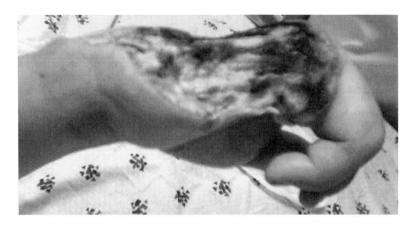

FIGURE 36.3. This patient's right hand after undergoing ray amputation of the fourth and fifth digits. The wound was left to heal by secondary intention.

REFERENCES

1. Feingold DS. The diagnosis and treatment of gangrenous and crepitant cellulitis. *Curr Clin Top Infect Dis* 1981;2:259–277.
2. Pitt DF. Management of gangrene in diabetic extremities. *Can J Surg* 1984;27:386–389.
3. Swartz MN. Myositis. In: Mandell GL, Bennett JE, Dolin R, eds. *Mandell, Douglas, and Bennett's principles and practice of infectious diseases,* 5th ed. New York: Churchill Livingstone, 2000: 1058–1066.
4. Stevens DL. Infections of the skin, muscle, and soft tissues. In: Braunwald E, Fauci AS, Kasper DL, et al., eds. *Harrison's principles of internal medicine,* 15th ed. New York: McGraw-Hill, 2001: 821–825.
5. Gonzalez MH. Necrotizing fasciitis and gangrene of the upper extremity. *Hand Clin* 1998;14:635–645.
6. Nichols RL, Smith JW. Anaerobes from a surgical perspective. *Clin Infect Dis* 1994;18(Suppl 4):S280–S286.
7. Chapnick EK, Abter EI. Necrotizing soft-tissue infections. *Infect Dis Clin North Am* 1996;10:835–855.
8. Giuliano A, Lewis F Jr, Hadley K, et al. Bacteriology of necrotizing fasciitis. *Am J Surg* 1977;134:52–57.
9. Swartz MN. Cellulitis and subcutaneous tissue infections. In: Mandell GL, Bennett JE, Dolin R, eds. *Mandell, Douglas, and Bennett's principles and practice of infectious diseases,* 5th ed. New York: Churchill Livingstone, 2000:1037–1057.
10. Stone HH, Martin JD Jr. Synergistic necrotizing cellulitis. *Ann Surg* 1972;175:702–711.

37

A YOUNG WOMAN WITH RIGHT-UPPER-QUADRANT PAIN AND FEVER

ANGELA M. MARSCHALK
NATALIE G. CORREIA

CASE PRESENTATION

A 24-year-old white woman from Ohio was admitted to our institution with 2 to 3 weeks of right-upper-quadrant pain, fever, rigors, and anorexia. She had been treated with amoxicillin/clavulanic acid 3 weeks earlier for a nonproductive cough and pleuritic chest pain believed to be due to an upper respiratory infection. Her past medical history was significant for chronic sinusitis and recent cervical cryotherapy for carcinoma *in situ*. Her only other medication was oral contraceptives, which she had been taking for 4 years. She was in a monogamous relationship with her boyfriend. She denied tobacco and illicit drug use. She consumed 10 to 15 alcoholic drinks per week. She did not have any risk factors for sexually transmitted diseases, including human immunodeficiency virus (HIV) and viral hepatitis. She had not traveled outside of the United States in the preceding 6 years.

Her physical examination was remarkable for hepatosplenomegaly and tenderness in the right upper quadrant. Laboratory work-up revealed leukocytosis (white blood cell count, 25 K/μL), anemia (hemoglobin, 8 g/dL), slightly elevated alkaline phosphatase, and an elevated erythrocyte sedimentation rate (61 mm/hr). A right-upper-quadrant ultrasound showed three cystic lesions in the right lobe of the liver.

QUESTIONS/DISCUSSION

Which of the following is the most likely diagnosis?

A. Malignancy
B. Cavernous hemangioma
C. Hepatic adenoma
D. Focal nodular hyperplasia
E. Abscess

Tumors within the liver are more often malignant than benign (1). Primary malignant tumors of the liver usually present in the setting of known chronic liver disease. A careful history should be taken to identify risk factors for chronic liver disease, such as viral hepatitis, hereditary hemochromatosis, and alcohol abuse, all of which can predispose patients to developing hepatocellular carcinoma. Signs and symptoms of hepatocellular carcinoma include abdominal pain, a palpable abdominal mass, ascites, jaundice, and constitutional symptoms. Hepatocellular carcinoma carries a poor prognosis, which is related to tumor size, residual liver function, and the presence of extrahepatic disease. Metastatic tumors are the most common malignant neoplasms of the liver in the United States. Metastases are most frequently found in patients with documented primary tumors in the gastrointestinal tract, lung, or breast.

Cavernous hemangiomas consist of ectatic dilated vascular spaces. They are the most common type of benign liver tumor and do not possess malignant potential. Hemangiomas are seen predominantly in women as an incidental finding. Large hemangiomas can occasionally cause symptoms due to bleeding or thrombosis within the lesion or stretching of the Glisson capsule. Since standard computed tomography (CT scan) of the abdomen is relatively insensitive for detecting hemangiomas, dual or triphasic scans are required to image the lesions properly (2,3). Magnetic resonance imaging (MRI) is the most expensive available imaging modality, but also has the greatest sensitivity and specificity, 85% to 95% (4). Nuclear blood pool scanning is less expensive than MRI but is only as sensitive and specific as MRI for lesions larger than 3 cm in diameter (5).

Hepatic adenomas are benign epithelial tumors that usually occur in the noncirrhotic liver. There is a strong association between the development of adenomas and the use of oral contraceptives. Most hepatic adenomas are found in women of reproductive age while on estrogens. Glycogen storage diseases and the use of androgens are also associated with hepatic adenomas (6). Greater than 50% of patients with hepatic adenomas present with symptoms of upper abdominal fullness or pain. Hepatic adenomas have the potential to transform into hepatocellular carcinoma or to rupture and cause life-threatening bleeding. Consequently, the discovery of a hepatic adenoma generally results in surgical resection. Alternatively, if patients with hepatic adenomas are taking oral contraceptives, the medication may be discontinued and the patient observed for regression of the adenoma.

Focal nodular hyperplasia (FNH) is the second most common benign lesion in the liver. Found in up to 3% of the population, FNH is a hepatic pseudotumor that is believed to arise from hamartomatous change within the liver. Patients with FNH tend to have other vascular malformations, which suggests a systemic propensity for vascular anomalies (7,8). Similar to hepatic adenomas, FNH occurs most commonly in women between the ages of 20 and 50. Although patients with FNH are typically asymptomatic, abdominal pain may occur in a minority of patients. An association between FNH and oral contraceptives/estrogens has not been clearly established. Because FNH appears to lack malignant potential, asymptomatic lesions may be observed.

Liver abscesses result from either local spread of contiguous infections within the peritoneal cavity or hematogenous seeding. The predominant symptoms of pyogenic liver abscesses include dull right-upper-quadrant pain, malaise, weakness, anorexia, and weight loss. Patients are often febrile and have rigors. When an abscess is located near the dome of the liver, patients may experience respiratory symptoms such as cough and pleuritic pain that radiates to the right shoulder as a result of diaphragmatic irritation. Tender hepatomegaly and/or splenomegaly are common findings on examination; movement and percussion often accentuate the tenderness. Alkaline phosphatase is the most frequently abnormal serum liver enzyme. Ultrasound shows single or multiple round or oval areas that are hypoechoic in relation to the surrounding liver. Amebic liver abscesses result from ingestion of cysts of *Entamoeba histolytica*. The clinical presentation of an amebic liver abscess is often more acute than that seen with a pyogenic liver abscess. Amebic abscesses are more likely to present with single lesions in the right lobe of the liver. Amebic serologies may aid in establishing the diagnosis.

All of the preceding diagnoses should be considered in the evaluation of this patient. While the patient's gender, age, and risk factors are suggestive of the diagnosis of a hepatic adenoma or FNH, this patient's presentation with fever and leukocytosis make the diagnosis of pyogenic liver abscess most likely. Fever and leukocytosis are uncommonly associated with the other conditions.

Which of the following is the most appropriate next step in the evaluation of these liver lesions?

A. **Computed tomography (CT scan) of the abdomen**
B. **Technetium (Tc) sulfur colloid scanning**
C. **Fine-needle aspiration (FNA)**
D. *Entamoeba histolytica* **serology**
E. **Nuclear blood pool scan**

Ultrasonography, CT, MRI, and 99-technetium scintigraphy are all highly sensitive techniques for the detection of liver abscesses (9). Ultrasonography is the initial imaging modality of choice and may distinguish solid from fluid-filled lesions. Contrast-enhanced CT scan offers improved accuracy over ultrasonography, with sensitivity approaching 100%. CT is the procedure of choice when it is critical to determine the exact location of an abscess and its relationship to adjacent structures. Hepatic abscesses usually appear hypodense on CT scan, and up to 20% of abscesses may display a rim of contrast enhancement. Sonography and CT scan, as opposed to ^{99}Tc-labeled scintigraphy, can often distinguish an abscess from a tumor or other solid focal lesions. Technetium sulfur colloid scanning was the first reliable noninvasive imaging modality, with a sensitivity of 70% to 80%. It is no longer commonly utilized.

Nuclear blood pool scans are used in the diagnosis of hemangiomas, which have a characteristic appearance on ^{99}Tc-labeled red blood cell scan with progressive filling of the lesion from the periphery and prolonged return of the isotope in the tumor. The specificity for peripheral lesions larger than 2 cm is greater than 90%.

Fine-needle aspiration (FNA) biopsy is commonly used to assist in the diagnosis of a variety of liver lesions. Its overall accuracy exceeds 90%. However, since FNA is an invasive test, it does involve some risk. Another potential drawback of FNA is its potential to be nondiagnostic in the evaluation of hepatic adenomas and FNH. Overall, FNA may not be as cost-effective as some noninvasive modalities.

Amebic serology can be of considerable assistance in differentiating amebic from pyogenic abscesses. Serologic tests indicative of prior or current amebiasis are positive in more than 90% of amebic liver abscesses (10).

Given the high suspicion for a pyogenic liver abscess, CT scan and/or MRI of the abdomen to characterize the lesions further is the appropriate next step in the work-up. This patient's CT scan (Fig. 37.1) revealed three dominant large cystic lesions (not simple cysts) within the right lobe of the liver with adjacent daughter cysts. Surrounding each cyst was a thin, rimlike area of inflammation with increased enhancement in relation to the surrounding liver. These findings were consistent with abscesses. Although the patient did not give a history of travel to an endemic area, serology for *Entamoeba histolytica* was performed and was negative.

Which of the following is the most common mechanism by which pyogenic liver abscesses develop?

A. **Appendicitis with rupture**
B. **Suppurative pyelophlebitis**
C. **Biliary seeding**
D. **Hematogenous seeding**

The pathogenesis of pyogenic liver abscesses has changed over the past several decades, particularly in the

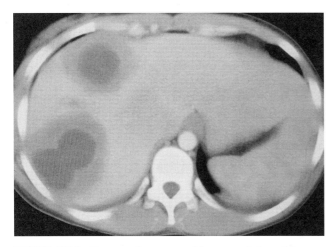

FIGURE 37.1. Computed tomographic scan of the abdomen revealing three dominant large cystic lesions within the right lobe of the liver with adjacent daughter cysts. Surrounding each cyst was a thin, rimlike area of inflammation with increased enhancement in relation to the surrounding liver. These findings were most consistent with abscesses.

last 10 years, with the advent of more aggressive treatment of pancreatic and biliary malignancies and more widespread use of diagnostic and therapeutic endoscopy. Pyogenic liver abscess has recently been noted as an infectious complication following liver transplantation, and patients with chronic granulomatous disease have a high frequency of liver abscesses (11). Of the intraabdominal processes leading to generalized peritonitis and abscess formation, appendicitis with rupture had been the most common mechanism by which liver abscesses formed (12). However, infections of the biliary tract, such as cholangitis and cholecystitis, are now the most common causes of liver abscess (13,14). Therefore, biliary seeding is the most common mechanism by which pyogenic liver abscesses develop.

Suppurative pyelophlebitis, which usually arises from infection in the female genital tract or elsewhere in the peritoneal cavity, is another frequent source for bacterial seeding of the liver (15). Less commonly, hematogenous seeding results in the development of liver abscesses. However, if a solitary organism is isolated from a liver abscess, an evaluation to identify a source for hematogenous seeding should be performed. Any systemic bacteremia can spread to the liver. In about 50% of cases of liver abscess, no obvious source is identified; these cases are classified as cryptogenic abscesses (16–18). Oral flora has been proposed as a potential source in cryptogenic cases.

In this case, extensive work-up, including CT scan of the abdomen and pelvis and pelvic examination with cultures for gonorrhea and chlamydia, did not reveal an intraabdominal or biliary source for the liver abscesses. Multiple sets of blood cultures remained negative.

Which of the following is least commonly associated with pyogenic liver abscesses?

A. Enterococci/Enterobacteriaceae
B. Anaerobes
C. Staphylococci and streptococci
D. *Candida* species
E. Mycobacteria

Mixed facultative and anaerobic species are most frequently isolated from liver abscesses. When the biliary tree is the source of infection, Enterobacteriaceae (mostly *E. coli, Klebsiella, Proteus,* and *Pseudomonas* species) and enterococci are common isolates. Since anaerobes are not common constituents of the gallbladder, they are not generally associated with liver abscesses arising from biliary infections unless previous surgery or stenting of the biliary tree has been performed. In liver abscesses that develop from pelvic and other intraperitoneal sources, the organisms isolated are similar to those found in nonvisceral intraabdominal abscesses. Cultures from these abscesses often grow mixed flora, including aerobic and anaerobic species, especially *Bacteroides fragilis.* With hematogenous spread of infection, a single organism is most commonly isolated, including *Staphylococcus aureus* and streptococci such as *Streptococcus milleri.* Fungal abscesses of the liver, including those with *Candida* species, may occur in immunocompromised hosts, particularly in those with hematologic malignancies. Mycobacteria are not common pathogens of liver abscesses. The correct answer is thus choice E.

Blood cultures are positive in about 50% of patients (18,19). Multiple samples of blood for anaerobic and aerobic cultures must be obtained, as they are often the only cultures obtained prior to antibiotic administration (20,21). The diagnosis ultimately relies upon obtaining purulent material from the abscess cavity. Gram stain of the purulent fluid may provide the only clue to a mixed infection in patients already receiving antibiotics. Prompt delivery of anaerobic specimens under proper conditions is essential.

Which of the following is not an appropriate empiric antibiotic regimen for pyogenic liver abscesses?

A. Ticarcillin/clavulanic acid
B. Piperacillin/tazobactam
C. Gentamicin and metronidazole
D. Levofloxacin
E. Imipenem

Drainage and antibiotic therapy are the cornerstones of treatment for liver abscesses. Although conservative medical therapy without definitive drainage is a reasonable option in selected patients, this option has been employed less frequently since the development of minimally invasive strategies for abscess drainage (22). Most reports have emphasized the necessity of some type of drainage procedure to ensure a favorable outcome (23,24). Catheters are left in place until drainage has slowed to a minimum; this typically occurs 5 to 7 days after placement. Multiple studies have shown that percutaneous catheter drainage with antimicrobial therapy is 69% to 90% successful (25,26). Surgical intervention is usually reserved for patients who have failed percutaneous drainage, those who require surgical management of concurrent intraabdominal disease, and some with multiple large abscesses (27).

The choice of empiric antibiotic therapy in liver abscesses depends upon the probable source of infection. If the biliary tree is the suspected source, the combination of ampicillin and gentamicin, which covers both enterococci and Enterobacteriaceae, is recommended. If an intraabdominal source other than the gallbladder is likely, an antibiotic regimen that covers anaerobes should be started. Metronidazole provides excellent coverage against most anaerobes, although resistance of some anaerobes to metronidazole has developed (28). Other agents with excellent anaerobic coverage include cefoxitin and clindamycin. The combination of gentamicin and metronidazole is recommended as the initial choice for liver abscesses with a probable intraabdominal source. Agents such as imipenem, meropenem, ticarcillin/clavulanic acid, and piperacillin/tazobactam are highly active, but are more expensive. Levofloxacin is not active against anaerobes. Therefore, by itself, it is an inappropriate empiric antibiotic choice for liver abscesses. Choice D is the correct answer.

An extended period of antibiotic therapy is the standard. Treatment should continue until the CT scan shows complete resolution of the abscess cavity, which often requires weeks to months of therapy (28). Complications of pyogenic liver abscesses include empyema, pleuropericardial effusion, portal or splenic vein thrombosis, rupture into the pericardium, thoracic and abdominal fistula formation, and sepsis (12).

CONCLUSION

After obtaining multiple samples for anaerobic and aerobic cultures, this patient was empirically treated with piperacillin/tazobactam. She underwent ultrasound-guided percutaneous drainage with pigtail catheter placement on the second day of her hospitalization. Only one of the three dominant cysts was amenable to this approach, with 30 mL of foul-smelling pus drained from that lesion. Gram stain of the drainage material revealed many polymorphonuclear cells, but no organisms were seen. The procedure was complicated by the development of a small right pneumothorax and a right-sided empyema, which required the placement of a chest tube and later pleuroscopic evacuation. Because of a lack of clinical response, the patient underwent on hospital day 4 open surgical drainage of the two dominant cysts not amenable to percutaneous drainage. The causative

organism(s) and the underlying mechanism of these pyogenic abscesses were never identified. After surgical drainage, the patient experienced rapid clinical improvement. After 10 days in the hospital, the patient was discharged home on home intravenous antibiotic therapy with piperacillin/tazobactam and continuous percutaneous drainage of her abscesses. The chest tube and the percutaneous catheters were removed 14 days after hospital discharge. The patient completed a 4-week course of intravenous antibiotics followed by 2 more weeks of oral amoxicillin/clavulanic acid. Upon completion of antibiotic therapy, a repeat CT scan showed complete resolution of the abscess cavities.

REFERENCES

1. Schwartz JM, Outwater EK. Approach to the patient with a focal liver lesion. *UpToDate Online* 10.2, 2002.
2. Leslie DF, Johnson CD, Johnson CM, et al. Distinction between cavernous hemangiomas of the liver and hepatic metastases on CT: value of contrast enhancement patterns. *Am J Roentgenol* 1995;164:625–629.
3. Yamashita Y, Ogata I, Urata J, et al. Cavernous hemangioma of the liver: pathologic correlation with dynamic CT findings. *Radiology* 1997;203:121–125.
4. Mitchell DG, Saini S, Weinreb J, et al. Hepatic metastases and cavernous hemangiomas: distinction with standard- and triple-dose gadoteridol-enhanced MR imaging. *Radiology* 1994;193:49–57.
5. Farlow DC, Chapman PR, Gruenewald SM, et al. Investigation of focal hepatic lesions: Is tomographic red blood cell imaging useful? *World J Surg* 1990;14:463–467.
6. Ishak KG, Rabin L. Benign tumors of the liver. *Med Clin North Am* 1975;59:995–1013.
7. Haber M, Reuben A, Burrell M, et al. Multiple focal nodular hyperplasia of the liver associated with hemihypertrophy and vascular malformations. *Gastroenterology* 1995;108:1256–1262.
8. Ndimbie OK, Goodman ZD, Chase RL, et al. Hemangiomas with localized nodular proliferation of the liver: a suggestion on the pathogenesis of focal nodular hyperplasia. *Am J Surg Pathol* 1990;14:142–150.
9. Stenson WF, Eckert T. Pyogenic liver abscess. *Arch Intern Med* 1983;143:126–128.
10. Barnes PF, De Cock KM, Reynolds TN, et al. A comparison of amebic and pyogenic abscess of the liver. *Medicine* 1987;66:472–483.
11. Kusne S, Dummer JS, Singh N, et al. Infections after liver transplantation: an analysis of 101 consecutive cases. *Medicine* 1988;67:132–143.
12. Srivastava ED, Mayberry JF. Pyogenic liver abscess: a review of aetiology, diagnosis and intervention. *Dig Dis* 1990;8:287–293.
13. Rubin RH, Swartz MN, Malt R. Hepatic abscess: changes in clinical, bacteriologic and therapeutic aspects. *Am J Med* 1974;57:601–610.
14. Miedema BW, Dineen P. The diagnosis and treatment of pyogenic liver abscesses. *Ann Surg* 1984;200:328–335.
15. Zaleznik DF, Kasper DL. Intraabdominal infections and abscesses. In: Braunwald E, Fauci AS, Kasper DL, et al., eds. *Harrison's principles of internal medicine,* 15th ed. New York: McGraw-Hill, 2001:829–834.
16. Johannsen EC, Sifri CD, Madoff LC. Pyogenic liver abscesses. *Infect Dis Clin North Am* 2000;14:547–563.

17. The liver in infections. In: Sherlock S, Dooley P, eds. *Diseases of the liver and biliary system,* 11th ed. Oxford: Blackwell Science, 2002:495–526.
18. Sabbaj J, Sutter VL, Finegold SM. Anaerobic pyogenic liver abscess. *Ann Intern Med* 1972;77:627–638.
19. Lazarchick J, De Souza e Silva NA, Nichols DR, et al. Pyogenic liver abscess. *Mayo Clin Proc* 1973;48:349–355.
20. McDonald MI, Corey GR, Gallis HA, et al. Single and multiple pyogenic liver abscesses: natural history, diagnosis and treatment, with emphasis on percutaneous drainage. *Medicine* 1984;63: 291–302.
21. Seeto RK, Rockey DC. Pyogenic liver abscess: changes in etiology, management, and outcome. *Medicine* 1996;75:99–113.
22. Huang CJ, Pitt HA, Lipsett PA, et al. Pyogenic hepatic abscess: changing trends over 42 years. *Ann Surg* 1996;223:600–607.
23. Gerzof SG, Johnson WC, Robbins AH, et al. Intrahepatic pyogenic abscesses: treatment by percutaneous drainage. *Am J Surg* 1985;149:487–494.
24. Altemeier WA, Schowengerdt CG, Whiteley DH. Abscesses of the liver: surgical considerations. *Arch Surg* 1970;101:258–266.
25. Bertel CK, van Heerden JA, Sheedy PF 2nd. Treatment of pyogenic hepatic abscesses: surgical vs percutaneous drainage. *Arch Surg* 1986;121:554–558.
26. Chou FF, Sheen-Chen SM, Chen YS, et al. Single and multiple pyogenic liver abscesses: clinical course, etiology and results of treatment. *World J Surg* 1997;21:384–388.
27. Chou FF, Sheen-Chen SM, Chen YS, et al. Prognostic factors for pyogenic abscess of the liver. *J Am Coll Surg* 1994;179:727–732.
28. Zaleznik DF. Pyogenic liver abscess. *UpToDate Online* 10.2, 2002.

38

A 42-YEAR-OLD WOMAN WITH FEVER, COUGH, AND DYSPNEA

MOHAMMED ALGHOUL
J. WALTON TOMFORD

CASE PRESENTATION

A 42-year-old woman presented with a 5-day history of worsening shortness of breath, fever, cough productive of yellowish sputum, and right-sided pleuritic chest pain. She also noted 2 days of moderately severe epigastric pain, which was aggravated by food intake and associated with two episodes of nausea and vomiting. Ten days before this presentation, the patient presented with life-threatening angioedema secondary to ramipril. This episode required mechanical ventilation for 3 days; she was in the intensive care unit (ICU) for 4 days. During her ICU stay, she developed a right-lower-lobe (RLL) infiltrate. Endotracheal tube

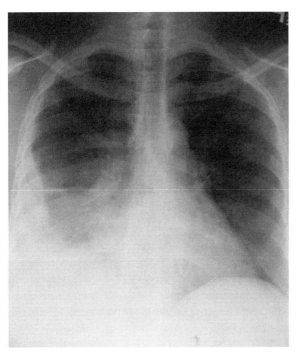

FIGURE 38.1. Chest x-ray obtained on admission showing a right-sided pleural effusion.

cultures grew *Haemophilus influenzae*. She was discharged on amoxicillin/clavulanic acid 875 mg twice a day.

The patient had a history of type 2 diabetes mellitus and hypertension. She had never received an influenza or pneumococcal vaccination. She smoked two packs of cigarettes per day for 20 years. She also had a history of alcohol and cocaine abuse. She denied any history of recent travel outside of the Cleveland area or exposure to tuberculosis.

Physical examination revealed a tachypneic patient with a respiratory rate of 24 breaths per minute without cyanosis. Her temperature was 38.5°C, blood pressure 104/67 mm Hg, pulse 115 beats per minute, and pulse oximetry 91% on room air. Chest examination revealed use of accessory muscles. Auscultation revealed dullness to percussion, bronchial breath sounds, and coarse inspiratory crackles over the right lower lung fields. Her abdomen was distended, with epigastric tenderness and tender hepatomegaly. Bowel sounds were normal, and there was no evidence of ascites. An erythematous skin ulceration was noted over the upper lip. There was no lower-extremity swelling.

Laboratory data on presentation included a white blood count of 17.4 K/µL with 78% neutrophils and 14% lymphocytes. Hemoglobin was 12.1 g/dL, and platelets were 170 K/µL. Metabolic profile revealed sodium of 126 mmol/L, blood urea nitrogen of 25 mg/dL, creatinine of 0.7 mg/dL, glucose of 401 mg/dL, alanine aminotransferase of 95 U/L, aspartate aminotransferase of 20 U/L, and alkaline phosphatase of 228 U/L. A chest x-ray revealed a right-sided pleural effusion (Fig. 38.1).

QUESTIONS/DISCUSSION

All the following are potentially part of the appropriate management of this patient except:

A. Empiric antibiotic treatment with ceftriaxone and azithromycin

B. **Diagnostic thoracentesis**
C. **Right lateral decubitus chest x-ray**
D. **Blood cultures**

This patient's clinical picture is suggestive of an infectious process. The symptoms of shortness of breath, fever, and cough productive of purulent sputum in the presence of leukocytosis and a RLL infiltrate on chest x-ray are consistent with pneumonia. The history of recent hospitalization, ICU admission, and intubation makes the diagnosis of either nosocomial or aspiration pneumonia most likely.

Blood cultures can have diagnostic and prognostic value, and should be obtained in this patient. Bacteremia in nosocomial pneumonia predicts a more complicated course and the need for more aggressive treatment (1). The causative pathogen is isolated from blood cultures in only 8% to 20% of all patients with pneumonia (1).

The possibility of a parapneumonic effusion needs to be considered in this patient with radiographic evidence of a right-sided pleural effusion. If a parapneumonic effusion is present, it is essential to determine promptly whether the effusion is complicated or uncomplicated. A delay in proper drainage of a complicated parapneumonic effusion may substantially increase morbidity. An appropriate first step is to estimate the amount of pleural fluid present with a decubitus chest radiograph. If the pleural fluid is less than 10 mm thick, then the effusion will likely resolve with appropriate systemic antibiotics alone and a diagnostic thoracentesis need not be performed (2). However, if the effusion is thicker than 10 mm, a diagnostic thoracentesis should be performed. A decubitus film can also help assess if fluid is free-flowing or loculated. Ultrasound is an effective adjunct in distinguishing pleural fluid loculations from parenchymal infiltrates. Ultrasound can detect as little as 5 mL of loculated pleural effusion (3).

Patients with a parapneumonic effusion requiring thoracentesis should ideally undergo the thoracentesis before starting antibiotic therapy. Intravenous antibiotics achieve the same concentration in the pleural fluid as they do in blood. Therefore, antibiotics can affect Gram stain results and delay the recovery of pathogens from pleural fluid cultures. However, waiting for a decubitus film and preparing for a thoracentesis should not delay the institution of appropriate antibiotics in cases where the patient is critically ill or appears toxic. The presence of a parapneumonic effusion should not alter the selection of empiric antibiotics. If Gram stain identifies a pathogen, then antibiotic therapy should be tailored to treat that organism.

Ceftriaxone and azithromycin are appropriate treatment for community-acquired pneumonia, rather than aspiration and/or nosocomial pneumonia, as was suspected in this patient. Initial antimicrobial selection should include coverage for anaerobes and viridans streptococci, both of which can cause aspiration pneumonia. Neither ceftriaxone nor azithromycin provides optimal anaerobic coverage. Since this patient most likely developed pneumonia during her recent hospitalization, she should also be treated empirically for nosocomial pneumonia pending culture results. Initial antibiotic therapy should cover Gram-negative bacilli, including *Pseudomonas aeruginosa,* anaerobes, streptococci, and methicillin-susceptible *Staphylococcus aureus.* A broad-spectrum penicillin in combination with a β-lactamase inhibitor is appropriate empiric therapy (4). Clindamycin can be utilized in cases of suspected aspiration pneumonia; however, most of the antibiotics used to treat nosocomial pneumonia also have good anaerobic coverage (5). Atypical organisms such as *Legionella* can cause nosocomial pneumonia in the setting of ICU outbreaks. Ceftriaxone and azithromycin do not provide adequate coverage against *P. aeruginosa.*

Case Continued: The patient was started on intravenous fluids and was treated empirically with piperacillin/tazobactam for suspected aspiration and/or nosocomial pneumonia. The patient remained dyspneic, tachycardic, and febrile. A thoracentesis yielded 10 mL of thick white fluid. Pleural fluid analysis revealed a pH of 7.18, white blood count of 20,948/μL, protein of 5.2 g/dL, glucose of 39 mg/dL, and lactate dehydrogenase (LDH) of 8,943 U/L.

Which of the following is the most appropriate next step in the management of this patient?

A. **Chest tube insertion**
B. **Change piperacillin/tazobactam to imipenem**
C. **Repeat thoracentesis**
D. **None of the above**

In addition to starting appropriate antibiotics, clinicians need to decide if patients with parapneumonic effusions need tube thoracostomy drainage. The decision to drain a parapneumonic effusion depends on multiple factors, including pleural fluid analysis, pleural fluid culture, the radiographic size of the effusion, and the general condition of the patient. Important components of pleural fluid analysis include pH, glucose, LDH, protein, and Gram stain with culture. Pleural fluid pH is a more sensitive indicator of complicated effusions than glucose because a decrease in pleural fluid pH typically precedes a decrease in glucose (2). The pleural fluid should also be visually inspected for the presence of pus.

Deciding which effusions require tube drainage is somewhat controversial. Some authors advocate draining pleural effusions with a pH less than 7.3 in high-risk patients and less than 7.2 in low-risk patients (3). If the pleural fluid pH is above 7.2, the pleural fluid glucose is above 40 mg/dL, and the pleural fluid LDH is below 1,000 U/L, most authors would typically consider definitive drainage to be unnecessary (3). If the pleural fluid pH is below 7.0 and/or the pleural fluid glucose is below 40 mg/dL, then tube thoracostomy should be performed immediately because such effusions are almost always complicated (3).

Other absolute indications for definitive pleural fluid drainage include a positive Gram stain and/or culture, frank pus, and the presence of an air–fluid level in the pleural space, which is suggestive of a bronchopleural fistula or ruptured esophagus. Radiographic evidence of loculated pleural fluid is not an absolute indication for chest tube drainage unless a thoracentesis demonstrates that the pleural fluid within the loculation is complicated (3). However, the presence of multiple loculations increases the likelihood that tube drainage will be required (3).

In this case, insertion of a chest tube is appropriate, since pus was drained during the thoracentesis. A repeat thoracentesis would not provide any new information. Switching antibiotics is not likely to change this patient's clinical course without definitive drainage of the effusion being performed first.

Case Continued: A chest tube was inserted, with drainage of 100 mL of purulent fluid. Despite this the patient's condition further deteriorated. Vancomycin was added to piperacillin/tazobactam. Following the thoracentesis, a chest x-ray revealed the presence of a nodular mass (Fig. 38.2). The following day, a repeat chest x-ray and computed tomography (CT) of the chest revealed a right-sided parenchymal mass with an air–fluid level, both of which were thought to be consistent with a lung abscess (Figs. 38.3 and 38.4).

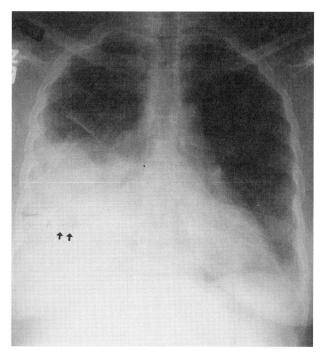

FIGURE 38.3. Chest x-ray obtained 1 day after thoracentesis revealing an air–fluid level (*arrows*) within the right-sided nodular mass.

Which of the following microorganisms is least likely to be the cause of this patient's pulmonary process?

A. *Staphylococcus aureus*
B. *Pseudomonas aeruginosa*
C. *Klebsiella pneumoniae*
D. *Haemophilus influenzae*
E. *Prevotella intermedia*
F. *Streptococcus milleri*

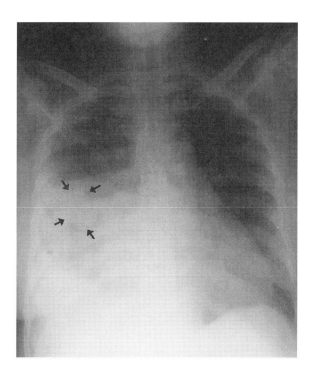

FIGURE 38.2. Chest x-ray obtained following a thoracentesis showing a nodular mass in the right lower lobe as outlined by the *arrows*.

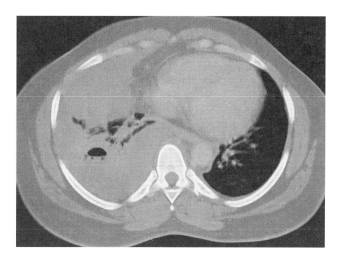

FIGURE 38.4. Computed tomography of the chest revealing a right-sided mass with an air–fluid level, most consistent with a lung abscess.

Staphylococcus aureus is a common aerobic cause of lung abscesses and necrotizing pneumonia, which can develop within 3 to 5 days (5). In particular, patients with diabetes mellitus, coma, head trauma, renal failure, or recent influenza have an increased risk of pulmonary infection with *S. aureus.* Other patients at risk for *S. aureus* lung infections include patients on mechanical ventilation for more than 5 days, those on prior antibiotics or corticosteroids, and those with a prolonged ICU stay (4). The prevalence of *S. aureus* pneumonia remains controversial. Some authors believe that unless a chest radiograph reveals cavitation within 72 hours or tissue culture grows *S. aureus,* the diagnosis of *S. aureus* pneumonia should not be a significant consideration (5). In this patient with risk factors for *S. aureus* lung infection, the development of a lung abscess due to *S. aureus* needs to be considered.

Pseudomonas aeruginosa and *Klebsiella pneumoniae* can both cause necrotizing pneumonia and lung abscesses. These microorganisms are among the most virulent. *P. aeruginosa* can cause rapid cavitation within 72 hours, whereas *K. pneumoniae* typically causes cavitation within 5 to 7 days (5). Coverage for *Pseudomonas* should always be considered in pneumonias acquired in the ICU, especially in high-risk patients with or without radiographic evidence of cavitation.

Haemophilus influenzae rarely causes lung abscesses and is the least likely causative pathogen in this patient. A positive endotracheal aspirate (ETA) culture, as in this patient, may lead clinicians to consider *H. influenzae* the most likely causative organism. However, the ETA culture is the least accurate test in the evaluation of pneumonia, since it mainly reflects upper and lower airway colonization, which is very common in intubated patients (5). The presence of cavitation on this patient's CT scan should guide therapy toward organisms known to cause cavitation and abscess formation, rather than *H. influenzae.*

Prevotella intermedia is an anaerobic bacterium that normally inhabits gingival crevices. Anaerobes have considerable propensity for causing necrotizing pneumonia and lung abscesses. They usually cause lung abscesses following aspiration in high-risk patients, such as alcoholics, patients under general anesthesia, and intubated patients. These patients also frequently have periodontal disease, especially gingivitis. Infection with anaerobes such as *P. intermedia* is usually indolent and is often polymicrobial. The most common anaerobic organisms producing lung abscesses are *Peptostreptococcus, Prevotella, Fusobacterium,* and *Bacteroides* species (usually not *B. fragilis*).

Members of the *Streptococcus milleri* group are viridans streptococci that are classified as Lancefield group C or G. These organisms are widely distributed commensals found in the oropharynx, auditory canal, gastrointestinal tract, genitourinary tract, and umbilicus. Organisms in the *Streptococcus milleri* group include *Streptococcus angiosus, Streptococcus constellatus,* and *Streptococcus intermedius.* These organisms are virulent and can cause serious suppurative infections, with a predisposition for abscess formation in the brain, liver, lungs, teeth, subphrenic region, pelvis, and subcutaneous tissues (6). *Streptococcus milleri* is a possible cause of this patient's pulmonary infection.

Case Conclusion

Despite the insertion of a chest tube and 4 days of broad-spectrum antibiotics, the patient's condition continued to deteriorate. She remained febrile and became progressively dyspneic. She was taken to the operating room on the fifth day. A right thoracotomy revealed a RLL abscess. The patient underwent pleurectomy, decortication, drainage of lung abscess, and RLL wedge resection. Pleural fluid culture grew *Streptococcus milleri.* Her clinical condition improved after surgery. She was discharged from the hospital on intravenous oxacillin 3 g every 8 hours to complete a total of 14 days of antibiotic treatment.

CONCLUSION

Streptococcus milleri is increasingly recognized as a pathogen that can lead to the development of lung abscess and empyema (6). Pulmonary infections with *Streptococcus milleri* usually follow aspiration of oral and gastric contents. Direct implantation during surgery, extension of a liver abscess, and hematogenous spread are other routes by which lung infection develops. *Streptococcus milleri* is underdiagnosed because these organisms are frequently considered part of the normal flora in sputum cultures.

Pulmonary infections with *Streptococcus milleri* are five times more common in men than in women (6,7). Predisposing factors for *Streptococcus milleri* empyema and lung abscess include periodontal disease, sinusitis, prior pneumonia, recent antibiotic therapy, thoracic surgery, malignancy, alcohol abuse, intubation, neurologic disease predisposing to aspiration, and diabetes mellitus (6).

Streptococcus milleri lung infections are often mixed infections with anaerobes. *In vitro* studies have shown that anaerobes enhance the growth of *Streptococcus milleri* and suppress the host's bactericidal activity. Therefore, antibiotic coverage against anaerobes needs to be considered when treating *Streptococcus milleri* lung infections (8).

One of the key principles in the management of *Streptococcus milleri* infections is the initiation of early and adequate drainage, since this microorganism is associated with an increased risk of empyema and lung abscess. Serial chest radiographs may reveal lung abscess formation, especially in the presence of a history of aspiration and a lack of clinical improvement. Penicillin is the antibiotic of choice (7,9).

Clinicians need to recognize patients at risk for aspiration and/or nosocomial pneumonia and initiate appropriate antimicrobial therapy. When patients do not improve on appropriate therapy, complications of lung infections, such as empyema and lung abscess, need to be considered. These processes may need combined medical and surgical treatment. In cases of lung abscess formation, clinicians need to consider both anaerobic and aerobic pathogens. In this case, the patient developed a severe necrotizing pneumonia due to *Streptococcus milleri,* which required surgical treatment.

REFERENCES

1. Hospital-acquired pneumonia in adults: diagnosis, assessment of severity, initial antimicrobial therapy, and preventive strategies. A consensus statement, American Thoracic Society, November 1995. *Am J Respir Crit Care Med* 1996;153:1711–1725.
2. Light RW. Parapneumonic effusions and empyema. In: Light RW, *Pleural diseases,* 4th ed. Philadelphia: Lippincott Williams & Wilkins, 2001:151–181.
3. Heffner JE, Klein J. Parapneumonic effusions and empyema. *Semin Respir Crit Care Med* 2001;22:591–604.
4. Cross JT Jr, Campbell GD Jr. Therapy of nosocomial pneumonia. *Med Clin North Am* 2001;85:1583–1594.
5. Cunha BA. Nosocomial pneumonia: diagnostic and therapeutic considerations. *Med Clin North Am* 2001;85:79–114.
6. Wong CA, Donald F, Macfarlane JT. *Streptococcus milleri* pulmonary disease: a review and clinical description of 25 patients. *Thorax* 1995;50:1093–1096.
7. Marinella MA, Harrington GD, Standiford TJ. Empyema necessitans due to *Streptococcus milleri. Clin Infect Dis* 1996;23:203–204.
8. Shinzato T, Saito A. The *Streptococcus milleri* group as a cause of pulmonary infections. *Clin Infect Dis* 1995;2(Suppl 3): S238–S243.
9. Hocken DB, Dussek JE. *Streptococcus milleri* as a cause of pleural empyema. *Thorax* 1985;40:626–628.

39

A 54-YEAR-OLD WOMAN WITH HEADACHE, FEVER, AND CONFUSION

MARTIN E. LASCANO
M. FERNANDA BONILLA
PETER J. MAZZONE

CASE PRESENTATION

A 54-year-old woman was brought to the emergency department (ED) by her daughter after she was found to be confused at home 1 hour earlier. She was well until 2 days before presentation when she developed malaise, sore throat, dry cough, and nasal congestion. She also noted chills and low-grade fevers, although no temperature was recorded. For these symptoms, the patient took acetaminophen 500 mg every 6 hours without significant improvement. One night before presentation, she developed a diffuse headache, which worsened throughout the night. Her daughter noted that she was confused, disoriented, and acting inappropriately, which prompted her to bring the patient to the ED.

Her past medical history was significant for hypertension, type 2 diabetes mellitus, and hypercholesterolemia, all of which were well controlled on medications. The patient did not have any history of tobacco, alcohol, or illicit drug use. None of her medications were new, and the patient did not have any sick contacts during the preceding weeks.

Physical examination revealed an ill-appearing patient, who was lethargic but arousable, confused, and would not answer questions or follow commands. Vital signs included a temperature of 38.3°C, heart rate of 90 beats per minute, respiratory rate of 20 breaths per minute, and blood pressure of 156/84 mm Hg. Pupils were equal, round, and reactive to light; funduscopic examination did not reveal any papilledema. The oropharynx was dry and slightly erythematous without plaques. Her neck was rigid without jugular venous distension. The lungs were clear to auscultation. Cardiac examination did not reveal any murmurs or gallops. The abdomen was soft and nontender, without organomegaly. There was no peripheral edema. The skin was warm and dry without any rashes or lesions. There was no lymphadenopathy. On neurologic examination, she moved all extremities symmetrically, and her deep tendon reflexes were 2+ throughout. Brudzinski, Kernig, and Babinski signs were absent.

Two sets of blood cultures were drawn, and initial laboratory testing revealed a urinalysis with glucose greater than 1,000 mg/dL, negative leukocyte esterase and nitrites, and no cells or casts on microscopic examination. Electrolytes included sodium of 140 mmol/L, potassium of 4.2 mmol/L, chloride of 98 mmol/L, bicarbonate of 23 mmol/L, blood urea nitrogen of 9 mg/dL, creatinine of 0.6 mg/dL, and glucose of 307 mg/dL. Liver function tests were within normal limits. Complete blood count revealed a white blood cell count of 14.63 K/μL (neutrophils, 86%; lymphocytes, 10%; monocytes, 4%), hemoglobin of 15.2 g/dL, hematocrit of 42.3%, and platelets of 272 K/μL. A urine toxicology screen was negative. A chest x-ray did not show any signs of acute disease. A noncontrast computed tomography (CT) scan of the brain showed no evidence of acute intracranial hemorrhage, intracranial mass, hydrocephalus, or other underlying structural abnormalities.

QUESTIONS/DISCUSSION

What is the most appropriate next step in this patient's diagnostic evaluation?

A. Contrast-enhanced CT scan of the brain
B. Magnetic resonance imaging (MRI) of the brain
C. Lumbar puncture (LP) with cerebrospinal fluid (CSF) analysis
D. Electroencephalogram
E. No further diagnostic testing

This patient's clinical presentation is highly suggestive of intracranial pathology, and infectious etiologies should be at the top of the differential diagnosis. Infections of the central nervous system (CNS) can occur at a variety of anatomic sites, including the meninges, subdural and epidural spaces, and the brain parenchyma. A variety of pathogens—including viruses, bacteria, mycobacteria, fungi, protozoa, and helminths—can cause CNS infections. Depending upon the specific pathogen, the pace of the illness can vary from an acute, fulminant presentation, as occurs in bacterial meningitis, to a more indolent illness, such as fungal meningitis, which presents and evolves over weeks to months. Common signs and symptoms of CNS infections include fever, headache, and delirium.

Bacterial meningitis is a medical emergency and if suspected, immediate steps should be taken to establish a specific diagnosis. The most important factor associated with delayed diagnosis and therapy is the decision to perform a CT scan of the brain before a lumbar puncture (LP) (1). The controversy surrounding this issue stems from concern of precipitating herniation with LP in patients with a subclinical increase in intracranial pressure. Patients in whom CT should be considered before LP are those at greatest risk of having an unrecognized structural abnormality, notably individuals more than 60 years of age, immunocompromised hosts, and those with focal neurologic findings, severely depressed sensorium, or a history of central nervous system disease or seizure within 1 week of presentation (2). The absence of these clinical characteristics has a negative predictive value of 97% in excluding elevated intracranial pressure. Therefore, the decision to perform neuroimaging before LP should be guided by clinical findings; neuroimaging should not be done routinely in cases of suspected meningitis. If the patient is to undergo CT scan, blood cultures should be drawn and empiric antibiotics should be started before imaging. LP should be performed immediately thereafter if no intracranial mass lesion is demonstrated.

In this patient's case, the appropriate initial evaluation had been initiated, including complete blood count and blood cultures. Although there was no definitive indication for neuroimaging, the CT scan of the brain performed was normal. In this setting, further imaging studies are unnecessary. The next step should be to perform a lumbar puncture with analysis of the CSF.

Case Continued: Within 45 minutes of the [p]... at the ED, a lumbar puncture was perform[ed]... pressure was 270 mm H_2O, and the CSF... appearance. Analysis revealed red blood cells of 48/µL, white blood cells of 1,050/µL (neutrophils, 93%; monocytes, 7%), protein of 81 mg/dL, and glucose of 121 mg/dL.

Which of the following is this patient's most likely diagnosis?

A. Viral meningitis
B. Fungal meningitis
C. Bacterial meningitis
D. Mycobacterial meningitis
E. Noninfectious meningeal irritation

Bacterial meningitis is an acute suppurative infection within the subarachnoid space. Definitive diagnosis is based on morphologic and chemical CSF analysis as well as evidence of bacterial growth from blood and/or CSF samples. Table 39.1 summarizes the different categories into which CNS infections may be divided based on CSF findings. Although the patient in this case clearly fits into the category of bacterial meningitis, a definitive diagnosis requires the isolation of a causative organism. It is important to recognize that although her CSF glucose was normal, her CSF/serum glucose ratio was less than 40%, which is typical of bacterial meningitis.

Case Continued: Gram stain of the CSF revealed many Gram-positive cocci in pairs, many polymorphonuclear leukocytes (PMNs), and few mononuclear cells. Fluid was also sent for bacterial culture.

Based on the Gram stain, which of the following antibiotic regimens is most appropriate in this patient?

A. Penicillin G
B. Ceftriaxone
C. Ceftriaxone and vancomycin
D. Ampicillin and cefotaxime
E. Cefepime

TABLE 39.1. CEREBROSPINAL FLUID ANALYSIS IN MENINGITIS

Measurement	Normal	Bacterial Meningitis	Aseptic Meningitis (Viral)	Granulomatous Meningitis (Mycobacterial, Fungal)	Spirochetal Meningitis
Opening pressure (mm H_2O)	70–180	Markedly elevated	Slightly elevated	Moderately elevated	Normal to slightly elevated
White blood cells (cells/µL)	0–5 lymphocytes	200–20,000 neutrophils	25–2,000, mostly lymphocytes	100–1,000, mostly lymphocytes	100–1,000, mostly lymphocytes
Glucose (mg/dL)	45–85	<45	Normal or low	<45	Normal
Protein (mg/dL)	15–45	>50	>50	>50	>50

Gram stain remains a very useful and rapid technique for initial assessment of CSF in patients with suspected bacterial meningitis. It is positive in 70% to 90% of cases (3). Positive CSF cultures, which are found in 80% to 90% of cases, establish the definitive diagnosis. Therapy should not be delayed while awaiting culture results. Instead, empiric antibiotics should be started as soon as possible, directed toward the most common microorganisms for each age group (Table 39.2). In most adult patients, the recommended initial empiric regimen is either ceftriaxone or cefotaxime, plus ampicillin in patients more than 50 years of age (1,4). In areas with a high prevalence of penicillin-resistant pneumococci, the addition of vancomycin is warranted (5,6). Epidemiologic surveillance data from 1995 revealed that bacterial meningitis has become predominantly a disease of the adult population, with a median age of 25 years. This trend is due to a dramatic decrease in the incidence of meningitis due to *Haemophilus influenzae* type B (Hib) since the inception of conjugated vaccination in children. Currently, the most commonly implicated bacteria are *Streptococcus pneumoniae* (47% of cases), *Neisseria meningitidis* (25%), and *Streptococcus agalactiae* (12%) (7). In patients with depressed cellular immunity, *Listeria monocytogenes* should be considered as a possible pathogen. At-risk groups include patients older than 50 years of age and those with impaired cell-mediated immunity due to chronic illness, pregnancy, organ transplantation, alcoholism, malignancy, or immunosuppressive therapy.

Based on the Gram stain findings, the patient in this case most likely has bacterial meningitis due to *S. pneumoniae.* Since the presence of penicillin-resistant pneumococcus is a concern in many communities, the most appropriate antibiotic regimen, pending culture results, is ceftriaxone or cefotaxime plus vancomycin. If the Gram stain had been unrevealing, including ampicillin as part of the initial regimen to target *Listeria monocytogenes* would have been appropriate.

Case Continued: The patient was admitted to a telemetry unit after starting intravenous ceftriaxone and vancomycin. Six hours after admission, she had a witnessed generalized tonic–clonic seizure lasting 2 minutes. She was transferred to the medical intensive care unit (ICU) for closer observation after receiving a loading dose of intravenous fosphenytoin.

Should this patient receive adjuvant therapy with dexamethasone?

A. Yes
B. No

The understanding of the pathophysiology of pneumococcal meningitis has significantly improved over the past few years. Animal studies suggest that activation of host inflammatory pathways rather than direct damage from the invading organism is responsible for much of the cerebral damage (8). Ischemia and the formation of oxygen free radicals are important contributors to cortical necrosis. Neuronal apoptosis in the hippocampus may be responsible for the development of cognitive impairment and learning disabilities in patients following an episode of bacterial meningitis (9). Antiinflammatory treatment with corticosteroids has emerged as a possible tool to reduce these deleterious responses to infection. Some evidence in children with Hib meningitis suggests a reduction in the incidence of neurologic sequelae, particularly deafness, with early adjuvant treatment with dexamethasone (8). Conversely, antiinflammatory treatment with steroids has been shown to aggravate hippocampal damage in pneumococcal meningitis, which may lead to learning deficits (10). There is also a suggestion that the permeability of the blood–brain barrier and penetration of the CSF by certain antibiotics, such as vancomycin, is reduced by dexamethasone (4,6). Compelling data showing benefits of adjuvant corticosteroids in adult patients was recently published (8a). Therefore, adjuvant steroids are routinely recommended in this population. Novel approaches to adjuvant therapy targeting the inhibition of matrix metalloproteinases and tumor necrosis factor-α converting enzyme are being studied and may help prevent long-term sequelae (9).

Seizures are seen in 20% to 30% of patients with bacterial meningitis (3). They tend to occur more frequently in

TABLE 39.2. RECOMMENDED EMPIRIC ANTIBIOTICS FOR PATIENTS WITH SUSPECTED BACTERIAL MENINGITIS

Patient Group	Likeley Pathogens	Emperic Antibiotics
18 to 50 years	S. pneumoniae, N. meningitidis	Cefotaxime or ceftriaxone
>50 years	S. pneumoniae, N. meningitidis, L. monocytogenes, Gram-negative bacilli	Ampicillin + cefotaxime or ceftriaxone
Impaired cellular immunity	L. monocytogenes, Gram-negative bacilli, S. pneumoniae	Ampicillin + ceftazidime
Postneurosurgical intervention/shunt devices	S. aureus, S. pneumoniae, Gram-negative bacilli	Vancomycin + ceftazidime
High-prevalence area for penicillin-resistant S. pneumoniae	Multiresistant pneumococci	Cefotaxime or ceftriaxone + vancomycin

cases of *S. pneumoniae* or Hib, with *N. meningitidis* a less common etiologic agent. The presence of seizures within 24 hours of admission has been shown to be a predictor of mortality in bacterial meningitis (72% mortality in those with seizures versus 18% in those without seizures) (11). Sequelae, including decreased perceptual performance ability and decreased spelling skills, occur more frequently in children with Hib meningitis accompanied by seizures (12).

Chemoprophylaxis in bacterial meningitis is aimed at the prevention of secondary cases in close contacts once an index case is detected. There are clear indications for the use of chemoprophylaxis for household members and close contacts in meningococcal meningitis, In Hib meningitis, chemoprophylaxis is appropriate for members of households in which there is at least one child under age 2 (13). However, for pneumococcal meningitis, the risk of infection for household contacts is low, approaching that of the general population. Therefore, prophylaxis is not routinely recommended in this setting for immunocompetent individuals.

Case Conclusion

While in the ICU, the patient had no further seizure activity. An electroencephalogram was within normal limits, showing no epileptiform discharges. Blood and CSF cultures grew *S. pneumoniae,* susceptible to ceftriaxone. Vancomycin was discontinued, and the patient continued to receive intravenous ceftriaxone 2 g every 12 hours. By the second day of hospitalization, the patient's delirium was completely resolved. She remained afebrile, and her neurologic examination did not reveal any focal deficits. She was transferred back to a regular nursing unit and was discharged home on hospital day 4. She completed a 10-day course of intravenous ceftriaxone, with follow-up arranged with her primary care physician within 1 week.

CONCLUSION

Bacterial meningitis is the most severe and frequent type of CNS infection. It carries a mortality of up to 20%, and up to 50% of survivors may develop significant neurologic sequelae. This is particularly true in pneumococcal meningitis, which accounts for most cases across all age groups. If bacterial meningitis is suspected, the diagnosis should be pursued aggressively. Initial evaluation should include a detailed history and physical examination, complete blood count, blood cultures, and lumbar puncture with CSF analysis and Gram stain.

The cornerstone of treatment is prompt initiation of empiric antibiotics directed against the most common

microorganisms for each age group. Therapy should be tailored with the aid of the Gram stain; definitive treatment and the duration of therapy are determined by the culture results. Chemoprophylaxis for close contacts, if appropriate, should be instituted once the etiologic agent is confirmed.

Recent improvements in antibiotic therapy have failed to produce significant changes in the outcome of the disease. Therefore, it is essential to focus efforts on a better understanding of the pathogenesis of brain damage that results from meningitis in order to prevent neurologic sequelae. At present, the most promising approach to prevention is likely through universal vaccination for *Streptococcus pneumoniae,* as one would hope for similar reductions in disease prevalence as has occurred with Hib vaccination.

REFERENCES

1. Quagliarello VJ, Scheld WM. Treatment of bacterial meningitis. *N Engl J Med* 1997;336:708–716.
2. Hasbun R, Abrahams J, Jekel J, et al. Computed tomography of the head before lumbar puncture in adults with suspected meningitis. *N Engl J Med* 2001;345:1727–1733.
3. Kaplan SL. Clinical presentations, diagnosis, and prognostic factors of bacterial meningitis. *Infect Dis Clin North Am* 1999;13: 579–594.
4. Sáez-Llorens X, McCracken GH Jr. Antimicrobial and anti-inflammatory treatment of bacterial meningitis. *Infect Dis Clin North Am* 1999;13:619–636.
5. Freidland IR, Istre GR. Management of penicillin-resistant pneumococcal infections. *Pediatr Infect Dis J* 1992;11:433–435.
6. Paris MM, Ramilo O, McCracken GH Jr. Management of meningitis caused by penicillin-resistant *Streptococcus pneumoniae. Antimicrob Agents Chemother* 1995;39:2171–2175.
7. Schuchat A, Robinson K, Wenger JD, et al. Bacterial meningitis in the United States in 1995. *N Engl J Med* 1997;337:970–976.
8. Should we use dexamethasone in meningitis? The Meningitis Working Party of the British Paediatric Immunology and Infectious Diseases Group. *Arch Dis Child* 1992;67:1398–1401.
8a. de Gans J, van de Beek D. Dexamethasone in adults with bacterial meningitis. *N Engl J Med* 2002;347:1549–1556.
9. Meli DN, Christen S, Leib SL, et al. Current concepts in the pathogenesis of meningitis caused by *Streptococcus pneumoniae. Curr Opin Infect Dis* 2002;15:253–257.
10. Zysk G, Bruck W, Gerber J, et al. Anti-inflammatory treatment influences neuronal apoptotic cell death in the dentate gyrus in experimental pneumococcal meningitis. *J Neuropathol Exp Neurol* 1996;55:722–728.
11. Durand ML, Calderwood SB, Weber DJ, et al. Acute bacterial meningitis in adults: a review of 493 episodes. *N Engl J Med* 1993;328:21–28.
12. Taylor HG, Schatschneider C, Watters GV, et al. Acute-phase neurologic complications of *Haemophilus influenzae* type b meningitis: association with developmental problems at school age. *J Child Neurol* 1998;13:113–119.
13. Cuevas LE, Hart CA. Chemoprophylaxis of bacterial meningitis. *J Antimicrob Chemother* 1993;31(Suppl B):79–91.

40

A 61-YEAR-OLD WOMAN WITH PERSISTENT PNEUMONIA

BENJAMIN J. FREDA
JEFFREY T. CHAPMAN
ROBIN K. AVERY

CASE PRESENTATION

A 61-year-old woman was transferred from Puerto Rico for further evaluation of persistent fever, anorexia, malaise, and right-lower-lobe pneumonia. Her past medical history was significant for gastroesophageal reflux disease, status post Nissen fundoplication, and hypothyroidism. She was well until 6 weeks before admission, when she developed fevers, fatigue, and cough productive of yellowish-brown sputum. She received a 10-day course of clarithromycin, with clinical improvement within several days. Three weeks later, the same symptoms recurred. She was treated with moxifloxacin for 10 days without improvement. A chest radiograph at that time showed bibasilar interstitial and alveolar infiltrates. She had no known sick contacts and no history of tobacco use, immunodeficiency, or pulmonary disease. She denied any human immunodeficiency virus (HIV) risk factors. She was in a monogamous relationship and denied any history of blood transfusions.

She was hospitalized in Puerto Rico and was treated with several antibiotics, including cefepime, levofloxacin, and—immediately before transfer—fluconazole and imipenem. Pulmonary function tests showed a reduced diffusion capacity, and computed tomography (CT) of the chest showed bibasilar reticulonodular infiltrates. Purified protein derivative (PPD) without anergy panel was reported as negative. Blood, sputum, and urine cultures were negative. Her fevers continued.

The patient presented to our institution with a temperature of 37.7°C, pulse of 94 beats per minute, respiratory rate of 18 per minute, blood pressure of 99/50 mm Hg, and pulse oximetry of 95% on room air. Physical examination revealed a thin woman in no respiratory distress, with decreased breath sounds at both bases; there was no evidence of consolidation or pleural effusion on examination. Cardiac and abdominal examinations were normal. There was no lymphadenopathy or clubbing.

The patient was continued on imipenem and fluconazole, and vancomycin was added upon transfer to our institution.

QUESTIONS/DISCUSSION

Which of the following is the most appropriate reason to add vancomycin to this patient's antibiotic regimen?

A. Coverage for methicillin-resistant *Staphylococcus aureus* (MRSA) pneumonia
B. Increased coverage for hospital-acquired Gram-negative pneumonia
C. Coverage for penicillin-resistant *Streptococcus pneumoniae* pneumonia
D. Bactericidal action against enterococcal pneumonia

Vancomycin does not cover Gram-negative organisms. Enterococci such as *E. faecalis* and *E. faecium* do not usually cause primary pulmonary infections. They more commonly lead to urinary tract infections, nosocomial bacteremia, and abdominal infections. Furthermore, vancomycin is bacteriostatic, not bactericidal, against enterococci.

MRSA pneumonia is unlikely in this patient, as it often progresses in a fulminant manner with systemic toxicity, dyspnea, and chest pain. Occasionally, the presentation can be less acute. Her prior hospitalizations and broad-spectrum antibiotic therapy may have increased her risk for colonization with MRSA (1), but she had not required endotracheal intubation and did not have an indwelling vascular catheter. In this patient, the possibility of MRSA pneumonia could be considered a secondary reason for adding vancomycin but would not be the primary consideration.

Vancomycin was added to this patient's regimen to cover for possible penicillin (PCN)-resistant *Streptococcus pneumoniae*. A recent national survey by the Centers for Disease Control showed that about 24% of pneumococcal isolates were resistant to PCN (2). Resistance to penicillin appears

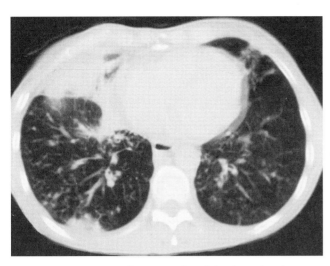

FIGURE 40.1. Computed tomography of the chest showing scattered, bilateral, small parenchymal nodules with bibasilar and right middle lobe infiltrates and small bilateral pleural effusions. The right middle lobe infiltrate had areas of necrosis and microabscess formation.

to develop as a result of altered PCN-binding proteins. High levels of resistance may cross over to include all β-lactam antibiotics, including the newer third- and fourth-generation agents. The clinical significance of this resistance is not entirely known. The addition of β-lactamase inhibitors offers no advantage. Newer-generation fluoroquinolones, such as moxifloxacin and levofloxacin, have excellent activity against PCN-resistant pneumococci. However, the concern for other bacteria developing quinolone resistance should limit the routine use of these antimicrobials. All pneumococci are susceptible to vancomycin, making vancomycin the drug of choice in the setting of potential drug-resistant pneumococcal pneumonia. The routine use of vancomycin in the treatment of pneumonia should be discouraged to limit the development of vancomycin-resistant enterococci.

Vancomycin was added on admission; however, the patient continued to have fevers up to 39.2°C. Her oxygenation remained stable on room air. Sputum Gram stain showed many neutrophils without any organisms. A repeat CT scan of the chest showed scattered, bilateral, small parenchymal nodules with bibasilar and right middle lobe infiltrates and small bilateral pleural effusions (Fig. 40.1). The right middle lobe infiltrate had areas of necrosis and microabscess formation. There was no lymphadenopathy or bronchiectasis.

The differential diagnosis for this chronic, progressive, necrotizing, nodular pneumonic process includes all of the following except:

A. Microscopic polyangiitis
B. *Nocardia* pneumonia

C. Bronchiolitis obliterans with organizing pneumonia (BOOP)
D. Allergic bronchopulmonary aspergillosis (ABPA)
E. *Mycobacterium avium* complex (MAC) pneumonia

ABPA is a disorder that occurs in less than 1% of patients with preexisting asthma. *Aspergillus fumigatus* colonizes the airways, producing an IgE-mediated immediate hypersensitivity-type reaction in the lung parenchyma and airways (3). Patients typically present with worsening asthma, low-grade fever, and eosinophilia in the sputum and/or blood. Radiographic changes include migratory pulmonary infiltrates, more often in the upper lobes, and central bronchiectasis. Treatment of ABPA includes corticosteroids, and adjunctive therapy with itraconazole is considered for patients requiring frequent or prolonged courses of steroids (4). This patient's clinical and radiographic presentation is not consistent with ABPA.

Microscopic polyangiitis is a systemic, necrotizing small vessel vasculitis that predominantly affects glomerular and pulmonary capillaries (5). Systemic symptoms such as fever and malaise are usually present. More than 90% of patients eventually develop renal disease. Other common clinical manifestations include arthralgias and purpura. Radiographic findings include diffuse interstitial changes and/or infiltrates that can cavitate. Some patients develop pulmonary hemorrhage and hemoptysis.

BOOP is a syndrome of unknown etiology in which foci of organizing pneumonia develop. Pathologic specimens reveal proliferation of granulation tissue within small airways and chronic inflammation in surrounding tissue (6). BOOP may be a reaction to various lung injuries, including infection, medications, connective-tissue disease, radiation therapy, and transplantation. Many cases are idiopathic; one study showed that 14 of 25 biopsy-proven cases were not associated with another clinical condition (7). Patients often present with a protracted flulike illness with fever, cough, and mild dyspnea; a restrictive pattern is seen on pulmonary function testing. Chest radiographs show bilateral patchy infiltrates that may mimic multifocal pneumonia. High-resolution CT scans may show patchy airspace consolidation and small nodular opacities. Cavities and effusions are rarely present. Treatment is with an extended course of corticosteroids.

Nocardia pneumonia typically presents in a subacute fashion over days to weeks. Cough with purulent sputum is the primary symptom, and patients typically have systemic complaints, such as fever, anorexia, and malaise. Patients with deficiencies in cell-mediated immunity (HIV, hematologic malignancies, and high-dose corticosteroids) are at particular risk for nocardial infections. However, a significant number of infections occur in patients without predisposing conditions. Radiographic studies show infiltrates with variable appearance. Multiple small nodules, which can cavitate, and pleural effusions often accompany infiltrates; empyema can also occur (8). Clinical specimens may show branching Gram-positive bacilli that may stain weakly acid-fast. Treatment is usually with an extended course of a sulfonamide. In sulfa-intolerant patients, imipenem, amikacin, or ceftriaxone may be used. Infection is usually fatal if untreated.

Mycobacterium avium complex (MAC) pulmonary infections have been described in a variety of patients. Cavitary disease typically occurs in patients with underlying lung disease, immunodeficiency, or malignancy. Severely immunocompromised patients may also develop disseminated disease. MAC pulmonary infections typically occur in older men with chronic obstructive pulmonary disease (COPD) presenting with worsening cough, upper lobe infiltrates, and cavities. MAC pneumonia can also occur in patients without immunodeficiency or underlying lung disease. Most of these cases have been described in nonsmoking women more than 50 years of age, particularly in association with pectus excavatum and scoliosis. Symptoms of cough, fever, weight loss, and profound fatigue usually progress over several days to weeks. In one study, cough had been present for a mean of 26 weeks before MAC pneumonia was diagnosed (9). Radiographic appearance is variable, with most cases showing interstitial changes, small nodules, or right-middle-lobe infiltrates on CT scan. MAC pneumonia has also been reported in patients with cystic fibrosis and in other patients with bronchiectasis.

Case Continued: The patient's laboratory studies included negative blood, urine, and sputum cultures and a negative enzyme-linked immunosorbent assay (ELISA) for HIV. Complete blood cell count revealed white blood cells of 12.4 K/µL with a normal differential, hemoglobin of 10.2 g/dL, and platelets of 553 K/µL. Electrolytes, blood urea nitrogen, creatinine, and transaminases were all normal; albumin was 2.4 g/dL. Sedimentation rate and C-reactive protein were elevated at 106 mm/hr and 16.7 mg/dL, respectively. Antinuclear antibody, fungal serologies, antineutrophil cytoplasmic antibody, *Legionella* urinary antigen, and *Chlamydia* and *Mycoplasma* IgM were all negative. A repeat PPD was nonreactive with reactive controls.

The patient continued to have fevers, and a bronchoscopy without a biopsy was performed with washings from bronchoalveolar lavage (BAL) sent for cytology, staining, and culture. The bronchoscopy revealed copious purulent secretions but no endobronchial abnormalities. The Gram stain from the BAL showed many neutrophils and no organisms. The *Legionella* direct fluorescence antigen (DFA) and stains for fungi, acid-fast bacilli (AFB), *Pneumocystis carinii,* and *Nocardia* were negative. Cultures for herpes simplex, cytomegalovirus (CMV), and respiratory viruses showed no growth.

The patient reported feeling better over the next 2 days. Her appetite improved, and she was afebrile both the day of and the day after her bronchoscopy. The following day, her fevers returned, and she complained of night sweats. Chest radiograph showed small bilateral effusions. Imipenem and

fluconazole were stopped, and piperacillin/tazobactam and doxycycline were added to vancomycin. Her fevers and fatigue continued, and 1 day later, azithromycin was started in place of doxycycline due to gastrointestinal intolerance. Vancomycin was also discontinued at this time; trimethoprim/sulfamethoxazole was added to cover for possible *Nocardia* while further culture results were pending.

At this point, the most appropriate diagnostic or therapeutic maneuver would be:

A. Antiglomerular basement membrane antibodies (anti-GBM)
B. Thoracentesis to rule out complicated parapneumonic effusion
C. Initiation of 1 mg/kg/day of prednisone for suspected chronic eosinophilic pneumonia (CEP)
D. Bone marrow biopsy to rule out disseminated mycobacterial infection

Circulating anti-GBM antibodies are detected in more than 90% of patients with Goodpasture syndrome (10). Most patients have glomerulonephritis and hemoptysis. Progressive renal failure often occurs within weeks. There are diffuse alveolar infiltrates on chest radiograph. Therapy consists of corticosteroids, plasmapheresis, and cytotoxic agents. Measuring anti-GBM antibodies is not indicated in this patient, since she did not have clinical, radiographic, or laboratory evidence of either pulmonary hemorrhage or glomerulonephritis.

Chronic eosinophilic pneumonia (CEP) is characterized by bilateral peripheral alveolar infiltrates, with a predilection for the upper lobes (a photonegative of pulmonary edema). Pathology reveals aggregates of histiocytes, eosinophils, and giant cells. Patients present with cough, fever, weight loss, and dyspnea (11). Symptoms evolve over weeks to months. Peripheral eosinophilia is present in most patients. Clinical response to corticosteroids is usually immediate. This patient did not have clinical, laboratory, or radiographic evidence of CEP. Moreover, initiation of high-dose steroid therapy before ruling out an infectious process would not be recommended in this patient.

Bone marrow biopsy would likely offer little assistance at this time. Other diagnostic studies aimed at lung parenchyma and pleural fluid likely would provide more information. Bone marrow biopsy with appropriate stains and cultures is helpful in the setting of suspected disseminated mycobacterial disease, which is unlikely in this apparently immunocompetent patient without evidence of bone marrow suppression.

Thoracentesis is appropriate at this point to rule out an empyema or complicated parapneumonic effusion in this patient with pleural effusion and nonresolving pneumonia. Experts recommend thoracentesis for all parapneumonic effusions larger than 10 mm on lateral decubitus radiograph (12). Although CT scan was not suspicious for loculations or empyema, pleural fluid analysis could provide a diagnosis if this patient's syndrome represents an infectious or malignant process. Moreover, if the Gram stain was positive or other features suggestive of complicated parapneumonic effusion were present (pH less than 7.0 and/or glucose less than 40 mg/dL), tube thoracostomy would be necessary, in addition to antibiotics.

A thoracentesis and repeat bronchoscopy with transbronchial biopsy of the right middle and lower lobes were performed. Bronchoscopy did not reveal any endobronchial lesions. Gram stain of the BAL was negative. Thoracentesis revealed 25 mL of straw-colored fluid with lactate dehydrogenase 164 U/L (serum = 229 U/L), total protein of 1.7 g/dL, glucose of 68 mg/dL, and pH of 7.38. These findings were consistent with an exudate and an uncomplicated parapneumonic effusion. Pleural fluid Gram stain and cytology were negative. Transbronchial biopsy of the right middle and lower lobe showed acute and organizing bronchopneumonia without granuloma, viral inclusions, or neoplasm. Acid-fast and methenamine silver stains were negative. The patient's fever and night sweats resolved, and her appetite started to improve.

At this point, all AFB stains were negative from both BALs and a sputum sample. Two weeks after the initial bronchoscopy, the BAL grew an acid-fast bacillus, which was later identified as *Mycobacterium avium intracellulare* (MAI) by gene probe. MAI was also later cultured from one sputum sample and the BAL from her second bronchoscopy. Cultures for fungi, viruses, *Legionella*, CMV, and *Nocardia* were negative at 29 days.

Pending susceptibility testing, which of the following treatment regimens is appropriate?

A. Rifampin 600 mg daily, azithromycin 250 mg daily and ethambutol (25 mg/kg for first 2 months, then 15 mg/kg) for 1 year

B. Isoniazid 300 mg daily with supplemental pyridoxine for 9 months

C. Rifampin 600 mg daily and clarithromycin 500 mg twice a day for 9 months

D. No treatment is necessary, as this MAI likely represents airway colonization

E. Rifampin 600 mg daily, clarithromycin 500 mg twice a day, and ethambutol (25 mg/kg for first 2 months, then 15 mg/kg) for 6 months

Therapy for MAC pulmonary infections is potentially toxic and not well tolerated by many patients. Therefore, the decision to treat is based on the combination of clinical, bacteriologic, and radiographic evidence of disease (Table 40.1). Patients with MAC pulmonary infections and no underlying immunodeficiency or lung disease can develop progressive disease resulting in death. Current American Thoracic Society guidelines recommend therapy for all patients meeting diagnostic criteria of MAC pulmonary disease (13).

Treatment of MAC pulmonary disease in non-HIV patients should include a macrolide, a rifamycin, and ethambutol for at least 1 year after cultures have cleared. Accept-

TABLE 40.1. AMERICAN THORACIC SOCI GUIDELINES FOR THE DIAGNOSIS OF NONTUBERCULOUS MYCOBACTERIAL PU... DISEASE IN PATIENTS SERONEGATIVE FOR HIV[a]

I. Clinical criteria
   A. Compatible signs/symptoms (cough, fatigue, fever, weight loss, hemoptysis, dyspnea) with documented deterioration in clinical status if an underlying condition is present *and*
   B. Reasonable exclusion of other diseases (tuberculosis, cancer, histoplasmosis)
II. Radiographic criteria
   A. Any of the following chest x-ray abnormalities[b]
      1. Infiltrates with or without nodules (persistent ≥2 months or progressive)
      2. Cavitation
      3. Nodules alone (multiple)
   B. Either of these high-resolution CT abnormalities
      1. Multiple small nodules
      2. Multifocal bronchiectasis with or without small lung nodules
III. Bacteriologic criteria
   A. At least three available sputum/bronchial wash samples within 1 year:
      1. Three positive cultures with negative acid-fast bacilli (AFB) smears *or*
      2. Two positive cultures and one positive AFB smear *or*
   B. Single available bronchial wash and inability to obtain sputum samples
      1. Positive culture with 2+, 3+, or 4+ growth *or*
      2. Positive culture with a 2+, 3+, or 4+ AFB smear *or*
   C. Tissue biopsy
      1. Any growth on bronchopulmonary tissue biopsy
      2. Granuloma and/or AFB on lung biopsy with one or more positive cultures on sputum/bronchial wash

[a]For a diagnosis of pulmonary disease, all three criteria are necessary.
[b]If baseline films are more than 1 year old, then there should be evidence of progression.
From Diagnosis and treatment of disease caused by nontuberculous mycobacteria. Medical Section of the American Lung Association. *Am J Respir Crit Care Med* 1997;156:S1–S25.

able regimens include azithromycin (250 mg daily) or clarithromycin (500 mg twice daily), rifabutin (300 mg daily) or rifampin (600 mg daily), and ethambutol (25 mg/kg daily for first 2 months, then 15 mg/kg daily thereafter) (13). Streptomycin may be added in patients with cavitary disease. Isoniazid is not recommended due to the development of resistance by most nontuberculous mycobacteria. Fluoroquinolones can also be used in the management of MAC pulmonary disease. Most patients have symptomatic improvement after 3 to 6 months of therapy (14).

Sputum cultures should be monitored monthly for clearance, and macrolide resistance should be suspected if there is new or persistent growth. Patients should be monitored closely for drug toxicities, including hepatitis, leukopenia, nausea and diarrhea (rifampin), vestibular and renal dysfunction (streptomycin), and impaired visual acuity (ethambutol).

The diagnosis of MAC pulmonary disease in non-HIV patients requires clinical, bacteriologic, and radiographic evidence of disease. This patient had a chronic course, necrotizing and nodular infiltrates, and multiple cultures positive for MAI. Furthermore, an extensive evaluation did not reveal other etiologies for her infiltrates, such as fungi, *Nocardia,* or noninfectious causes. She also had a clinical response to 10 days of treatment with clarithromycin early in the course of her disease. Because of significant gastrointestinal intolerance, this patient's regimen was modified to include ethambutol, ciprofloxacin, and clarithromycin. Subsequent sensitivities revealed that the MAI isolate was sensitive to ciprofloxacin, ethambutol, and clarithromycin but was resistant to imipenem.

CONCLUSION

The evaluation of nonresolving pneumonia requires that the clinician recognize the time required for symptomatic and radiographic improvement of pneumonia caused by common and uncommon pathogens. In addition, patients may respond differently, depending on age, comorbidities, and severity of the pneumonia. The clinician should consider inadequate antimicrobial selection/drug levels or treatment duration, noninfectious mimics of pneumonia, and complications of pneumonia (e.g., empyema) in the differential diagnosis of nonresolving pneumonia.

REFERENCES

1. Vlahakis SR, Steckelberg JM. Methicillin-resistant *Staphylococcus aureus:* a practical primer. *Emerg Med* 2001;33:45–59.
2. Whitney CG, Farley MM, Hadler J, et al. Increasing prevalence of multidrug-resistant *Streptococcus pneumoniae* in the United States. *N Engl J Med* 2000;343:1917–1924.
3. Wardlaw A, Geddes DM. Allergic bronchopulmonary aspergillosis: a review. *J R Soc Med* 1992;85:747–751.
4. Stevens DA, Schwartz HJ, Lee JY, et al. A randomized trial of itraconazole in allergic bronchopulmonary aspergillosis. *N Engl J Med* 2000;342:756–762.
5. Bacon PA, Adu D. Microscopic polyangiitis: clinical aspects. In: Hoffman GS, Weyand CM, eds. *Inflammatory diseases of blood vessels.* New York: Marcel Dekker, 2002:355–363.
6. Reynolds HY, Noble PW, Matthay RA. Diffuse interstitial and alveolar inflammatory diseases. In: George RB, Light RW, Matthay MA, et al, eds. *Chest medicine: essentials of pulmonary and critical care medicine,* 4th ed. Philadelphia: Lippincott Williams & Wilkins, 2000:262–313.
7. Alasaly K, Muller N, Ostrow DN, et al. Cryptogenic organizing pneumonia: a report of 25 cases and a review of the literature. *Medicine* 1995;74:201–211.
8. Haglund L, Deepe GS Jr. *Nocardia.* In: *Current therapy in infectious disease,* 2nd ed. St Louis: CV Mosby, 2001:525–527.
9. Prince DS, Peterson DD, Steiner RM, et al. Infection with *Mycobacterium avium* complex in patients without predisposing conditions. *N Engl J Med* 1989;321:863–868.
10. Appel GB, Radhakrishnan J, D'Agati V. Secondary glomerular disease. In: Brenner BM, ed. *Brenner and Rector's The Kidney,* 6th ed. Philadelphia: WB Saunders, 2000:1350–1448.
11. Jederlinic PJ, Sicilian L, Gaensler EA. Chronic eosinophilic pneumonia: a report of 19 cases and a review of the literature. *Medicine* 1988;67:154–162.
12. Light RW, Girard WM, Jenkinson SG, et al. Parapneumonic effusions. *Am J Med* 1980;69:507–512.
13. Diagnosis and treatment of disease caused by nontuberculous mycobacteria. Medical Section of the American Lung Association. *Am J Respir Crit Care Med* 1997;156:S1–S25.
14. Havlir DV, Ellner JJ. *Mycobacterium avium* complex. In: Mandell GL, Bennett JE, Dolin R, eds. *Mandell, Douglas, and Bennett's principles and practice of infectious diseases,* 5th ed. Philadelphia: Churchill Livingstone, 2000:2616–2630.

41

A 73-YEAR-OLD MAN WITH FEVER AND CHILLS

MOHAMMED S. GHANAMAH
RITESH GUPTA

CASE PRESENTATION

A 73-year-old man presented with a 5-day history of fever up to 38.1°C and shaking chills. The patient also noted a chronic nonproductive cough and a 4-week history of low back pain. He denied chest pain, shortness of breath, orthopnea, paroxysmal nocturnal dyspnea, palpitations, nausea, vomiting, diarrhea, dysuria, or urgency. He did note the presence of mild bilateral lower extremity edema.

The patient's past medical history was significant for coronary artery disease and hypertension. Four months before this presentation, the patient underwent coronary artery bypass grafting (CABG) and a bioprosthetic aortic valve replacement for aortic insufficiency. His postoperative course included a lumbar laminectomy performed 1 month before this presentation. The patient's medications on admission included aspirin, atorvastatin, metoprolol, and ramipril. He had not received any antibiotics before his presentation. He was an ex-smoker and denied any history of intravenous drug abuse.

Upon admission, physical examination revealed a temperature of 38.5°C, pulse of 84 beats per minute, and blood pressure of 100/55 mm Hg. The patient was not in distress and was oriented to person, place, and time. His oropharynx was dry, without evidence of dental caries. Examination of the neck did not reveal jugular venous distension. Auscultation of the lungs revealed bibasilar crackles. Cardiac examination revealed a regular rhythm without any gallops. There was a grade III/VI systolic ejection murmur heard best at the right sternal border. The murmur did not radiate but was thought to be louder when compared with his most recent physical examination. Examination of the back revealed swelling and erythema at the laminectomy site; there was no drainage from the wound. No skin rashes were present.

Laboratory studies on admission included a white blood cell count of 33,000/μL with a differential of 89% neu-

trophils, 5% lymphocytes, and 5% monocytes. Hemoglobin was 8.4 g/dL, and platelets were 155 K/μL. His electrolytes and renal function were normal. Troponin T was 0.2 ng/mL, total creatine kinase was 223 U/L, and the CK–MB was 12 ng/mL. Urinalysis showed 1+ blood, trace leukocyte esterase, and five to ten white blood cells per high-power field. An electrocardiogram (ECG) showed first-degree atrioventricular (AV) block with nonspecific ST–T changes (Fig. 41.1). ST elevation was not present. The first-degree AV block was not seen on prior ECGs. A chest x-ray revealed borderline cardiomegaly, without evidence of any pulmonary infiltrates.

QUESTIONS/DISCUSSION

At this point, which of the following needs to be considered in the differential diagnosis?

A. **Infection involving the laminectomy site**
B. **Pneumonia**
C. **Infective endocarditis**
D. **Acute myocardial infarction**
E. **Urinary tract infection**
F. **All of the above**

An infection involving the laminectomy site needs to be considered, given this patient's recent surgery and the presence of swelling and erythema at the incision site. A local infection with subsequent bacteremia, vertebral osteomyelitis, or epidural abscess could explain the patient's presentation.

Older patients with pneumonia may not present with many of the features commonly associated with pneumonia. These patients may only present with fever and/or chills. The absence of a productive cough, shortness of breath, or pleuritic chest pain does not preclude the diagnosis of pneumonia. In this patient, the absence of signs of consolidation—including dullness to percussion, decreased

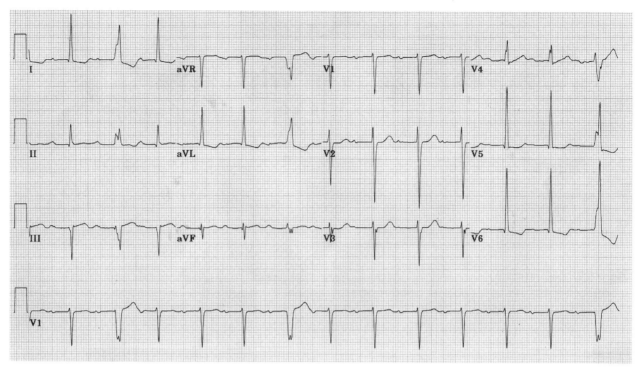

FIGURE 41.1. Electrocardiogram (ECG) showing first-degree atrioventricular (AV) block with nonspecific ST–T changes. The first-degree AV block was not seen on prior ECGs.

air entry, and bronchial breath sounds—makes pneumonia less likely but does not rule it out.

Infective endocarditis needs to be considered in any patient with fever and a paucity of localizing symptoms. Patients can present acutely, with progressive symptoms over a period of days. Patients who present in a subacute fashion often have nonspecific symptoms, such as fatigue, low-grade fevers, night sweats, and weight loss. This patient did not have evidence of peripheral stigmata of endocarditis, such as Janeway lesions, Osler nodes, and splinter hemorrhages. Moreover, the patient did not have renal failure or change in mental status, both of which are suggestive of embolic disease. However, given this patient's recent history of aortic valve replacement, prosthetic valve endocarditis needs to be considered, especially with the presence of a louder systolic murmur.

Acute myocardial infarction can cause fever, and it must be considered in this patient, since he had elevated cardiac enzymes. However, the patient was not having any chest pain, and several ECGs did not show evidence of ischemia. Serial cardiac enzymes remained positive in this case.

Urinary tract infections can present in older patients with only changes in mental status. While the presence of localizing symptoms such as urgency, frequency, and dysuria increases the likelihood of a urinary tract infection, the absence of those symptoms does not exclude the diagnosis. Fever and chills may be suggestive of pyelonephritis

or bacteremia. Since this patient had evidence of pyuria on urinalysis, a urinary tract infection needs to be considered in the differential diagnosis.

All of the preceding need to be included in the differential diagnosis at this point.

Which of the following tests is/are appropriate to help establish the diagnosis?

A. **Blood cultures**
B. **Transthoracic echocardiogram**
C. **Computed tomography (CT) of lumbosacral spine**
D. **Urine culture**
E. **All of the above**

Blood cultures are essential in the diagnosis and management of patients with fever and chills. In the absence of prior antibiotic therapy, blood cultures will be positive in 90% or more of patients with infective endocarditis (1,2). About 25% to 30% of patients with pneumonia have bacteremia at the time of presentation (3). Identification of an organism on blood cultures can help guide antimicrobial therapy. Positive blood cultures associated with a urinary tract infection can indicate a more serious infection, such as pyelonephritis, a renal cortical abscess, or a perinephric abscess. Similarly, bacteremia with laminectomy site infection suggests the need to rule out vertebral osteomyelitis or an epidural abscess.

Patients with fever in whom infective endocarditis is a possibility should undergo a transthoracic echocardiogram to look for valvular abnormalities, vegetations, and possible complications, such as a valve ring abscess.

CT of the lumbosacral spine is useful to evaluate the laminectomy site for the presence of a fluid collection. It can also assess for vertebral osteomyelitis or an epidural abscess. Magnetic resonance imaging (MRI) is typically the imaging study of choice to assess the spine and vertebrae, but was contraindicated in this patient because of the metal implant used for his laminectomy.

Urine culture is often helpful to confirm the presence of a urinary tract infection, especially in cases such as this one in which the diagnosis is unclear. A urine culture can also identify the microorganism and provide information about the sensitivity of an organism to various antibiotics.

After blood cultures were drawn, the patient was started on empiric treatment for infective endocarditis with vancomycin, gentamicin, and rifampin. Urine culture was negative. Transthoracic echocardiography revealed normal left ventricular function and thickened redundant mitral leaflets but did not show any vegetations. Computed tomography of the lumbosacral spine revealed a superficial fluid collection at the laminectomy site but no evidence of osteomyelitis. CT-guided drainage of the fluid collection was performed; the culture of the fluid was negative for bacteria.

After 2 days, blood cultures returned positive for coagulase-negative staphylococci, which were subsequently identified as *Staphylococcus epidermidis.* The organism was sensitive to oxacillin. Consequently, vancomycin was switched to oxacillin, while both gentamicin and rifampin were continued. However, the patient remained febrile.

At this point, which of the following tests is appropriate?

A. **CT of the abdomen and pelvis**
B. **Transesophageal echocardiogram**
C. **CT of the chest**
D. **None of the above**

At this point, pneumonia, urinary tract infection, myocardial infarction, and laminectomy site infection were not considered likely causes of the patient's fever. Although the transthoracic echocardiogram did not reveal evidence of vegetations, this clinical setting mandates further investigation into the diagnosis of infective endocarditis. In addition, the presence of a new first-degree heart block on ECG raises suspicion for the presence of invasive infection into the perivalvular tissues. Therefore, a transesophageal echocardiogram is the appropriate next test. Given the decreased likelihood of a complicated urinary tract infection or a pulmonic process, neither a CT of the abdomen and pelvis nor a CT of the chest is the appropriate next test in this patient.

In cases highly suspicious for endocarditis, a negative transthoracic echocardiogram (TTE) should be followed by a transesophageal echocardiogram (TEE). Transesophageal echocardiography can detect vegetations as small as 1 to 1.5 mm, whereas TTE typically fails to detect lesions smaller than 2 to 3 mm (4). The sensitivity of detecting vegetations by TTE is 65%, whereas TEE has greater than 90% sensitivity (5). A negative TEE provides strong evidence against the presence of endocarditis. TEE is also superior to TTE in the detection of abscesses, fistulas, and paraprosthetic leaks (5).

This patient underwent a TEE, which showed multiple aortic valve vegetations with severe paravalvular aortic insufficiency into an abscess cavity (Fig. 41.2). In retrospect, the elevated cardiac enzymes on presentation were thought to be a result of the invasive annular and myocardial infection, which is quite common in prosthetic valve endocarditis.

Prosthetic valve endocarditis (PVE) carries mortality rates as high as 20% to 40% (6). PVE is usually divided into early and late infection. Early infection is typically described as occurring in the initial 2 months after surgery, when organisms reach the valve prosthesis by direct contamination intraoperatively or via hematogenous spread. Perivalvular infection, abscess formation, and dehiscence of sutures with resulting paravalvular regurgitant flow frequently complicate early PVE. The most frequently encountered pathogens in the first 2 months following surgery are coagulase-negative staphylococci, followed by *Staphylococcus aureus,* Gram-negative bacilli, enterococci, and fungi (6).

The pathogenesis of late-onset PVE resembles that of native valve endocarditis. The pathogens responsible for late PVE tend to be bacteremic isolates that adhere to microthrombi that form on the prosthetic valve. The perivalvular tissues are less likely to be affected in late pros-

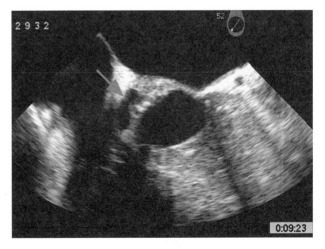

FIGURE 41.2. Transesophageal echocardiogram demonstrating multiple aortic valve vegetations (*arrow*).

thetic valve endocarditis because endothelialization of the sewing ring and the sutures limits access to these tissues. When PVE presents 3 to 12 months after surgery, the causative organisms are usually coagulase-negative staphylococci, *S. aureus,* and to a lesser extent, enterococci and streptococci. The same organisms causing native valve endocarditis usually cause cases of endocarditis occurring more than 12 months after surgery (6).

Which of the following treatment strategies is appropriate for this patient?

A. **Oxacillin alone for 6 weeks**
B. **Conservative therapy with oxacillin, gentamicin, and rifampin for 6 weeks**
C. **Cardiac surgery consultation for urgent debridement and redoing of aortic valve replacement (AVR), along with oxacillin, gentamicin, and rifampin**
D. **None of the above**

Uncomplicated infective endocarditis can be treated with 4 to 6 weeks of appropriate intravenous antibiotic therapy. Bactericidal agents must be used to sterilize the vegetations. Home intravenous antibiotic therapy is used more frequently and has been shown to be cost-effective and successful in carefully selected patients (7). Gentamicin and rifampin are indicated for patients with persistent bacteremia or severely ill patients. These agents work synergistically to enhance the bactericidal action of other antimicrobial agents. Medical therapy alone is not appropriate for this patient since he has evidence of extravalvular extension of infection.

Extravalvular extension of infective endocarditis is an indication for surgical intervention. Infection extending beyond the valve leaflets occurs in 10% to 20% of patients with native valve endocarditis and in more than 50% of those with prosthetic valve endocarditis (6). Persistent fever, the appearance of conduction defects on ECG, and pericarditis all suggest perivalvular extension, which can be confirmed by echocardiography. Ideally, surgery should be performed after several days of appropriate antimicrobial therapy. However, when extension of infection occurs, the prospect of cure with medical therapy alone diminishes substantially (5).

In addition to extravalvular extension of endocarditis, surgical intervention is warranted in several other instances. Surgery should be considered in cases of persistent bacteremia despite appropriate intravenous antibiotic therapy. In recurrent endocarditis with the same organism, it is often necessary to remove the vegetation, debride the valve, and repair or replace the valve. Because fungal endocarditis is characterized by large vegetations and severe valvular damage, surgery is the only effective therapy in most cases. Recurrent systemic emboli (mycotic aneurysms in the brain, emboli to large arteries, and renal emboli) and pul-

monary emboli with right-sided endocarditis are also indications for surgery. New onset of heart failure due to severe valvular regurgitation, myocarditis, or valve destruction is also considered an indication for valve replacement. The presence of large vegetations is a controversial indication for surgery.

In this patient, cardiothoracic surgery was consulted. Although subsequent blood cultures did not reveal any growth, the patient remained febrile on appropriate antibiotic coverage. He received continuous cardiac monitoring because of the risk for progression of the conduction defect. A redo AVR with debridement of the aortic annulus and annular abscess was performed. The patient had an uncomplicated postoperative course.

CONCLUSION

Clinicians need to maintain a healthy suspicion for the diagnosis of infective endocarditis. In this patient, the history of recent valve replacement surgery, the presence of a new first-degree heart block, and fever made infective endocarditis a distinct possibility. A negative transthoracic echocardiogram is insufficient to exclude endocarditis when there is a high clinical suspicion for the disease. As in this case, transesophageal echocardiography is often required to make a definitive diagnosis. When patients with infective endocarditis do not improve on appropriate intravenous antibiotic therapy, complications, such as a valvular abscess, need to be considered and surgical consultation should be sought.

REFERENCES

1. Karchmer AW. Infective endocarditis. In: Braunwald E, Fauci AS, Kasper DL, et al., eds. *Harrison's principles of internal medicine,* 15th ed. New York: McGraw-Hill, 2001:809–816.
2. Bayer AS. Infective endocarditis. *Clin Infect Dis* 1993; 17: 313–320.
3. Woodhead MA, Macfarlane JT, McCracken JS, et al. Prospective study of the aetiology and outcome of pneumonia in the community. *Lancet* 1987;1:671–674.
4. Schiller NB. Clinical decision making in patients with endocarditis: the role of echocardiography. In: Otto CM, ed. *The practice of clinical echocardiography.* Philadelphia: WB Saunders, 1997: 389–403.
5. Yu VL, Fang GD, Keys TF, et al. Prosthetic valve endocarditis: superiority of surgical valve replacement versus medical therapy only. *Ann Thorac Surg* 1994;58:1073–1077.
6. Karchmer AW. Infections of prosthetic valves and intravascular devices. In: Mandell GL, Bennett JE, Dolin R, eds. *Mandell, Douglas, and Bennett's principles and practice of infectious diseases,* 5th ed. Philadelphia: Churchill Livingstone, 2000:903–917.
7. Kubak BM, Nimmagadda AP, Holt CD. Advances in medical and antibiotic management of infective endocarditis. In: Childs JS, ed. *Cardiology clinics: diagnosis and management of infective endocarditis,* vol. 14. Philadelphia: WB Saunders, 1996:405–436.

42

A 49-YEAR-OLD MAN WITH COUGH, FEVER, AND NIGHT SWEATS

SUZANNE M. BRECKENRIDGE
J. WALTON TOMFORD

CASE PRESENTATION

A 49-year-old man presented to the emergency department (ED) with a 3-week history of a cough productive of whitish sputum. The patient stated that he had intermittently experienced these symptoms during the preceding few months. He also complained of dyspnea on exertion, anorexia, occasional nonbiliary emesis, and drenching night sweats. He reported intermittent low-grade fevers during the preceding year. He denied any sick contacts, chills, chest pain, sore throat, diarrhea, hemoptysis, dysuria, hematuria, abdominal pain, weakness, or headaches.

The patient stated that he was in the ED 2 weeks earlier with similar symptoms and was treated with azithromycin. At that time, his examination was notable for right-sided rales and his chest radiograph revealed bilateral hilar adenopathy and a right-upper-lobe infiltrative process. His symptoms persisted, prompting him to return to the ED.

The patient's past medical history was notable for human immunodeficiency virus (HIV) and hepatitis C, both diagnosed 2 years before this presentation. At that time, the patient was admitted for pneumonia. His CD4 count was 355 cells/μL, and the viral load was 55,000 copies/mL. The patient did not have a history of opportunistic infections and had not taken any antiretroviral therapy. Six months before being diagnosed with HIV, the patient was seen for an upper respiratory infection; chest x-ray at that time was suspicious for a left hilar mass. The patient was lost to follow-up before his appointment with a pulmonologist.

Upon admission, the patient was not taking any medications. He admitted to a history of tobacco use but stated that he had quit approximately 5 years earlier. He occasionally used alcohol and denied any intravenous drug use. He was homeless. He did not have a history of prior purified protein derivative (PPD) testing, nor did he recall any history of exposure to tuberculosis.

On physical examination, the patient was a healthy-appearing, well-developed man in no acute distress. Vital signs included a temperature of 38.3°C, heart rate of 107 beats per minute, respiratory rate of 20 per minute, blood pressure of 130/70 mm Hg, and pulse oximetry of 97% on room air. His throat was clear, without evidence of thrush or other oral lesions. He had anterior cervical adenopathy and diffuse axillary and inguinal adenopathy. Cardiac examination revealed tachycardia with a regular rhythm; no murmurs were heard. Lung examination revealed scattered rhonchi and decreased breath sounds in the right base. Abdominal examination was benign. He did not have any peripheral edema or clubbing.

Laboratory testing revealed serum sodium of 129 mmol/L, potassium of 5.2 mmol/L, and creatinine of 1.8 mg/dL. Complete blood count did not reveal evidence of leukocytosis. An arterial blood gas on room air revealed pH of 7.44, PCO_2 of 31 mm Hg, PO_2 of 76 mm Hg, and bicarbonate of 20 mmol/L. His CD4 count was 155 cells/μL, and the viral load was 244,000 copies/mL. Chest radiography was significant for right-middle- and upper-lobe infiltrates, a small right pleural effusion, and bilateral hilar adenopathy.

QUESTIONS/DISCUSSION

Which of the following is the most likely diagnosis in this patient?

A. **Influenza**
B. *Pneumocystis carinii* **pneumonia**
C. **Community-acquired pneumonia**
D. **Tuberculosis (TB)**

Influenza is a viral syndrome typically characterized by fever, chills, myalgias, and malaise. It typically has a paucity of findings on chest radiography. Symptoms associated with influenza typically resolve within 1 week. The more prolonged nature of this patient's symptoms makes influenza less likely.

Pneumocystis carinii pneumonia (PCP) should be considered in any patient with HIV and respiratory symptoms. Fever, progressive dyspnea, hypoxia, and cough typically characterize PCP. In contrast to this patient's radiographic presentation with focal infiltrates, patients with PCP typically have interstitial infiltrates on chest radiography.

Patients with community-acquired pneumonia often present much like this patient, with fever, dyspnea, and productive cough. However, this patient was treated with appropriate antibiotics for community-acquired pneumonia without resolution of his symptoms. Therefore, although the patient may have pneumonia with a resistant organism, other etiologies must be considered.

Pulmonary tuberculosis develops due to infection with *Mycobacterium tuberculosis*, which is an obligate aerobic bacillus that is transmitted via aerosolization of respiratory droplets. The deposition of these bacilli into terminal alveoli results in primary pulmonary tuberculosis. The signs and symptoms of primary pulmonary tuberculosis can vary widely, with fever the most common symptom. Other common symptoms include pleuritic chest pain, cough, and fatigue, all of which can be self-limited. Physical examination is often normal. Chest radiography most often reveals unilateral hilar adenopathy, followed by pulmonary infiltrates and pleural effusions (1).

In contrast, reactivation tuberculosis occurs in patients previously infected with *M. tuberculosis.* Presenting symptoms include cough (either dry or productive), hemoptysis, dyspnea, night sweats, pleuritic chest pain, anorexia, and weight loss. Chest radiographs of patients with reactivation TB often reveal upper-lobe infiltrates ranging in appearance from fluffy infiltrates to cavitary lesions. Reactivation TB most commonly involves the posterior and apical segments of the right upper lobe, as well as the left upper lobe. It can also affect the superior segments of the lower lobes (2).

Given this patient's history of HIV, his symptoms, the prolonged duration of symptoms, and radiographic findings, tuberculosis was considered the most likely diagnosis. Patients with HIV can present with typical or atypical signs and symptoms of TB. Individuals with HIV who are newly infected with tuberculosis have increased vulnerability to progressive disease, as well as a greater incidence of extrapulmonary involvement and miliary spread (1,3).

Case Continued: The patient was admitted to the hospital and was placed in respiratory isolation because of the high suspicion for tuberculosis. He continued to have fevers and productive cough despite appropriate antibiotic coverage for community-acquired pneumonia. Blood cultures were negative, but multiple sputum samples revealed acid-fast bacilli. The patient was started on appropriate antituberculous therapy. Sputum cultures subsequently grew *Mycobacterium tuberculosis.*

In this patient, which of the following is consistent with a positive reaction to PPD testing?

A. 2 mm of induration
B. 5 mm of induration
C. 10 mm of induration
D. 15 mm of induration

The diagnosis of latent TB infection is made via intradermal injection of PPD. The diameter of the area of induration is measured 48 to 72 hours following injection. The interpretation of the test is based on both the diameter and the clinical scenario. A positive PPD does not necessarily signify active tuberculosis; rather, it indicates that the patient has been infected with *M. tuberculosis* in the past. An area of induration of 5 mm is considered a positive reaction in patients who are at greatest risk for developing TB. These patients include those with HIV/acquired immunodeficiency syndrome (AIDS), organ transplant recipients, patients on chronic immunosuppression, close contacts, and those with chest radiographs suspicious for prior TB infection. Ten millimeters of induration is considered positive in patients with moderate potential for TB infection. This group includes immigrants, laboratory personnel working with mycobacteria, intravenous drug abusers, and medical personnel. A 15-mm area of induration is considered positive in patients without risk factors (2). AIDS patients, patients on immunosuppression, and healthy patients sometimes fail to mount a response to a PPD due to defects in cell-mediated immunity. In this patient with HIV, induration of 5 mm would be considered positive.

Active tuberculous infection is diagnosed by identification of acid-fast bacilli (AFB) on sputum smear and confirmation on sputum culture. Approximately 40% to 50% of patients have smears negative for AFB; sputum culture has a greater diagnostic yield (4). Furthermore, patients with HIV are less likely to have positive sputum smears. Cultures can take 3 to 6 weeks to grow *M. tuberculosis*; therefore, prompt treatment needs to be initiated when the clinical suspicion for TB is high. If sputum studies are unrevealing and the clinical suspicion for tuberculosis remains high, bronchoscopy with bronchoalveolar lavage needs to be considered as a next step in the diagnostic evaluation.

Which of the following regimens is the most appropriate treatment for this patient?

A. Isoniazid (INH) alone for 6 months
B. INH and rifampin for 6 months
C. INH, rifampin, and ethambutol for 6 months
D. INH and rifampin for 6 months, ethambutol, and pyrazinamide for the first 2 months

The duration of therapy for tuberculosis depends on the medications used, drug sensitivities, and the clinical response to therapy. Current recommendations from the Centers for Disease Control include a regimen of isoniazid

(INH), rifampin, ethambutol, and pyrazinamide (choice D). In the absence of any drug resistance, treatment with INH and rifampin for a period of 9 months is appropriate. If pyrazinamide is used for the first 2 months, the duration of treatment may be decreased to 6 months. If culture sensitivities are not known, ethambutol or streptomycin is usually added until susceptibilities are confirmed (5). Multidrug therapy and directly observed treatment (DOT) for the treatment of active tuberculosis are essential in preventing the emergence of drug-resistant strains. Isoniazid alone is appropriate for patients with a positive PPD in whom active tuberculosis has been excluded. Recent recommendations favor a 9-month duration of treatment with INH (6).

Patients receiving treatment for active tuberculosis need to be closely monitored for adverse reactions to antituberculous medications. INH is associated with the development of hepatitis and peripheral neuropathy. Patients should have baseline liver function tests and have them rechecked on a monthly basis while on INH. Treatment with INH should be discontinued if the transaminases increase to three to five times the upper limits of normal. To prevent neuropathy, patients should receive pyridoxine supplementation during treatment.

Patients on rifampin need to be monitored closely for potential drug–drug interactions. Rifampin increases the clearance of medications metabolized by the cytochrome P450 system. Medications whose serum levels are decreased by rifampin include warfarin, oral contraceptives, theophylline, dapsone, ketoconazole, and protease inhibitors. Pyrazinamide may cause hyperuricemia. Streptomycin is potentially both ototoxic and nephrotoxic. Renal function should be carefully monitored. Ethambutol can cause optic neuritis; baseline visual acuity and color testing should be performed.

Patients with HIV/AIDS pose multiple challenges to the successful treatment of tuberculosis. The bioavailability of some antiretroviral agents decreases with the use of rifampin, resulting in subtherapeutic levels of antiretrovirals and/or toxic levels of rifampin. Rifabutin, which is a less potent inducer of the cytochrome P450 pathway than rifampin, can be used as a substitute (7). In addition, patients with HIV may develop malabsorption, which results in inadequate absorption of antituberculous medications and treatment failure. These patients should be monitored closely to prevent the development of drug resistance secondary to subtherapeutic levels (8).

Case Conclusion

The patient was started on INH, rifampin, ethambutol, and pyrazinamide. Culture susceptibilities revealed nonresistant *Mycobacterium tuberculosis*. The patient was transferred to a TB clinic for directly observed therapy.

CONCLUSION

Tuberculosis remains an important cause of pulmonary infection, especially in patients with HIV disease. Clinicians need to maintain a healthy suspicion for TB, especially when patients present with suggestive symptoms and radiographic findings. Although PPD testing is important in the diagnosis of tuberculosis, patients with HIV can have nonreactive PPD skin tests. A number of treatment regimens are used to treat TB. Regardless of the specific regimen used, multidrug therapy is essential to treat TB appropriately and prevent resistance.

REFERENCES

1. Barnes PF, Bloch AB, Davidson PT, et al. Tuberculosis in patients with human immunodeficiency virus infection. *N Engl J Med* 1991;324:1644–1650.
2. Diagnostic Standards and Classification of Tuberculosis in Adults and Children. This official statement of the American Thoracic Society and the Centers for Disease Control and Prevention was adopted by the ATS Board of Directors, July 1999. This statement was endorsed by the Council of the Infectious Disease Society of America, September 1999. *Am J Respir Crit Care Med* 2000;161:1376–1395.
3. Alpert PL, Munsiff SS, Gourevitch MN, et al. A prospective study of tuberculosis and human immunodeficiency virus infection: clinical manifestations and factors associated with survival. *Clin Infect Dis* 1997;24:661–668.
4. Garay SM. Tuberculosis and HIV infection. *Semin Respir Crit Care Med* 1995;16:187.
5. Core curriculum on tuberculosis. The Centers for Disease Control and Prevention, www.cdc.gov, 2002.
6. Targeted tuberculin testing and treatment of latent tuberculosis infection. *Am J Respir Crit Care Med* 2000;161(4 Pt 2):S221–S247.
7. Prevention and treatment of tuberculosis among patients infected with human immunodeficiency virus: Principles of therapy and revised recommendations. Centers for Disease Control and Prevention. *MMWR Recomm Rep* 1998;47(RR-20):1–58.
8. Patel KB, Belmonte R, Crowe HM. Drug malabsorption and resistant tuberculosis in HIV-infected patients. *N Engl J Med* 1995;332:336–337.

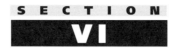

MISCELLANEOUS

43

A 78-YEAR-OLD WOMAN WITH PROGRESSIVE LOWER-EXTREMITY AND FACIAL WEAKNESS

AHMED K. ABDEL LATIF
LARA E. JEHA
BRYAN E. TSAO

CASE PRESENTATION

A 78-year-old woman presented with a 2-week history of progressive lower-extremity weakness. During this period, she noted difficulty walking, followed by an inability to stand. These symptoms progressed to complete paralysis of the lower extremities, with associated low back pain and increased constipation. The patient denied any associated sensory changes. After 1 week of symptoms, the patient developed right facial weakness, dysarthria, and dysphagia. Upon presentation, she also noticed the development of shortness of breath.

The patient's past medical history was significant for hypothyroidism, emphysema, vitamin B_{12} deficiency, and bilateral cataracts. The patient was receiving levothyroxine and monthly vitamin B_{12} injections. The patient had an upper respiratory tract infection 4 weeks before the start of her presenting symptoms. She denied any history of trauma, cancer, chemical or heavy metal exposure, substance abuse, or alcohol abuse. There was no history of tick bites, intake of canned food, skin rash, or family history of similar illnesses.

Physical examination revealed a temperature of 36.4°C, pulse of 82 beats per minute, blood pressure of 155/91 mm Hg, respiratory rate of 20 per minute, and pulse oximetry of 96% on room air. The patient was alert and fully oriented. Examination of the heart, lungs, abdomen, skin, and vascular systems was unremarkable. Cranial nerve examination revealed bilateral upper and lower facial weaknesses, which was worse on the right; depressed gag reflex; and minimal elevation of the palate. The remainder of her cranial nerve examination was normal. Motor examination revealed flaccid tone throughout. Strength was 4/5 in the proximal upper extremities and 5–/5 distally. Lower-extremity strength was 2/5 proximally and 3+/5 distally. Sensory examination was notable for absent vibratory sensation at the ankles and markedly diminished proprioception at the toes. Deep tendon reflexes were absent in the lower extremities and decreased in the upper extremities. Gait was not assessed due to the patient's weakness. Rectal examination revealed normal sphincter tone.

Complete blood count, electrolytes, calcium, magnesium, creatine kinase, and thyroid stimulating hormone were unremarkable except for a sodium of 117 mmol/L. Computed tomography (CT scan) of the brain was normal. Chest x-ray did not reveal any infiltrates, and plain films of the lumbar spine and hips were normal.

QUESTIONS/DISCUSSION

Based on the history, physical examination, and initial laboratory data, what is the most likely explanation of this patient's findings?

A. **Acute transverse myelitis**
B. **Myasthenia gravis**
C. **Guillain–Barré syndrome (GBS)**
D. **Spinal cord compression (SCC)**
E. **None of the above**

The differential diagnosis for patients presenting with flaccid paraplegia is wide and potentially complex. However, the diagnostic approach can be simplified by localizing the symptoms within the neuroaxis. The lower motor neuron system (from proximal to distal) consists of the anterior horn cell, peripheral nerve (including nerve roots), neuromuscular junction, and muscle.

■ *Anterior horn cell:* Spinal cord compression, transverse myelitis, and spinal cord infarction comprise some of the emergent causes of acute flaccid paralysis. The West Nile virus has recently been described as causing a poliomyelitis-like syndrome that results in flaccid paralysis (1). Electrodiagnostic data suggest that the virus has this effect by acting on the anterior horn cell.

- *Peripheral nerve:* Causes of acute-onset neuropathies include GBS, vasculitis, toxins (thallium, selenium), infection [human immunodeficiency virus (HIV)-related, diphtheria, Lyme disease], porphyria, granulomatous disease (sarcoidosis), and paraneoplastic syndromes.
- *Neuromuscular junction:* Myasthenia gravis, botulism, tick-borne paralysis, and Lambert–Eaton myasthenic syndrome interfere with function at the neuromuscular junction. In addition, electrolyte abnormalities, including hypermagnesemia and hypophosphatemia, can mimic these disorders.
- *Muscle:* Myopathies that present with acute weakness include those associated with metabolic conditions (thyroid disease, storage diseases), toxins (medications and alcohol), and inflammatory conditions (polymyositis).

The key features necessary to differentiate among these etiologies are the following:

- Establishing the onset, pattern, and progression of weakness.
- Determining the extent of cranial nerve and autonomic involvement.
- Determining the presence or absence of sensory findings.

Appropriate laboratory, radiographic, and electrodiagnostic studies are often helpful to establish a diagnosis and exclude other causes.

Acute transverse myelitis is an acute inflammatory disorder of the spinal cord. The clinical picture consists of variable sensory loss, paresthesias, motor weakness, and sphincter disturbances. The disease may be partial or complete. Hyperreflexia, rather than areflexia or hyporeflexia, is typically present. In 40% of cases, an infection precedes symptoms and likely triggers myelitis through an autoimmune process (2). Cranial nerve abnormalities are not typically present. Magnetic resonance imaging (MRI) is the preferred imaging study to diagnose transverse myelitis. MRI commonly shows variable swelling of the spinal cord and diffuse or multifocal enhancement of the cord, which is suggestive of disruption of the blood–brain barrier. Cerebrospinal fluid shows pleocytosis with a mononuclear predominance and normal or slightly elevated protein. Moderate and severe cases are treated with corticosteroids and supportive care. In this patient, the presence of persistent areflexia and cranial nerve and bulbar symptoms makes transverse myelitis unlikely.

Myasthenia gravis (MG) is an autoimmune disease that affects the neuromuscular junction and produces symptoms of weakness and fatigability. The hallmark of the disease is autoantibodies directed toward the postsynaptic acetylcholine receptors at the neuromuscular junction. The disease is limited to the motor system, with weakness initially affecting the facial and bulbar muscles, followed by involvement of the proximal skeletal muscles (3). Fatiguing weakness and cranial nerve dysfunction, characterized by symptoms such as diplopia, dysarthria, and dysphagia, are often prominent features. MG can occasionally cause muscle weakness involving the diaphragm and respiratory muscles, which leads to respiratory compromise. Deep tendon reflexes and the sensory systems are unaffected. Cerebrospinal fluid analysis is typically normal. The diagnosis of MG is made clinically but can be confirmed by the detection of acetylcholine receptor antibodies and by certain electrodiagnostic criteria that are characteristic of MG. Mild cases are treated with acetylcholinesterase inhibitors, oral steroids, and other immunosuppressants. Plasmapheresis and intravenous immunoglobulins are used in more severe cases. Although MG can present with lower extremity weakness, the presence of prominent sensory deficits and loss of reflexes make the diagnosis of myasthenia gravis unlikely in this patient.

Spinal cord compression (SCC) can develop as a result of structural (degenerative or neoplastic disease) or infectious causes (epidural abscess). Spinal cord compression typically manifests as back pain, followed by acute or subacute neurologic deficits, including sensory loss and weakness below the level of the compression and sphincter dysfunction. MRI with and without contrast is the gold standard for the radiographic diagnosis of cord compression. In patients with contraindications to MRI, CT myelogram provides excellent images for epidural masses. Both extradural processes, such as metastatic tumors and lymphoma, and intradural processes, such as meningiomas and neurofibromas, can cause radicular symptoms and cord compression. Oral or intravenous corticosteroids are used to treat spinal cord compression. Biopsy is indicated in selected cases. Treatment, including the judicious use of radiotherapy and surgery, is tailored to the pathologic diagnosis. Although spinal cord compression can cause flaccid paralysis and areflexia, the pattern of cranial nerve involvement, as well as normal sphincter tone, makes SCC an unlikely diagnosis in this patient.

In this patient, the presence of back pain, flaccid proximal weakness, areflexia, and cranial nerve involvement following a respiratory infection is most likely consistent with an acquired demyelinating neuropathy such as GBS.

With a yearly incidence of two to four cases per 100,000 people, GBS is the most common cause of acute generalized paralysis in the Western world (4). There is a peak of GBS in early adulthood and late adolescence, with a second peak in the elderly (5).

Which of the following pathogens most commonly precedes GBS?

A. Cytomegalovirus
B. *Campylobacter jejuni*

C. *Mycoplasma pneumoniae*
D. Epstein–Barr virus

Up to 75% of cases of GBS have a history of a preceding infectious process, most notably respiratory and gastrointestinal infections. Approximately 20% to 30% of cases are associated with an antecedent *Campylobacter jejuni* infection, the pathogen that most commonly precedes GBS (2). Infections with cytomegalovirus, Epstein–Barr virus, varicella-zoster virus, and *Mycoplasma pneumoniae* have also been reported to precede GBS (2). The interval between pathogen exposure and the onset of GBS symptoms ranges from 1 to 3 weeks (5). Despite initial reports describing swine influenza vaccine as a prominent predisposing pathogen for GBS, subsequent investigations have shown that the incidence of GBS following swine influenza vaccine was one additional case per million individuals vaccinated (2).

Although the specific etiology of GBS remains unknown, it likely develops due to an autoimmune process mediated through both cellular and humoral pathways. An antecedent immune challenge with infection (bacterial or viral) or immunization is thought to trigger an autoimmune response with early activation of lymphocytes surrounding blood vessels, spinal roots, and peripheral nerves. The most likely target of this abnormal immune response is surface myelin components, resulting in segmental demyelination with preservation of the axon. IgM antibodies against surface myelin components can be detected in 20% to 50% of cases of GBS following *Campylobacter* infection (2).

Demyelination disrupts electrical conductance, which results in both sensory and motor symptoms. In severe cases of GBS, axonal loss occurs as a result of intense peripheral nerve edema and inflammation, leading to slower recovery and more residual deficits. In milder cases without axonal loss, patients have a greater chance of early recovery.

The diagnosis of GBS should be suspected in patients presenting with acute onset of flaccid paralysis, hypo- or areflexia, and/or cranial nerve deficits. Although GBS is classically described as presenting with ascending numbness followed by weakness, the disease primarily affects motor nerves. Therefore, patients may not have significant sensory disturbances. Weakness typically develops over hours to days and is followed by loss of reflexes within days. The proximal pattern of weakness associated with GBS is atypical for most neuropathies. The cranial nerves, especially nerves VII, IX, and X, are also frequently involved, resulting in diplopia, facial weakness, and dysphagia. Diaphragmatic weakness results in dyspnea. Most patients who require hospitalization do so because of an inability to clear secretions, protect the airway, and/or maintain ventilation; up to 30% of patients with GBS eventually require ventilatory support (5). Autonomic system involvement is prominent in two-thirds of patients with GBS, manifested by labile blood pressure, bowel and bladder dysfunction, and cardiac dysrhythmias (4). As seen in this case, pituitary axis dysfunction can develop in the context of the syndrome of inappropriate antidiuretic hormone (SIADH) secretion, resulting in hyponatremia (6).

Variants of GBS include acute motor–sensory axonal neuropathy (AMSAN), acute motor axonal neuropathy, Miller–Fisher syndrome (characterized by areflexia, ophthalmoplegia, and ataxia), pure sensory GBS, pharyngeal–cervical–brachial variant, and acute pandysautonomia (7–9).

Which of the following cerebrospinal fluid (CSF) profiles is most commonly seen in GBS?

A. **Elevated white blood cell count and decreased protein**
B. **Elevated white blood cell count and protein**
C. **Elevated protein, glucose, and white blood cell count**
D. **Elevated protein and normal white blood cell count**

The diagnosis of GBS is often established on clinical grounds. Laboratory and electrodiagnostic findings can help support the diagnosis, but treatment should not be delayed if these tests are unavailable or pending. Criteria proposed by Asbury and Cornblath (10) were designed to simplify the diagnosis of GBS. Table 43.1 summarizes these guidelines (5).

Cerebrospinal fluid (CSF) studies are crucial in the diagnostic work-up of GBS. However, clinicians should recognize that the sensitivity of CSF studies is lowest in the first week after onset of symptoms (52%) but increases to 78% in the second week and to 93% subsequently (11). Typical

TABLE 43.1. DIAGNOSTIC CRITERIA FOR TYPICAL GUILLAIN–BARRÉ SYNDROME

Features Required for Diagnosis
  Progressive weakness in all four extremities
  Hypo/areflexia
Features Strongly Supporting Diagnosis
  Relative symmetry of symptoms
  Cranial nerve involvement, especially of the facial nerve
  Recovery beginning 2 to 4 weeks after progression ceases
  Autonomic dysfunction
  Cerebrospinal fluid with high protein and low cell count
    (cytoalbuminologic dissociation)
  Typical demyelinating electrodiagnostic features
  Rapid progression of symptoms over days to 4 weeks
  Absent/mild sensory symptoms or signs
  Absence of fever at onset
Features Excluding Diagnosis
  History of recent diphtherial infection
  Purely sensory symptoms without motor symptoms
  Abnormal porphyrin metabolism
  Diagnosis of botulism, myasthenia gravis, poliomyelitis, or
    toxic neuropathy

Modified from Hahn AF. Guillain–Barré syndrome. *Lancet* 1998;352:635–641.

CSF findings in patients with GBS include an elevated protein (greater than 45 mg/dL) with a normal white blood cell count (less than 6 cells/μL). This combination is referred to as cytoalbuminologic dissociation. CSF protein above 250 mg/dL should raise suspicion for spinal cord compression. CSF pleocytosis greater than 50 cells/μL should raise suspicions for conditions such as HIV seroconversion states, Lyme disease, carcinomatous meningitis, and sarcoid meningitis (3).

The most sensitive and specific laboratory finding in GBS is the electrodiagnostic examination, which includes nerve conduction studies (NCS) and the needle electrode examination (NEE). The examination typically demonstrates evidence of acquired demyelination with occasional mild axonal damage. Although nerve conduction studies often confirm the presence of demyelination as soon as weakness develops, the needle electrode examination does not reliably demonstrate axonal loss for 3 weeks. Electrodiagnostic changes typical of GBS occur earlier and more frequently than do abnormal CSF findings (3). Normal electrodiagnostic studies more than 1 week after the onset of symptoms make the diagnosis of GBS less likely.

Case Continued: A lumbar puncture was performed and revealed a white blood cell count of 0 cells/μL, red blood cell count of 3 cells/μL, and protein of 90 mg/dL (normal, less than 45 mg/dL). Electrodiagnostic studies showed evidence of a generalized sensorimotor polyneuropathy with features of acquired segmental demyelination compatible with GBS. MRI of the spine did not reveal evidence of spinal cord compression.

The patient was transferred to the intensive care unit (ICU) for closer respiratory monitoring. She continued to have progressive weakness of the lower extremities, and weakness progressed to the upper extremities.

Which of the following is an effective treatment for GBS?

A. **Plasma exchange**
B. **Corticosteroids**
C. **Intravenous immunoglobulin**
D. **A and C**
E. **All of the above**

In addition to considering appropriate therapeutic options for GBS, clinicians need to monitor these patients closely due to their increased risk of respiratory compromise. The risks of hemodynamic instability, autonomic dysfunction, and arrhythmias also mandate the need for close cardiac monitoring. One-third of GBS patients require admission to an ICU (4).

Corticosteroids have not been of significant benefit compared to placebo in patients with GBS (12). Although a recent study by the Dutch Guillain–Barré Study Group

suggested that the combination of intravenous IgG and high-dose methylprednisolone may be beneficial, the utility of corticosteroids in GBS has not been demonstrated (13).

Plasma exchange (PE) has been shown to be an effective treatment for GBS. Multiple large multicenter trials in North America and Europe have demonstrated the benefit of plasma exchange (13,14). The duration of mechanical ventilation and time before patients could walk unassisted were reduced by 50% in patients undergoing PE compared to supportive care alone. These benefits were achieved without any increase in morbidity. Plasma exchange was less effective if it was started more than 2 weeks from the start of symptoms (5). Therefore, this treatment should be initiated as soon as possible. Plasma exchange requires the placement of a large-bore central venous catheter. Four to five treatments are typically given on alternate days for 7 to 10 days. Potential complications of plasma exchange include catheter-site infections and hemodynamic fluctuations. If blood pressure is labile, intravenous immunoglobulin may be a more appropriate treatment option.

Intravenous immunoglobulin (IVIG) is an effective and less complex alternative treatment for GBS. High-dose IVIG (0.4 g/kg of body weight for 5 days) has been proven as effective as plasma exchange, even in cases of severe GBS (15). The combination of plasma exchange and IVIG has not provided additional benefit than either of these therapies individually (16). Limited relapses are described in 10% of cases treated with IVIG. Serum IgA levels should be checked before starting IVIG because IVIG infusion in IgA-deficient patients may precipitate an anaphylactic reaction.

Both plasma exchange and intravenous immunoglobulins are effective treatments of GBS. Although controlled studies analyzing the treatment of variants of GBS are lacking, these patients should be treated similarly.

Prognosis and Outcome

The outcome and prognosis of GBS is variable, depending on the type and degree of underlying nerve damage. Most patients recover over a period of weeks or months (4). While the majority does not experience permanent disability, only 15% of patients do not have any residual deficits (2). Poor prognostic criteria include severely reduced amplitudes of muscle action potentials on electrodiagnostic examination, older age, ventilatory support for more than 1 month, severe proximal motor and sensory axonal damage, and severe progressive disease (2).

Case Conclusion

The patient's symptoms and weakness improved significantly after 6 sessions of plasmapheresis. She was discharged to a rehabilitation center for continued physical and occupational therapy.

CONCLUSION

Lower-extremity weakness is a common presentation to the emergency and outpatient departments. Because of the potentially life-threatening consequences of GBS, it should be considered in the differential diagnosis of acute progressive flaccid muscle weakness in association with areflexia. The diagnosis of GBS is based on the clinical picture, including a history of an antecedent event. Laboratory findings, including cerebrospinal fluid and electrodiagnostic findings, are confirmatory. Treatment for GBS should be started in the absence of confirmatory laboratory tests if the diagnosis is strongly suspected.

REFERENCES

1. Leis AA, Stokic DS, Polk JL, et al. A poliomyelitis-like syndrome from West Nile virus infection. *N Engl J Med* 2002; 347: 1279–1280.
2. Asbury AK, Hauser SL. Guillain Barré syndrome and other immune-mediated neuropathies. In: Braunwald E, Fauci AS, Kasper DL, et al., eds. *Harrison's principles of internal medicine,* 15th ed. New York: McGraw-Hill, 2001:2507–2512.
3. Drachman DB. Myasthenia gravis. *N Engl J Med* 1994;330: 1797–1810.
4. Ropper AH. The Guillain-Barré syndrome. *N Engl J Med* 1992; 326:1130–1136.
5. Hahn AF. Guillain-Barré syndrome. *Lancet* 1998;352:635–641.
6. Hoffmann O, Reuter U, Schielke E, et al. SIADH as the first symptom of Guillain–Barré syndrome. *Neurology* 1999;53:1365.
7. Feasby TE, Gilbert JJ, Brown WF, et al. An acute axonal form of Guillain–Barré polyneuropathy. *Brain* 1986;109:1115–1126.
8. Hughes RA, Hadden RD, Gregson NA, et al. Pathogenesis of Guillain-Barré syndrome. *J Neuroimmunol* 1999;100:74–97.
9. Fisher M. An unusual variant of acute idiopathic polyneuritis (syndrome of ophthalmoplegia, ataxia, and areflexia). *N Engl J Med* 1956;255:57–65.
10. Asbury AK, Cornblath DR. Assessment of current diagnostic criteria for Guillain–Barré syndrome. *Ann Neurol* 1990;27(Suppl): S21–S24.
11. Lyu RK, Tang LM, Cheng SY, %%. Guillain-Barré syndrome in Taiwan: a clinical study of 167 patients. *J Neurol Neurosurg Psychiatry* 1997;63:494–500.
12. Treatment of Guillain-Barré syndrome with high-dose immune globulins combined with methylprednisolone: a pilot study. Dutch Guillain Barré Study Group. *Ann Neurol* 1994;35:749–752.
13. Plasmapheresis and acute Guillain-Barré syndrome. The Guillain-Barré Syndrome Study Group. *Neurology* 1985;35:1096–1104.
14. Efficiency of plasma exchange in Guillain Barré syndrome: role of replacement fluids. French Cooperative Group on Plasma Exchange in Guillain-Barré syndrome. *Ann Neurol* 1987;22: 753–761.
15. Van der Meche FG, Schmitz PI. A randomized trial comparing intravenous immune globulin and plasma exchange in Guillain-Barré syndrome. Dutch Guillain-Barré Study Group. *N Engl J Med* 1992;326:1123–1129.
16. Randomised trial of plasma exchange, intravenous immunoglobulin, and combined treatments in Guillain-Barré syndrome. Plasma Exchange/Sandoglobulin Guillain-Barré Syndrome Trial Group. *Lancet* 1997;349:225–230.

44

A YOUNG WOMAN WITH DIZZINESS AND SYNCOPE

ANDRES A. GONZALEZ
FETNAT FOUAD-TARAZI

CASE PRESENTATION

A 20-year-old woman presented for evaluation of a 3-year history of dizziness. She described the symptoms as a "floating feeling" that would last for a few hours. The dizziness was usually most severe following exertion, during menses, or with hyperventilation. In association with these symptoms, she reported two unwitnessed syncopal episodes, during which she fainted "for a couple of seconds." One episode occurred while taking a hot shower and the other while getting out of bed swiftly. She had a history of frontotemporal headaches since starting college 3 years earlier. The headaches typically improved with acetaminophen, were not accompanied by an aura, and did not necessarily correlate with her dizziness. Her mother had a history of headaches and syncopal episodes as a teenager.

Comprehensive cardiac, otologic, and neurologic examinations were unremarkable. Complete blood count, electrolytes, and electrocardiogram (ECG) were within normal limits.

QUESTIONS/DISCUSSION

Which of the following is the next appropriate test in evaluating the patient's symptoms?

A. Exercise–echocardiogram
B. Head-up tilt-table test
C. Computed tomography (CT scan) of the brain
D. Magnetic resonance imaging (MRI) of the brain
E. Holter monitor

The initial diagnostic approach should be geared toward ruling out conditions that would prompt emergency treatment, such as hemorrhage, critical arrhythmias, and coronary events. A careful history is usually the most important initial diagnostic tool. Further diagnostic testing is usually guided by the clinical presentation and not by a preset algorithm. Initial testing should include glucose, electrolytes, and hematocrit. Cardiac enzymes should be ordered if a myocardial event is suspected. A toxicology panel should be done if alcohol or drug use is suspected. An ECG should be performed in every patient. Although routine electrocardiography rarely establishes a definitive diagnosis unless performed during symptoms, it occasionally provides clues that may guide further diagnostic studies (1).

Etiologies of syncope that may be diagnosed by an echocardiogram include hypertrophic obstructive cardiomyopathy (HOCM), valvular aortic stenosis, right ventricular hypertrophy (with pulmonary hypertension), and atrial myxoma. CT of the brain is indicated if stroke, seizure, or intracranial hemorrhage is suspected as the cause of syncope. MRI may provide greater sensitivity than CT if a thrombotic stroke is suspected. A Holter monitor or other types of continuous ECG monitoring may be helpful if the suspicion for arrhythmia is high, such as in patients with underlying structural heart disease or with a history of palpitations immediately preceding a syncopal event. Tilt testing is appropriate in patients in whom neurocardiogenic syncope is suspected. Before presentation, the patient had undergone MRI of the brain, which was normal, and had normal vestibular testing. Since most of the symptoms occurred during exercise, a stress echocardiogram was obtained, which was normal.

At this point, the patient's most likely diagnosis is:

A. Hypertrophic obstructive cardiomyopathy (HOCM)
B. Exercise-induced arrhythmia
C. Vestibular neuronitis
D. Neurocardiogenic syncope
E. Migraine-related dizziness

Syncopal or presyncopal symptoms frequently traverse the boundaries of cardiology, otolaryngology, neurology, and psychiatry. Elucidating the diagnosis is often aided by careful evaluation of the elements of the clinical presentation and the circumstances under which syncope occurred.

Hypertrophic obstructive cardiomyopathy usually presents as exertional syncope. On physical examination, a systolic murmur may be heard, which intensifies during Valsalva maneuvers. Patients with HOCM may have family members with HOCM or a history of sudden death. An echocardiogram with amyl nitrite and Valsalva maneuver can be diagnostic for HOCM.

Exercise-induced arrhythmias may be seen in young patients with right ventricular dysplasia. These patients may be asymptomatic until a syncopal event occurs. A family history of sudden death may be present. ECGs of patients with right ventricular dysplasia often show T-wave inversions in leads V_1 to V_3 and premature ventricular contractions with left bundle branch block configuration.

Vestibular neuronitis is usually associated with prolonged episodes of vertigo, with an associated "spinning" sensation, rather than lightheadedness. This condition is occasionally attributed to a viral infection. Patients with multiple sclerosis and posterior cerebrovascular ischemia can present similarly.

Neurally mediated syncope is usually one of the most common and most difficult-to-treat forms of syncope. It is a form of syncope that encompasses a variety of clinical syndromes, including vasovagal, vasodepressor, postmicturition, postdefecation, and postlaughter syncope. Neurally mediated syncope is sometimes preceded by postural orthostatic tachycardia syndrome (POTS) (2). Vasovagal reactions are the most common cause of neurally mediated syncope. Hot showers, crowded environments, alcohol, significant pain, prolonged standing, or stress may precipitate symptoms. Neurally mediated syncope occurs in the setting of increased sympathomimetic activity and venous pooling, which produces a vigorous contraction of a relatively underfilled heart. This activates ventricular mechanoreceptors and vagal afferent nerves, leading to a parasympathetic-mediated vasodilatation and bradycardia (3). Tilt testing will usually be diagnostic in cases of neurally mediated syncope.

Migraine-related dizziness (basilar artery migraine) predominantly affects young women and children. Symptoms vary from vertigo, tinnitus, and diplopia to symptoms as severe as ataxia and altered mental status. This disorder often affects both visual fields, which can help to differentiate it from migraine with aura.

Vestibular testing in this patient was normal, and she had no personal or family history of migraines or structural heart disease. The clinical presentation of this patient pointed to neurally mediated syncope, and she was subsequently scheduled for a tilt test.

Tilt Testing

With upright posture, approximately 500 to 700 mL of blood will pool in the lower extremities. The autonomic nervous system quickly compensates by pressor reflexes and increased heart rate via aortic and carotid reflexes.

There is also increased venous return by peripheral muscle contraction. The autonomic system may be dysfunctional in patients with diabetic autonomic neuropathies, multisystem atrophy (Shy–Drager syndrome), and idiopathic sympathetic dysfunction. Even in patients with debilitating illnesses, significant weight loss, and prolonged bed rest, the blood pressure may fall upon standing due to mechanisms totally or partially related to the inability of the autonomic system to maintain adequate vasoconstriction. Orthostatic intolerance may also be mediated by an increased adrenergic response, as seen in POTS.

Head-up tilt (HUT) testing has limited value in situational syncope (syncopal episodes that occur with defecation, cough, or vomiting). Moreover, "false-positive" responses to HUT have been observed in about 7% of subjects, especially in the later phases of the test (4). Tilt test duration is critical in maximizing the diagnostic yield in patients with syncope. The consensus is to perform a 45-minute test in order to increase sensitivity and specificity (5).

Tilt-Testing Patterns

The tilt test is designed to evaluate postural responses to blood pressure and heart rate. Several patterns can be seen:

- *Vasovagal response (VVR):* Drop in heart rate and blood pressure with presyncopal symptoms.
- *Vasodepressor response (VDR):* Symptomatic sudden drop in blood pressure in the absence of heart rate change.
- *Progressive orthostatic hypotension (POH):* Gradual decrease in blood pressure (systolic greater than 30 mm Hg and diastolic greater than 10 mm Hg) with increase in heart rate. This pattern is seen in patients with autonomic insufficiency as well as in other conditions.
- *Postural orthostatic tachycardia syndrome (POTS):* Symptomatic increase in heart rate of greater than 30 beats or greater than 120 beats per minute, without an associated drop in blood pressure.

This patient's upright tilt test is depicted in Fig. 44.1. Her blood pressure and heart rate responses are consistent with which pattern?

A. VVR
B. VDR
C. POH
D. POTS
E. POTS with VVR

The response seen in this patient is compatible with an elevation of her heart rate above 120 (POTS) followed by a sudden drop in both heart rate and blood pressure (VVR).

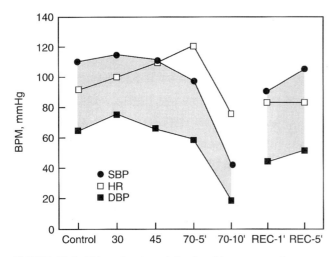

FIGURE 44.1. This patient's upright tilt table test. *BPM*, beats per minute; *DBP*, diastolic blood pressure; *HR*, heart rate; *SBP*, systolic blood pressure.

Postural Orthostatic Tachycardia Syndrome

Patients with postural orthostatic tachycardia syndrome are thought to have a subset of autonomic dysfunction (6). Patients may present with orthostatic intolerance (not hypotension), postural tachycardia, and/or palpitations. The pathogenesis of POTS is unclear but is thought to be linked to two underlying mechanisms: partial dysautonomia and hyperadrenergic orthostatic intolerance, the latter referring to sympathetic overcompensation in response to positional change (7). Hypovolemia, venous pooling, impaired brainstem regulation, and β-receptor hypersensitivity may also play a role.

Classic POTS is characterized by symptomatic orthostatic intolerance in the absence of hypotension and an increase in the heart rate to greater than 120 beats per minute or more than 30 beats per minute from baseline. POTS usually affects young females and may be seen in conjunction with some degree of exercise intolerance. Some patients with POTS also have an exaggerated response to isoproterenol infusions. These patients will manifest an accentuated emotional response during isoproterenol infusion, with symptoms such as tremulousness or profound anxiety, in addition to increased heart rate (8).

Historically, POTS has evolved from disorders previously termed *Da Costa syndrome,* the *effort syndrome,* and *soldier's heart syndrome* (9). There has also been an unclear relationship with preceding viral syndromes and immune-mediated disorders.

Vasovagal Response/Syncope

With current technology, it is possible to further characterize responses to HUT (POTS and VVR) in more physio-logic terms by measuring blood volumes and performing hemodynamic and autonomic testing.

- *Blood volume:* Radioactive iodinated serum albumin (RISA) is used to assess the degree of hypovolemia. Low blood volume may be due to diuretics, self-imposed salt restriction, or an idiopathic cause (10).
- *Circulatory dynamics:* With the 99m-technetium first-pass method, the isotope travels from a peripheral vein to the superior vena cava, lungs, and aortic circulation. Analysis of the left ventricle and right ventricle dilution curves allows determination of cardiac output, blood volumes and circulation kinetics. This test permits classification of the circulatory dynamics as normokinetic, hypokinetic, or hyperkinetic.
- *Autonomic testing:* A set of maneuvers is used to determine the integrity of the autonomic reflexes and localize autonomic insufficiency, if present. Valsalva maneuvers are used to assess the overall function of the baroreflex arc. The cold pressor test evaluates the efferent sympathetic pathways and medullary central mechanisms. Amyl nitrite and phenylephrine can evaluate baroreceptor sensitivity and the afferent pathway of the baroreflex arc.
- *Isoproterenol infusion testing:* This is performed in patients in whom a hyperdynamic β circulatory state is suspected.

CONCLUSION

This patient had a short pulmonary mean transit time, which was consistent with hyperkinetic circulation. She was also found to have increased venous pooling. Treatment for this patient included β-blockers and compression stockings. β-Blockers help blunt the autonomic hyperreactivity that occurs in response to the body's perceived hypovolemia. Compression stockings are useful in increasing venous return and reducing venous pooling, which may trigger an exaggerated adrenergic response. She was also advised to avoid prolonged standing and was referred to physical therapy to improve muscle tone. If these measures fail to improve symptoms, a mineralocorticoid such as fludrocortisone can be used.

REFERENCES

1. Jaeger F, Maloney J, Fouad-Tarazi F. Newer aspects in the diagnosis and management of syncope. In: Rapaport E, ed. *Cardiology update: reviews for physicians.* New York: Elsevier, 1990: 141–175.
2. Benditt DG, Remole S, Milstein S, et al. Syncope: causes, clinical evaluation, and current therapy. *Annu Rev Med* 1992;43: 283–300.
3. Fenton AM, Hammill SC, Rea RF, et al. Vasovagal syncope. *Ann Intern Med* 2000;133:714–725.

4. Fouad FM, Sitthisook S, Vanerio G, et al. Sensitivity and specificity of the tilt table test in young patients with unexplained syncope. *Pacing Clin Electrophysiol* 1993;16:394–400.
5. Benditt DG, Ferguson DW, Grubb BP, et al. Tilt table testing for assessing syncope. *J Am Coll Cardiol* 1996;28:263–275.
6. Grubb BP, Kosinski DJ, Boehm K, et al. The postural-orthostatic tachycardia syndrome: a neurocardiogenic variant identified during head-up tilt table testing. *Pacing Clin Electrophysiol* 1997;20:2205–2212.
7. Robertson D. The epidemic of orthostatic tachycardia and orthostatic intolerance. *Am J Med Sci* 1999;317:75–77.
8. Frohlich ED, Dustan HP, Page IH. Hyperdynamic beta-adrenergic circulatory state. *Arch Intern Med* 1966;117:614–619.
9. Low PA. Update on the evaluation, pathogenesis, and management of neurogenic orthostatic hypotension: Introduction. *Neurology* 1995;45(Suppl 5):S4–S5.
10. Fouad FM, Tadena-Thome L, Bravo EL, et al. Idiopathic hypovolemia. *Ann Intern Med* 1986;104:298–303.

45

A 47-YEAR-OLD MAN WITH PARESTHESIAS AND DIFFICULTY WALKING

BASUKI K. GUNAWAN
MICHAEL BAYTION
J. HARRY ISAACSON

CASE PRESENTATION

A 47-year-old man presented to the emergency department with a 3-month history of progressive difficulty walking. One year before presentation, he could run 3 to 5 miles a day, but upon presentation he had difficulty walking a city block or climbing a flight of stairs. He complained of pain and weakness in his lower extremities and poor balance. The patient described the pain as a "swelling pressure" and compared it to "walking on hot coals." The pain and weakness were localized to the anterior aspect of his thighs and plantar surface of his feet. The patient also experienced several months of fatigue and generalized pain in his tongue. His wife had noticed decreased calf muscle definition in both legs over the month before presentation and memory loss over several months.

His past medical history was significant for polio when the patient was 4 years old. A physical examination 5 years earlier revealed mild anemia. He was a nonsmoker and did not use alcohol. He had been a vegetarian for 16 years, eating a diet that mainly consisted of fruits, vegetables, and yogurt, but occasionally he had eaten chicken and fish. For years, he took multivitamins twice a day but stopped 3 months before presentation.

His physical examination was notable for a smooth, pale tongue. Neurologic examination revealed decreased two-point discrimination in the hands and feet and decreased proprioception in the lower extremities. There was marked hyporeflexia in all extremities with only the left patellar reflex elicited. Slight dysdiadochokinesis and slightly decreased coordination with the finger-to-nose test were noted. His gait was unstable, and he needed assistance with walking. Abnormal heel-to-toe walking and a positive Romberg sign were present. Generalized weakness was observed, but muscle strength was 5/5 in all four extremities. The remainder of his examination was normal.

QUESTIONS/DISCUSSION

What is the most likely cause of this patient's symptoms?

A. Thiamine deficiency
B. Diabetic neuropathy
C. Cerebellar neoplasm
D. Stroke
E. Vitamin B_{12} deficiency

Thiamine deficiency usually presents as Wernicke–Korsakoff syndrome (WKS) and/or polyneuropathy. The patient had ataxia and paresthesias, both of which may occur in patients with WKS. However, he did not have other features of WKS: nystagmus, oculomotor palsies, confusion, and psychosis. In developed countries, thiamine deficiency is rare in nonalcoholic patients. Diabetics often present with sensory neuropathy and decreased sensation in a stocking–glove distribution but seldom present with severe gait ataxia. In addition, the patient had no history of diabetes mellitus. Cerebellar lesions often present with gait ataxia but are usually accompanied by dysarthria, intention tremor, hypotonia, and oculomotor abnormalities. These lesions would not be expected to cause paresthesias or decreased proprioception. A stroke may cause a similar presentation only if affecting multiple areas. A stroke would be unlikely, given the gradual progression of neurologic manifestations in this patient.

The patient's history and physical examination are classic for vitamin B_{12} or cyanocobalamin deficiency. The neurologic manifestations result from axonal degeneration in peripheral nerves, in the posterior and lateral columns of the spinal cord, and in the brain. The manifestations typically consist of paresthesias, commonly in a stocking–glove distribution, decreased vibratory sense and proprioception, gait ataxia, and a positive Romberg sign. Weakness is commonly observed in the lower extremities due to both peripheral neuropathy and lesions in the lateral columns of the spinal cord. Reflexes may be decreased or increased, depending on the extent of peripheral neuropathy. When the brain is affected, manifestations include minor personality changes and memory loss. Severe disease may cause dementia and psychosis.

For patients with equivocal B_{12} levels (200 to 300 pg/mL), which of the following is most helpful in establishing a diagnosis of B_{12} deficiency?

A. **Macrocytic anemia**
B. **Blood smear showing macroovalocytes and hypersegmented neutrophils**
C. **Elevated methylmalonic acid and homocysteine levels**
D. **Decreased methylmalonic acid and homocysteine levels**

Macrocytic anemia is often found in B_{12} deficiency. However, more than 16% of patients with neurologic complaints related to B_{12} deficiency may have a normal hematocrit and mean corpuscular volume (MCV) (1). An MCV of greater than 130 fL is very specific for B_{12} deficiency but lacks sensitivity (2). Macroovalocytes and hypersegmented neutrophils are also often found in B_{12} deficiency but are neither sensitive nor specific for patients with mild B_{12} deficiency (3,4).

Most patients with B_{12} deficiency have levels less than 200 pg/mL, and only a small minority has levels greater than 300 pg/mL (5,6). For patients with B_{12} levels between 200 and 300 pg/mL, further work-up should include serum methylmalonic acid (MMA) and homocysteine (HCY) levels. B_{12} is a cofactor in two independent reactions: one involves the conversion of methylmalonyl-coenzyme A (CoA) to succinyl-CoA, and the other involves the synthesis of methionine from homocysteine and methyltetrahydrofolate. The lack of B_{12} halts these reactions and results in elevated levels of the metabolites MMA and HCY. In one study, 94.5% of patients with B_{12} deficiency were found to have elevated MMA and HCY, 3.9% were found to have elevated MMA with normal HCY levels, and 1.4% were found to have normal serum MMA and elevated HCY levels. Only 0.2% of patients had normal MMA and HCY levels (2). Therefore, the diagnosis of B_{12} deficiency is very likely if both MMA and HCY are elevated and unlikely if both levels are normal.

In this patient, laboratory studies revealed a hemoglobin level of 6.0 g/dL, a hematocrit of 16.7%, and MCV of 117.2 fL. A blood smear demonstrated macroovalocytosis with a hypersegmented neutrophil (Fig. 45.1). His B_{12} level was 54 pg/mL, MMA was 111,810 nmol/L (normal = 79 to 376 nmol/L), and HCY was 211.0 μmol/L (normal = 7.4 to 15.7 μmol/L).

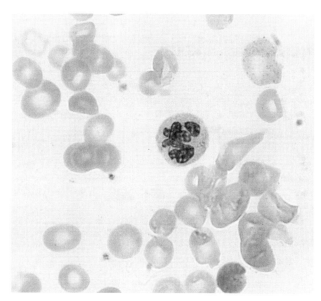

FIGURE 45.1. Slide of blood smear showing megaloblastosis with hypersegmented neutrophils.

Which of the following can cause B_{12} deficiency?

A. **Pernicious anemia**
B. **Ileal resection**
C. **Gastric resection**
D. **Chronic pancreatitis**
E. **All of the above**

B_{12} deficiency typically occurs due to malabsorption of B_{12}. Pernicious anemia is the most common cause. In normal individuals, B_{12} is bound to intrinsic factor in the stomach and absorbed in the distal ileum. Patients with pernicious anemia do not produce intrinsic factor secondary to parietal cell destruction or produce antiintrinsic factor antibodies that prevent the binding of B_{12}. Similarly, patients who have undergone gastric resection may have B_{12} deficiency due to decreased production of intrinsic factor. Since B_{12} is absorbed in the distal ileum, ileal resection results in reduced B_{12} absorption. Patients with chronic pancreatitis may not produce enough proteases required to digest proteins bound to B_{12}, which may prevent absorption. Insufficient dietary intake is another cause of B_{12} deficiency. Since B_{12} is normally found in animal products, vegans are susceptible to developing B_{12} deficiency. However, only strict vegans are susceptible, as B_{12} is also found in eggs, milk, other dairy products, and fortified foods. Other causes include severe gastritis, tropical sprue, celiac disease, Crohn disease, and blind loops. There have also been reports that acid-lowering agents, such as proton pump inhibitors and histamine-2 receptor blockers, can cause B_{12} malabsorption (7,8).

Case Continued. This patient had pernicious anemia, but his diet probably played a small role. His antiintrinsic factor antibodies and antiparietal cell antibodies tests were positive. Antiintrinsic factor antibodies are very specific and fairly sensitive for pernicious anemia; therefore, their presence establishes the diagnosis of pernicious anemia. Tests performed for antiparietal cell antibodies are not very specific and have a sensitivity that ranges from 55% to 85%, depending on the study (5,9). As a result, the use of antiparietal cell antibodies is debatable. If the etiology of vitamin B_{12} deficiency is still questionable, the Schilling test may be performed. However, many centers do not currently perform the Schilling test due to exposure to the radioactive cobalt used to tag the B_{12} and the relative effectiveness of the other tests mentioned previously.

Which of the following are effective treatment regimens for vitamin B_{12} deficiency?

A. **Monthly intramuscular B_{12} injection**
B. **Daily oral B_{12}**
C. **Daily sublingual B_{12}**
D. **Weekly intranasal B_{12}**
E. **All of the above**

The typical treatment for B_{12} deficiency is intramuscular B_{12} injection. Therapy may be required for life. Patients normally receive daily 1-mg injections for 1 week, followed by 1 mg weekly for 1 month, and 1 mg monthly afterward as maintenance treatment. Alternatively, B_{12} can be replaced with 2 mg oral B_{12} daily, which may result in better compliance from patients (10). Oral B_{12} is effective since an alternative pathway that does not require intrinsic factor absorbs a small amount of B_{12}. Sublingual B_{12}, 2 mg for 7 to 12 days (11), and intranasal B_{12} 500 μg weekly (12) have also proved to be efficacious for B_{12} replacement, but these forms of B_{12} administration are primarily used for the maintenance of B_{12} stores after initial treatment with intramuscular B_{12} injections. There is no indication for folate replacement unless patients also have folate deficiency. In fact, folate may exacerbate neuropathy when given without B_{12}.

How soon do neurologic symptoms typically improve after B_{12} replacement?

A. **1 day**
B. **3 days**
C. **2 weeks**
D. **3 months**
E. **1 year**

Once patients receive B_{12} replacement, paresthesias normally resolve within 2 weeks, followed by resolution of other neurologic signs and symptoms. Most patients improve within 3 months (1,13). In one study, 91% had more than 50% improvement and about half of the patients had complete recovery. In addition, only 7% had long-term moderate or severe neurologic disability (1). Patients may get worse during the first days or weeks before they get better.

CONCLUSION

Prognosis depends on the duration and severity of the neuropathy. Therefore, it is important to diagnose and treat B_{12} deficiency as early as possible.

REFERENCES

 1. Healton EB, Savage DG, Brust JC, et al. Neurologic aspects of cobalamin deficiency. *Medicine* 1991;70:229–245.
 2. Savage DG, Lindenbaum J, Stabler SP, et al. Sensitivity of serum methylmalonic acid and total homocysteine determinations for diagnosing cobalamin and folate deficiencies. *Am J Med* 1994; 96:239–246.
 3. Carmel R, Green R, Jacobsen DW, et al. Neutrophil nuclear segmentation in mild cobalamin deficiency: relation to metabolic tests of cobalamin status and observations on ethnic differences in neutrophil segmentation. *Am J Clin Pathol* 1996;106:57–63.
 4. Lindgren A, Swolin B, Nilsson O, et al. Serum methylmalonic acid and total homocysteine in patients with suspected cobalamin deficiency: a clinical study based on gastrointestinal histopathological findings. *Am J Hematol* 1997;56:230–238.
 5. Snow CF. Laboratory diagnosis of vitamin B_{12} and folate deficiency: a guide for the primary care physician. *Arch Intern Med* 1999;159:1289–1298.
 6. Lindenbaum J, Savage DG, Stabler SP, et al. Diagnosis of cobalamin deficiency: II. Relative sensitivities of serum cobalamin, methylmalonic acid, and total homocysteine concentrations. *Am J Hematol* 1990;34:99–107.
 7. Streeter AM, Goulston KJ, Bathur FA, et al. Cimetidine and malabsorption of cobalamin. *Dig Dis Sci* 1982;27:13–16.
 8. Marcuard SP, Albernaz L, Khazanie PG. Omeprazole therapy causes malabsorption of cyanocobalamin (vitamin B_{12}). *Ann Intern Med* 1994;120:211–215.
 9. Carmel R. Reassessment of the relative prevalences of antibodies to gastric parietal cell and to intrinsic factor in patients with pernicious anaemia: influence of patient age and race. *Clin Exp Immunol* 1992;89:74–77.
10. Kuzminski AM, Del Giacco EJ, Allen RH, et al. Effective treatment of cobalamin deficiency with oral cobalamin. *Blood* 1998; 92:1191–1198.
11. Delpre G, Stark P, Niv Y. Sublingual therapy for cobalamin deficiency as an alternative to oral and parenteral cobalamin supplementation. *Lancet* 1999;354:740–741.
12. Slot WB, Merkus FW, Van Deventer SJ, et al. Normalization of plasma vitamin B_{12} concentration by intranasal hydroxocobalamin in vitamin B_{12}-deficient patients. *Gastroenterology* 1997; 113:430–433.
13. Savage DG, Lindenbaum J. Neurological complications of acquired cobalamin deficiency: clinical aspects. *Baillieres Clin Haematol* 1995;8:657–678.

46

A 59-YEAR-OLD MAN WITH NONHEALING LOWER-EXTREMITY ULCERS

RONY M. ABOU-JAWDE
SARKIS B. BAGHDASARIAN
STEVEN K. SCHMITT
NATALIE G. CORREIA

CASE PRESENTATION

A 59-year-old white man presented with nonhealing, painful left-lower-extremity ulcers of 5 months' duration. Shortly before the first ulcer developed, the patient reported being bitten by a spider. After the bite, he developed a red, tender spot over his left lower shin that progressed to an open ulcer with purulent drainage. He denied fever or chills, but reported worsening lower-extremity edema, greater on the left leg, and severe pain at the ulcer site. The patient was treated with 4 weeks of intravenous antibiotics, wound care, and surgical debridement without significant improvement. While on antibiotics, the patient developed a new ulcer over the upper aspect of his left shin and a nodule over his right medial malleolus. Upon admission, his only complaints were painful ulcers, weakness, and fatigue.

The patient's past medical history was significant for rheumatic heart disease requiring an aortic valve replacement, culture-negative endocarditis, and bowel perforation due to diverticulitis. He denied any history of alcohol abuse or tobacco use. Family history was unremarkable.

On physical examination, the patient was afebrile with normal vital signs. He complained of pain but was not in acute distress. Head and neck, pulmonary, and abdominal examinations were unremarkable. Cardiac examination revealed regular rate and rhythm with a soft systolic ejection murmur at the left lower sternal border. The patient had two 5- × 9-cm ulcerations over the medial aspects of the upper and lower left tibia. The ulcerations had violaceous borders, punched-out-appearing bases, and minimal serous drainage (Fig. 46.1). In addition, a small, tender, erythematous nodule was present over the right medial malleolus.

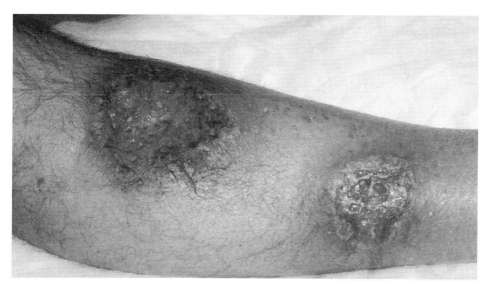

FIGURE 46.1. This patient presented with ulcerations on his left lower extremity. The ulcerations had violaceous borders, punched-out appearing bases, and minimal serous drainage.

The patient had minimal bilateral pitting edema and good capillary refill. Pulses in the distal lower extremities were 2+ bilaterally. There was no joint swelling or tenderness. Neurologic examination was nonfocal.

LABORATORY STUDIES

The patient's white blood cell count was 11.9 K/μL with 84% neutrophils. Hemoglobin was 9.4 g/dL, and platelets were 438 K/μL. His electrolytes and renal function were normal. Lower-extremity duplex ultrasound was negative for deep venous thrombosis. Plain films of the tibia and fibula were not suspicious for osteomyelitis. Transthoracic echocardiography did not demonstrate any vegetations, and blood cultures were negative. The dermatology service was consulted for a skin/ulcer biopsy.

QUESTIONS/DISCUSSION

Which of the following is the most likely cause of this patient's ulcers?

A. Peripheral arterial disease
B. Venous stasis
C. Vasculitis
D. Infection
E. Malignancy
F. C and E

Lower-extremity ulcers, especially nonhealing ulcers, can present a considerable diagnostic challenge. The differential diagnosis is wide and can involve a variety of complex disease processes.

Vascular disease, both venous and arterial, must be considered in any evaluation of nonhealing ulcers. In this patient, the presence of adequate peripheral pulses and brisk capillary refill make peripheral arterial disease a less likely cause of the patient's ulcers. Furthermore, the location of the ulcers and the associated inflammatory nodule on the right lower extremity are unlikely to be associated with an arterial process.

Patients with venous stasis can sometimes have ulcers located in the area of the lower shin. However, the presence of severe pain and the lack of significant edema in association with the ulcer make venous stasis less likely in this patient (1).

Infectious etiologies, including osteomyelitis, deep fungal infections, and septic emboli, also need to be considered. In this patient, the lack of response to a prolonged course of intravenous antibiotics and the apparent absence of vascular compromise make the diagnosis of an infectious ulcer unlikely.

Clinicians need to expand their differential diagnosis in cases such as this one, which is less likely to be due to a

venous, arterial, or infectious cause. Malignancy should be considered, with squamous cell carcinoma of the skin, basal cell carcinoma, and Kaposi sarcoma among the malignancies that can present in this manner. Other systemic processes, such as vasculitis, calciphylaxis, pyoderma gangrenosum, cryoglobulinemia, and bullous pemphigoid, also need to remain in the differential diagnosis of the patient with nonhealing ulcers (2). Therefore, pending more definitive data, both vasculitis and malignancy need to be considered among the most likely causes of this patient's ulcers.

In cases of nonhealing ulcers or ulcers of uncertain etiology, a biopsy from the wound edges or from a new ulcer is often indicated to rule out malignancy, vasculitis, or other processes, such as pyoderma gangrenosum and calciphylaxis (2).

A biopsy from this patient's left leg ulcer margin was consistent with pyoderma gangrenosum. Special stains of the biopsy tissue were negative for bacterial and fungal infections.

Pyoderma Gangrenosum

Pyoderma gangrenosum (PG) is a deforming ulcerative skin disease of unknown etiology. It typically presents with erythematous nodules or vesiculopustules on the lower extremities. These lesions often undergo rapidly destructive necrosis to form large ulcers with surrounding erythema (3).

Which of the following statements regarding pyoderma gangrenosum is incorrect?

A. It occurs with equal frequency in males and females.
B. It can develop following skin trauma.
C. Multiple myeloma is the systemic process most commonly associated with pyoderma gangrenosum.
D. Inflammatory bowel disease (IBD) is associated with both ulcerative and pustular forms of pyoderma gangrenosum.

The exact incidence of PG is difficult to determine because much of the literature is limited to small series or case reports (4). PG usually affects adults between the ages of 25 and 54 years and occurs with equal frequency in males and females (5). It can also affect children, especially in association with IBD, immunosuppression, or immunodeficiency (6). Adults can develop PG spontaneously, following trauma, or in association with a number of systemic diseases (5). Pyoderma gangrenosum can present in a variety of ways, some of which are more frequently associated with specific disease entities (Table 46.1) (4).

This patient most likely developed ulcerative pyoderma gangrenosum. An inflammatory pustule often precedes this form of pyoderma. However, some ulcerations develop from either an inflammatory nodule or trauma to normal skin (4). This patient initially developed an ulcer after skin trauma, namely, a spider bite, and then formed an ulcer from an inflamed nodule. Extremely painful and rapidly

TABLE 46.1. VARIANTS OF PYODERMA GANGRENOSUM AND ASSOCIATED DISEASES

Variant	Clinical Presentation	Associated Diseases
Ulcerative	Ulceration with purulent base and surrounding erythema. Rapid progression. Treatment: intense systemic immunosuppression	Arthritis, inflammatory bowel disease, monoclonal gammopathy
Pustular	Painful pustules on normal skin. Well controlled when underlying disease is treated.	Acute inflammatory bowel disease
Bullous	Painful bulla with rapid progression to erosive superficial ulcers. Requires systemic immunosuppression.	Myeloproliferative disorders
Vegetative	Slowly progressive, superficial ulcer. Nonpainful, solitary. Responds to topical treatment.	Rarely any associated diseases

progressive ulcers, which usually develop over several days to weeks, characterize ulcerative PG.

IBD, not multiple myeloma, is the disease entity most commonly seen in association with PG. Concomitant IBD is present in approximately one-third of patients with ulcerative PG (5). However, PG occurs in only 1.5% to 5% of all patients with IBD (7). Although pyoderma gangrenosum can precede, follow, or occur simultaneously with IBD, the two processes can develop independently from each other (4).

Case Continued. Since this patient had evidence of ulcerative pyoderma gangrenosum, he underwent further evaluation for the presence of underlying IBD, arthritis, or monoclonal gammopathy. The patient underwent a colonoscopy, which showed diverticulosis throughout the transverse colon, splenic flexure, descending, and sigmoid colon. Colonic biopsies showed chronic inflammation without evidence of IBD. The patient did not have any signs or symptoms of arthritis. Antinuclear antibody was negative, and rheumatoid factor was only minimally elevated at 23 IU/mL (normal: less than 20 IU/mL). Serum protein electrophoresis showed hypoalbuminemia and an electrophoretic pattern consistent with acute or subacute inflammation or infection. There was no evidence of a monoclonal gammopathy.

Which of the following treatment options is appropriate for pyoderma gangrenosum?

A. **Wound care and topical treatment**
B. **Systemic corticosteroids**
C. **Cyclosporine**
D. **All of the above**

The wide range of severity of disease in association with PG mandates a variety of treatment options. Therefore, all these treatment options are potentially appropriate for PG.

Pain relief, prevention or treatment of secondary wound infection, and appropriate wound care are the mainstays of local treatment. Wound care involves daily lavage with sterile saline or antiseptic solutions, the use of wet compresses or hydrocolloid occlusive dressings, and, on occasion, nonsensitizing topical antibacterial creams (4). Patients with less aggressive forms of PG may benefit from intralesional injections of triamcinolone hexacetonide (8). Other local treatment options include topical cromolyn sodium, hyperbaric oxygen, benzoyl peroxide and local irradiation of lesions (4). These local therapies are usually successful in treating the vegetative form of pyoderma gangrenosum.

Corticosteroids are the most frequently used systemic agent to treat the ulcerative, pustular, and bullous forms of pyoderma gangrenosum (4). High doses of oral prednisone (40 to 120 mg daily or a dose of approximately 1 mg/kg) are initially used for prompt control of the disease, which is defined as pain relief, reduction in erythema, and granulation at the ulcer base. High-dose corticosteroids are usually continued until the lesions are healed. Some patients require prolonged administration of low-dose corticosteroids to prevent recurrence (4). High-dose intravenous pulse steroids with 1 g of methylprednisolone for 1 to 5 days is an alternative dosing regimen designed to control ulcer pain and inflammation and reduce the likelihood of side effects associated with prolonged oral steroid therapy (9).

Immunosuppressive medications, including azathioprine, methotrexate, chlorambucil, and cyclosporine, have been used to manage pyoderma gangrenosum resistant to corticosteroid therapy. Cyclosporine has shown the most promise in the management of corticosteroid-resistant PG (10).

Oral dapsone and other oral sulfones have been used with variable success. Other antimicrobial agents, such as minocycline, have also been used to treat mild PG (11). Some treatment-resistant cases of pyoderma gangrenosum have been treated with variable success with plasmapheresis, interferon, and levamisole hydrochloride (4).

Case Conclusion

The patient was treated for the first 2 days with intravenous methylprednisolone 60 mg every 6 hours with marked improvement in pain and control of the local inflamma-

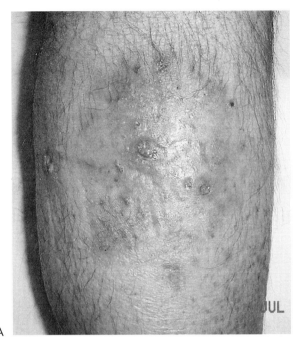
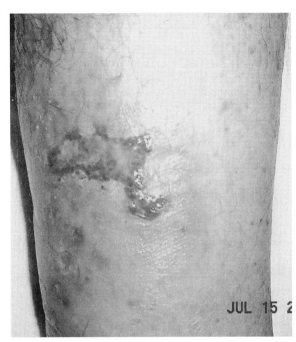

A   B

FIGURE 46.2. This patient's ulcerations after 1 month of treatment with corticosteroids. Both the ulcer in the upper tibial region (**A**) and the lower tibial region (**B**) experienced nearly complete resolution.

tion. He was discharged home on a daily dose of 40 mg of prednisone. Upon follow-up 1 month later, the patient had almost complete resolution of the ulcers on his left shin (Fig. 46.2) and the right inflammatory nodule.

CONCLUSION

This case details a presentation that clinicians in both inpatient and outpatient settings will encounter. The approach to ulcers of the extremities should include an assessment for common causes of ulcers, including infection, venous disease, arterial disease, and malignancy. If these conditions have been ruled out, less common causes such as vasculitis and, as in this case, pyoderma gangrenosum need to be considered. Nonhealing painful ulcers, especially on the lower extremities, should suggest the possibility of PG. When PG is suspected, a skin biopsy should be performed. Cultures to exclude infection also need to be obtained before initiating treatment. Systemic corticosteroids remain the most consistently effective treatment for pyoderma gangrenosum.

REFERENCES

1. Scardillo J. Unusual leg ulcers. *Ostomy Wound Manage* 1999;45:14.
2. Choucair MM, Fivenson DP. Leg ulcer diagnosis and management. *Dermatol Clin* 2001;19:659–678.
3. Holbrook MR, Doherty M, Powell RJ. Post-traumatic leg ulcer. *Ann Rheum Dis* 1996;55:214–215.
4. Powell FC, Su WP, Perry HO. Pyoderma gangrenosum: classification and management. *J Am Acad Dermatol* 1996;34:395–409.
5. Powell FC, Schroeter AL, Su WP, et al. Pyoderma gangrenosum: a review of 86 patients. *Q J Med* 1985;55:173–186.
6. Glass AT, Bancila E, Milgraum S. Pyoderma gangrenosum in infancy: the youngest reported patient. *J Am Acad Dermatol* 1991;25:109–110.
7. Johnson ML, Wilson HT. Skin lesions in ulcerative colitis. *Gut* 1969;10:255–263.
8. Gardner LW, Acker DW. Triamcinolone and pyoderma gangrenosum. *Arch Dermatol* 1972;106:599–600.
9. Johnson RB, Lazarus GS. Pulse therapy: therapeutic efficacy in the treatment of pyoderma gangrenosum. *Arch Dermatol* 1982; 118:76–84.
10. Matis WL, Ellis CN, Griffiths CE, et al. Treatment of pyoderma gangrenosum with cyclosporine. *Arch Dermatol* 1992;128:1060–1064.
11. Reynolds NJ, Peachey RD. Response of atypical bullous pyoderma gangrenosum to oral minocycline hydrochloride and topical steroids. *Acta Derm Venereol* 1990;70:538–539.

47

A 63-YEAR-OLD WOMAN WITH LEFT-SIDED WEAKNESS

ARMANDO PHILIP S. PAEZ
ANTHONY FURLAN

CASE PRESENTATION

A 63-year-old black woman with hypothyroidism and a 40-pack-year history of tobacco use presented to the emergency department after the sudden onset of left upper- and lower-extremity weakness. At home, the patient's daughter noticed her leaning to her left side while seated in a chair. The patient had difficulty moving her left arm and leg, and she noticed left arm numbness. She also developed slurred speech. She had never before experienced similar symptoms. The patient never lost consciousness and remained oriented to person, place, and time. She denied headache, dizziness, visual problems, involuntary movement, or urinary/fecal incontinence. Emergency Medical Services (EMS) brought the patient to the emergency department (ED). She arrived at the ED 2 hours after the onset of symptoms.

QUESTIONS/DISCUSSION

In this patient, which of the following should be performed first?

A. **Comprehensive history and physical examination**
B. **Carotid duplex ultrasound**
C. **Noncontrast computed tomography (CT) of the brain**
D. **Magnetic resonance imaging (MRI) of the brain**

Given this patient's presentation, the immediate concern was for an acute stroke, which is an emergency. With the advent of thrombolytic therapy for acute ischemic stroke, clinicians need to identify quickly those patients who can benefit from this therapy. A narrow 3-hour therapeutic window exists for administration of thrombolytics. This time frame is further limited by the time for transportation to the ED, basic laboratory work-up (especially to rule out bleeding tendencies), and a history and physical examina-

tion. In this setting, a well-focused history and physical examination that includes a thorough neurologic examination is more appropriate than a full and comprehensive evaluation, which can be done later. Relevant aspects of the history include the exact time the patient was last seen neurologically intact; symptoms consistent with or typical of stroke, such as hemiparesis, hemiparesthesia, aphasia, and slurring of speech; and evidence of any possible contraindications to thrombolytic therapy, such as recent trauma, surgical or invasive vascular procedures, intake of any anticoagulants, bleeding tendencies, or severe uncontrolled hypertension. The differential diagnosis of a stroke includes seizures, migraine auras, brain tumor, brain abscess, acute demyelinating diseases, hypoglycemia, syncope, drug overdose, and psychiatric causes. It is very important to rule out these possibilities before giving therapy for an acute stroke.

In a situation where obvious signs and symptoms of a stroke are present and thrombolytic therapy is being considered, neuroimaging to rule out intracranial bleeding should be performed as soon as possible. Because of its high sensitivity in identifying acute hemorrhage, noncontrast CT of the brain is the initial diagnostic study of choice (1,2). Although MRI is highly sensitive and specific, it is not as widely available as CT and may unnecessarily delay therapy. Carotid duplex ultrasound, although helpful in determining the etiology of a suspected stroke, is not indicated in screening patients for thrombolytic therapy.

In the initial hours of an acute stroke, which of the following can be seen on a CT scan of the brain?

A. **Effacement of the cerebral sulci**
B. **Evidence of subtle gray–white matter differentiation**
C. **Hyperdense middle cerebral artery**
D. **Normal findings**
E. **All of the above**

It is common to interpret a CT of the brain as normal in patients with an acute stroke, as it may take 6 hours or longer for signs of brain infarct to develop on CT. To trained eyes reading newer-generation CT scans, subtle changes such as sulcal effacement, disappearance of gray–white matter differentiation, and a hyperdense middle cerebral artery may be identifiable. These findings are early signs of brain ischemia (3,4). However, the most important information that can be obtained from CT is the absence of hemorrhage or other brain pathology, such as a tumor, that can mimic acute stroke.

With the advent of new imaging techniques, including fluid-attenuated inversion recovery imaging (FLAIR), diffusion-weighted imaging (DWI), and perfusion imaging (PI), MRI is more sensitive than CT in identifying early brain infarction. DWI is based on measurements of the Brownian movement of water molecule protons, which corresponds to a value known as the apparent diffusion coefficient (ADC). The ADC declines in ischemia, leading to the development of hyperintense signal intensity on DWI. Perfusion imaging (PI) estimates cerebral blood flow and can show a region of reduced microvascular perfusion after a stroke. An area of mismatch between DWI and PI that shows a larger abnormality on PI than on DWI is an infarct penumbra, which can potentially be salvaged by reperfusion therapy (5). Magnetic resonance angiography (MRA) will complement the study by imaging the vascular anatomy.

Case Continued. On physical examination, the patient had a blood pressure of 137/67 mm Hg, pulse of 78 beats per minute, respiratory rate of 16 per minute, and oxygen saturation of 99% on room air. She was alert and oriented to person, place, and time. She displayed good memory and attention. Moderate dysarthria was noted. There was preferential gaze to the right side, with a left partial hemianopsia. There was a left facial droop with a shallow nasolabial fold. The uvula was deviated slightly to the right on phonation, and the tongue was deviated to the left on protrusion. Sternocleidomastoid and trapezius muscle strength was normal. Motor examination showed 0 out of 5 strength in the left upper and lower extremities, except for 3 out of 5 strength on proximal hip flexion and abduction. Sensory deficits to light touch, pinprick, and proprioception in the left face and left upper extremity were present. Deep tendon reflexes were hyperreflexic, with Babinski sign present on the left side. Cardiac examination revealed regular rate and rhythm with normal first and second heart sounds; there were no murmurs, rubs, or gallops. Carotid pulses were normal, and no bruits were auscultated.

Serum electrolytes, blood glucose, complete blood count, and coagulation profile were all normal. CT of the brain showed effacement of the cerebral sulci over the right parietal region. There was also some loss of gray–white matter differentiation in the right supraparietal lobule, marginally extending into the precentral gyrus, suggesting an acute right middle cerebral artery (MCA) territory infarction (Fig. 47.1). There was no parenchymal hemorrhage, midline shift, or any extraaxial collection.

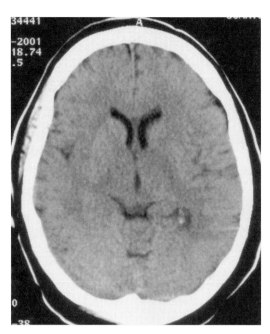

FIGURE 47.1. Noncontrast computed tomography of the brain showed effacement of the cerebral sulci over the right parietal region, loss of gray–white matter differentiation in the right supraparietal lobule. These findings were suggestive of an acute right middle cerebral artery territory infarction.

Apart from hyperthyroidism, tobacco use, and obesity, the patient did not have any other significant medical history. She had not undergone any recent invasive procedures or surgery. Her only home medication was levothyroxine 175 μg once a day. There was no history of aspirin or warfarin intake. She denied any alcohol or recreational drug use.

Is this patient a candidate for thrombolytic therapy?

A. Yes
B. No

Since the National Institute of Neurological Disorders and Stroke Recombinant Tissue Plasminogen Activator Stroke Trial (NINDS IV rt-PA Trial), all patients presenting with symptoms of a stroke within 3 hours of being seen neurologically intact should be treated with intravenous rt-PA as long as inclusion criteria (Table 47.1) are met and there are no contraindications (Table 47.2) (6). This patient

TABLE 47.1. INCLUSION CRITERIA FOR THROMBOLYTIC THERAPY

1. Ischemic stroke within 3 hr of onset, with clearly defined time of onset
2. Neurologic deficit measurable on the National Institutes of Health Stroke Scale and appropriate for such therapy
3. Computed tomography of the brain showing no evidence of intracranial hemorrhage or significant signs of early infarct

Data from refs. 6 and 20–22. (See Table 47.2 footnote for source information.)

TABLE 47.2. EXCLUSION CRITERIA FOR THROMBOLYTIC THERAPY

1. Stroke or serious head trauma within the preceding 3 months
2. Major surgery within 14 days
3. History of intracranial hemorrhage
4. Systolic blood pressure above 185 mm Hg or diastolic pressure above 110 mm Hg
5. Aggressive treatment required to reduce blood pressure to the specified limits
6. Gastrointestinal or urinary tract hemorrhage within the preceding 21 days
7. Arterial puncture within the preceding 7 days at a noncompressible site
8. Lumbar puncture within the preceding 7 days
9. Rapidly improving or minor neurologic symptoms
10. Symptoms suggestive of subarachnoid hemorrhage
11. Acute myocardial infarction (MI) or post-MI pericarditis
12. Seizure at the onset of the stroke
13. Pregnancy or lactation
14. Prothrombin time greater than 15 sec
15. Administration of heparin within the 48 hr preceding the onset of the stroke with an elevated partial thromboplastin time
16. Platelet count less than 100,000/mm^3
17. Glucose concentration below 50 mg/dL or above 400 mg/dL
18. Evidence of hemorrhage on head computed tomography (CT)
19. Evidence of major "early CT scan signs" of acute stroke: large middle cerebral artery involvement with hypodensity of the gray–white margins, or sulcal effacement in more than one-third of the middle cerebral distribution

Relative contraindication: Severe neurologic deficit, with National Institutes of Health Stroke Scale Score >22, especially in an elderly patient

Data from The National Institute of Neurological Disorders and Stroke rt-PA Stroke Study Group. Tissue plasminogen activator for acute ischemic stroke. *N Engl J Med* 1995;333:1581–1587; Adams HP Jr, Brott TG, Crowell RM, et al. Guidelines for the management of patients with acute ischemic stroke. A statement for healthcare professionals from a special writing group of the Stroke Council, American Heart Association. *Stroke* 1994;25:1901–1914; Adams HP Jr, Brott TG, Furlan AJ, et al. Guidelines of thrombolytic therapy for acute stroke: a supplement to the guidelines for the management of patients with acute ischemic stroke. *Circulation* 1996;94:1167–1174; and National Stroke Association (NSA). Stroke the first hours: the guidelines for acute treatment. Consensus Statement. 2000.

is a good candidate for thrombolytic therapy because she presented to the ED 2 hours after the onset of her neurologic symptoms, she had no hemorrhage seen on CT, and she had no other contraindications. The NINDS Trial showed that patients treated with rt-PA were at least 30% more likely to have minimal or no disability at 3 months, with an 11% to 12% absolute increase in neurologic recovery on the assessment scales. Moreover, the benefit was sustained at 12-month follow-up (7).

Although symptomatic intracerebral hemorrhage was significantly higher in the rt-PA group than in the placebo group, mortality was not increased. Since thrombolytic therapy in acute stroke carries an increased risk of brain hemorrhage, it is crucial in acute stroke management to follow closely the key components of the NINDS Trial (6,8,9). The National Institutes of Health (NIH) Stroke Scale is a standardized and validated tool that should be used in the initial evaluation and monitoring of progress. It is a 42-point scoring system that quantifies neurologic deficits in 11 categories (10,11). The NIH Stroke Scale assesses level of consciousness, attention, gaze, visual deficits, facial palsy, motor function, limb ataxia, sensory deficits, and language (Table 47.3). The rt-PA dose is 0.9 mg/kg, up to a maximum of 90 mg. Ten percent of the dose is given as a bolus, with the remainder given as an infusion over 60 minutes. Postthrombolytic therapy guidelines should always be followed, especially maintaining the blood pressure below 180/100 mm Hg (Table 47.4).

In selected patients beyond 3 hours but within 6 hours of the onset of neurologic deficits, intraarterial thrombolysis with prourokinase has demonstrated clinical efficacy (12). Hypothermia has shown some promise in decreasing infarct size and is currently being investigated in clinical trials. However, at present, there is no clinically proven neuroprotective agent that can limit brain infarcts.

Hospital Course

In the ED, the patient's NIH Stroke Scale (NIHSS) score was 17. After informed consent was obtained, the patient

TABLE 47.3. THE NATIONAL INSTITUTES OF HEALTH STROKE SCALE

1a. Level of consciousness (LOC)	0: Alert; keenly responsive
	1: Not alert, but arousable by minor stimulation to obey, answer, or respond
	2: Not alert, requires repeated stimulation to attend, or is obtunded and requires strong or painful stimulation to make movements (not stereotyped)
	3: Respond only with reflex motor or autonomic effects or totally unresponsive, flaccid, and areflexic
1b. LOC questions	0: Answers both questions correctly
	1: Answers one question correctly
	2: Answers neither question correctly
1c. LOC commands	0: Performs both tasks correctly
	1: Performs one task correctly
	2: Performs neither task correctly

Continued on next page

TABLE 47.3. *(CONTINUED)*

2. Best gaze	0: Normal
	1: Partial gaze palsy. This score is given when gaze is abnormal in one or both eyes, but forced deviation or total gaze paresis is not present
	2: Forced deviation, or total gaze paresis not overcome by the oculocephalic maneuver
3. Visual	0: No visual loss
	1: Partial hemianopia
	2: Complete hemianopia
	3: Bilateral hemianopia (blind, including cortical blindness)
4. Facial palsy	0: Normal symmetric movement
	1: Minor paralysis (flattened nasolabial fold, asymmetry on smiling)
	2: Partial paralysis (total or near total paralysis of lower face)
	3: Complete paralysis (absence of facial movement in the upper and lower face)
5 and 6. Motor Arm and Leg	0: No drift, arm holds 90 (or 45) degrees for full 10 sec
	1: Drift, arm holds 90 (or 45) degrees but drifts down before full 10 sec; does not hit bed or other support
	2: Some effort against gravity, arm cannot get to or maintain (if cued), 90 (or 45) degrees, drifts down to bed, but has some effort against gravity
	3: No effort against gravity, arm falls
	4: No movement
	x: Amputation, joint fusion
	5a: Left arm
	5b: Right arm
	0: No drift, limb holds 30 degrees position for full 5 sec
	1: Drift, leg falls by the end of the 5-sec period but does not hit bed
	2: Some effort against gravity, leg falls in bed by 5 sec but has some effort against gravity
	3: No effort against gravity, leg falls immediately
	4: No movement
	x: Amputation, joint fusion
	6a: Left leg
	6b: Right leg
7. Limb ataxia	0: Absent
	1: Present in one limb
	2: Present in two limbs
	x: Amputation or joint fusion
8. Sensory	0: Normal; no sensory loss
	1: Mild to moderate sensory loss; pinprick is less sharp or is dull on the affected side; or there is a loss of superficial pain with pinprick but patient is aware he/she is being touched
	2: Severe to total sensory loss; patient is not aware of being touched
9. Best language	0: No aphasia, normal
	1: Mild to moderate aphasia; some obvious loss of fluency or facility of comprehension, without significant limitation of ideas expressed or form of expression. Reduction of speech and/or comprehension, however, makes conversation about provided material difficult or impossible. For example, in conversation about provided materials, examiner can identify picture or naming card from patient's response
	2: Severe aphasia; all communication is through fragmentary expression; great need for inference, questioning, and guessing by the listener. Range of information that can be exchanged is limited; listener carries burden of communication. Examiner cannot identify materials provided from patient's response
	3: Mute, global aphasia; no usable speech or auditory comprehension
10. Dysarthria	0: Normal
	1: Mild to moderate; patient slurs at least some words and, at worst, can be understood with some difficulty
	2: Severe; patient's speech is so slurred as to be unintelligible in the absence of or out of proportion to any dysphasia, or is mute/anarthric
	x: Intubated or other physical barrier; explain
11. Extinction and inattention (neglect)	0: No abnormality
	1: Visual, tactile, auditory, spatial, or personal inattention or extinction to bilateral simultaneous stimulation in one of the sensory modalities
	2: Profound hemi-inattention or hemi-inattention to more than one modality. Does not recognize own hand or orients to only one side of space

Data from Brott T, Adams HP Jr, Olinger CP, et al. Measurements of acute cerebral infarction: a clinical examination scale. *Stroke* 1989;20:864–870; and Lyden P, Brott T, Tilley B, et al. Improved reliability of the NIH Stroke Scale using video training. NINDS TPA Stroke Study Group. *Stroke* 1994;25:2220–2226.

TABLE 47.4. GUIDELINES FOR MONITORING POSTTHROMBOLYTIC THERAPY

1. Vital signs and neurologic status should be closely monitored. Blood pressure should be maintained below 185/100 mm Hg.
2. A follow-up CT scan should be obtained 24 hr following administration of rt-PA to rule out intracranial hemorrhage. Patients with worsening neurologic status should have a CT scan on an emergent basis.
3. No anticoagulant or antiplatelet therapy should be initiated for 24 hr following the administration of rt-PA.

Data from refs. 6 and 20–22. (See Table 47.2 footnote for source information.)

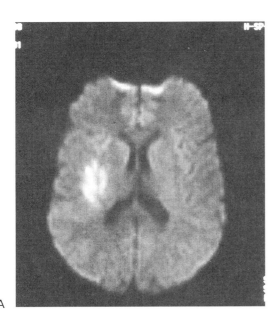

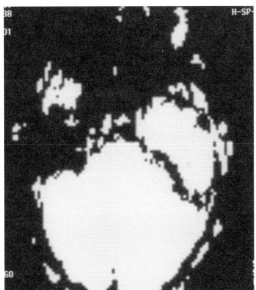

FIGURE 47.2. Diffusion-weighted image (**A**) and perfusion image (**B**). This patient's magnetic resonance imaging of the brain confirmed a right middle cerebral artery distribution infarct.

received rt-PA therapy based on the hospital stroke protocol. She was monitored in the neurologic intensive care unit (NICU) for 2 days, where blood pressure was maintained below 185/100 mm Hg. Normothermia was maintained, and hyperglycemia was avoided. MRI of the brain confirmed a right MCA distribution infarct (Fig. 47.2), and the MRA showed an occlusion of the right MCA just before the bifurcation (Fig. 47.3). Twenty-four hours after rt-PA infusion, the patient's NIHSS score was 8, with a persistent left hemianopsia, left facial droop, minimal weakness of the left upper extremity, mild sensory deficit, and slight dysarthria. Two days after admission, she was transferred to a regular nursing floor, where she started to receive physical therapy.

In this patient, which of the following is/are appropriate diagnostic or therapeutic strategies to help prevent a recurrent stroke?

A. Aspirin therapy
B. Smoking cessation
C. HMG–CoA reductase inhibitor
D. All of the above

This patient was further evaluated to identify factors contributing to her stroke. A carotid duplex ultrasound did not reveal any significant stenoses. In blacks, disease involving the intracranial vessels is more common than extracranial disease (13). A lipid profile showed total cholesterol of 271 mg/dL, high-density lipoprotein of 93 mg/dL, low-density lipoprotein of 161 mg/dL, and triglycerides of 83 mg/dL. Since therapy with aspirin and HMG–CoA reductase inhibitors has protective effects in the secondary prevention of stroke, this patient was started on atorvastatin 10 mg once a day and

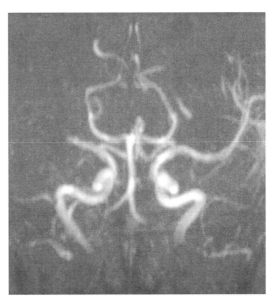

FIGURE 47.3. Intracranial magnetic resonance angiogram showed an occlusion of the right middle cerebral artery just before the bifurcation.

aspirin 81 mg once a day (14–16). Aspirin has a comparable effect to warfarin in preventing recurrences of acute ischemic stroke (17). The patient was advised to stop smoking, as tobacco use increases the likelihood of stroke (18). A transthoracic echocardiogram was unremarkable. Interestingly, hypertension, the most common and most important risk factor for stroke, was absent in this patient.

At the time of discharge, 7 days after the event, NIHSS score was 6 with improved dysarthria. The patient could sit at the edge of the bed and ambulate independently with a walker. At the subacute rehabilitation facility, she continued physical therapy. Twenty days after the acute event, repeat MRI of the brain showed recanalization of the occluded distal right MCA.

CONCLUSION

Although neurologists are primarily involved in the care of patients with acute strokes, internists also need to recognize the indications and contraindications for the administration of thrombolytic therapy. It is expected that acute stroke management will rapidly evolve as technological advances occur. Understanding stroke therapy and keeping up with the latest advances will help provide effective therapy and prevent serious complications. Efforts to address important issues in the management of acute stroke include recommendations for the establishment of primary stroke centers, as outlined by the Brain Attack Coalition, and the formulation and updates of specific guidelines for thrombolytic therapy (19–22). Online information about stroke can be found at *http://www.stroke-site.org*.

REFERENCES

1. Caplan LR, DeWitt LD, Breen JC. Neuroimaging in patients with cerebrovascular disease. In: *Neuroimaging*, 2nd ed. New York: McGraw-Hill, 1995:493–520.
2. Eckert B, Zeumer H. Brain computed tomography. In: *Cerebrovascular disease: pathophysiology, diagnosis, and management*. Boston: Blackwell Science, 1998:1241.
3. Von Kummer R, Nolte PN, Schnittger H, et al. Detectability of cerebral hemisphere ischaemic infarcts by CT within 6 h of stroke. *Neuroradiology* 1996;38:31–33.
4. Von Kummer R, Meyding-Lamade U, Forsting M, et al. Sensitivity and prognostic value of early CT in occlusion of the middle cerebral artery. *Am J Neuroradiol* 1994;15:9–18.
5. Fisher M, Albers GW. Applications of diffusion-perfusion magnetic resonance imaging in acute ischemic stroke. *Neurology* 1999;52:1750–1756.
6. The National Institute of Neurological Disorders and Stroke rt-PA Stroke Study Group. Tissue plasminogen activator for acute ischemic stroke. *N Engl J Med* 1995;333:1581–1587.
7. Kwiatkowski TG, Libman RB, Frankel M, et al. Effects of tissue plasminogen activator for acute ischemic stroke at one year. National Institute of Neurological Disorders and Stroke Recombinant Tissue Plasminogen Activator Stroke Study Group. *N Engl J Med* 1999;340:1781–1787.
8. Thrombolytic therapy with streptokinase in acute ischemic stroke. The Multicenter Acute Stroke Trial—Europe Study Group. *N Engl J Med* 1996;335:145–150.
9. Hacke W, Kaste M, Fieschi C, et al. Randomised double-blind placebo-controlled trial of thrombolytic therapy with intravenous alteplase in acute ischaemic stroke (ECASS II). Second European-Australasian Acute Stroke Study Investigators. *Lancet* 1998;352:1245–1251.
10. Brott T, Adams HP Jr, Olinger CP, et al. Measurements of acute cerebral infarction: a clinical examination scale. *Stroke* 1989;20: 864–870.
11. Lyden P, Brott T, Tilley B, et al. Improved reliability of the NIH Stroke Scale using video training. NINDS TPA Stroke Study Group. *Stroke* 1994;25:2220–2226.
12. Furlan A, Higashida R, Wechsler L, et al. Intra-arterial prourokinase for acute ischemic stroke. The PROACT II study: a randomized controlled trial: prolyse in acute cerebral thromboembolism. *JAMA* 1999;282:2003–2011.
13. Caplan LR, Gorelick PB, Hier DN. Race, sex and occlusive cerebrovascular disease: a review. *Stroke* 1986;17:648–655.
14. Byington RP, Davis BR, Plehn JF, et al. Reduction of stroke events with pravastatin: the Prospective Pravastatin Pooling (PPP) Project. *Circulation* 2001;103:387–392.
15. Di Mascio R, Marchioli R, Tognoni G. Cholesterol reduction and stroke occurrence: an overview of randomized clinical trials. *Cerebrovascular Dis* 2000;10:85–92.
16. A randomised, blinded, trial of clopidogrel versus aspirin in patients at risk of ischaemic events (CAPRIE). CAPRIE Steering Committee. *Lancet* 1996;348:1329–1339.
17. Mohr JP, Thompson JL, Lazar RM, et al. A comparison of warfarin and aspirin for the prevention of recurrent ischemic stroke. *N Engl J Med* 2001;345:1444–1451.
18. Kawachi I, Colditz GA, Stampfer MJ, et al. Smoking cessation and decreased risk of stroke in women. *JAMA* 1993;269: 232–236.
19. Alberts MJ, Hademenos G, Latchaw RE, et al. Recommendations for the establishment of primary stroke centers. Brain Attack Coalition. *JAMA* 2000;283:3102–3109.
20. Adams HP Jr, Brott TG, Crowell RM, et al. Guidelines for the management of patients with acute ischemic stroke. A statement for healthcare professionals from a special writing group of the Stroke Council, American Heart Association. *Stroke* 1994;25: 1901–1914.
21. Adams HP Jr, Brott TG, Furlan AJ, et al. Guidelines of thrombolytic therapy for acute stroke: a supplement to the guidelines for the management of patients with acute ischemic stroke. *Circulation* 1996;94:1167–1174.
22. National Stroke Association (NSA). Stroke the first hours: the guidelines for acute treatment. Consensus Statement. 2000.

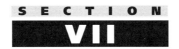

SECTION
VII

NEPHROLOGY

48

A 69-YEAR-OLD WOMAN WITH SUBCUTANEOUS NODULES AND ARTHRALGIAS

GAZALA N. KHAN
BYRON J. HOOGWERF

CASE PRESENTATION

A 69-year-old white woman presented with a symptom complex of generalized arthralgias, subcutaneous nodules, emesis, and ulcerative skin lesions. Her symptoms started approximately 2 weeks before presentation, when she had an insidious onset of nausea, emesis, and generalized arthralgias. Associated with these symptoms, she noticed multiple purplish nodules, predominantly in her lower extremities. These nodules were extremely painful and tender to touch. Subsequently, they ulcerated into nonhealing ulcers with black eschar formation.

The patient's past medical history was notable for type 2 diabetes mellitus for 30 years, chronic renal insufficiency (baseline creatinine of 1.9 mg/dL), hypothyroidism, hypercholesterolemia, a mitral valve replacement with St. Jude valve, and chronic anticoagulation for 7 years before presentation. Medications on admission included digoxin, extended-release metoprolol, levothyroxine, warfarin 2.5 mg once a day, amiodarone, iron sulfate, prednisone 5 mg once a day, allopurinol, and NPH insulin. The patient was married, with two healthy children. There was no history of tobacco or alcohol abuse. Family history was significant for type 2 diabetes mellitus in the patient's mother.

Physical examination revealed a moderately built white woman who appeared to be in mild distress. The patient's pulse was 85 beats per minute and regular, blood pressure was 128/76 mm Hg in the supine position, respiratory rate was 16 per minute, and pulse oximetry was 96% on room air. Cardiac examination revealed a grade II/VI holosystolic murmur that radiated to the left axilla. Pulses were normal, except for a diminished dorsalis pedis pulse on the left side. There were multiple violaceous, exquisitely tender nodules in a reticulate pattern, predominantly located on the distal lower extremities. Some of the nodules had focal central necrosis. Associated with these were cutaneous ulcers with an indurated, exquisitely tender base, with black eschar formation (Fig. 48.1). There was no associated pedal edema.

QUESTIONS/DISCUSSION

Which of the following should be included in the differential diagnosis of the skin lesions in this patient?

A. **Embolic phenomena**
B. **Calciphylaxis**
C. **Warfarin skin necrosis**
D. **Cutaneous anthrax**
E. **All of the above**

Embolic phenomena resulting from infective endocarditis and atheroembolism are typically associated with necrotic-appearing cutaneous ulcerations. Infective endocarditis can be associated with embolic phenomena such as Osler nodes, Janeway lesions, and splinter hemorrhages. However, corroborative evidence such as positive blood cul-

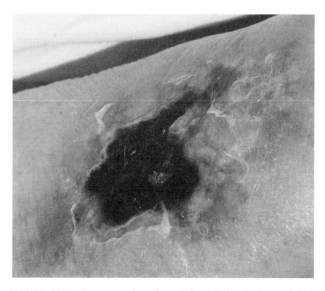

FIGURE 48.1. Cutaneous leg ulcer with an indurated, exquisitely tender base and black eschar formation.

tures and typical echocardiographic findings are needed to make the diagnosis. Also, lesions are typically not associated with eschar formation. On the other hand, atheroembolism is usually iatrogenic but can also be spontaneous. The clinical picture of atheroembolism can vary from mild livedo reticularis to severe limb pain, cyanosis, and eventual tissue loss with concurrent elevated plasma muscle enzymes and myoglobinuria, which can be associated with rising creatinine, oliguria, and urine eosinophils in renal atheroemboli. Cases of iatrogenic atheroembolism usually occur after aortic catheterization procedures. The diagnosis of cholesterol emboli can be confirmed by skin biopsy of peripheral lesions demonstrating cholesterol crystals in the capillaries.

Nodules due to calciphylaxis present as multiple, violaceous, exquisitely tender nodules that ulcerate with a tender indurated base and black eschar formation. The ulcers associated with calciphylaxis typically do not heal and are usually located on the lower extremities, buttocks, and abdomen. They are often seen in patients with end-stage renal disease (1,2).

Reactions similar to those described earlier also occur in warfarin-associated necrosis of the skin. These reactions usually develop 3 to 10 days after introduction of the medication, with women developing the reaction more frequently than men. Lesions are typically erythematous, indurated, and tender. These may either resolve or progress to hemorrhagic, bullous formations that ulcerate to form slow-healing eschars. They are usually associated with protein C deficiency from warfarin-induced inhibition of its vitamin K–dependent synthesis, with resultant hypercoagulability and microvascular thrombosis. Treatment involves administration of vitamin K and heparin.

Cutaneous anthrax usually develops as a small red macule that progresses to vesicular and pustular stages, and subsequently to ulcerations with black eschar formation. Early lesions may be pruritic, but cutaneous anthrax ulcers usually are painless and associated with brawny edema that can be extensive. Small satellite lesions surround the primary lesion, and again, are typically painless. Usually, a history of contact with animal products is present.

All the preceding choices should be included in the differential diagnosis of the skin lesions seen in this patient.

Hospital Course: Routine hematologic and biochemical investigations were performed (Table 48.1). These were remarkable for elevated blood urea nitrogen and creatinine, elevated parathyroid hormone, and elevated calcium–phosphorus product. Blood cultures were negative. A transesophageal echocardiogram was unremarkable. The patient was started on intravenous antibiotics for presumed culture-negative endocarditis. After 10 days in the hospital, the patient's condition deteriorated. A full-thickness skin biopsy was performed (Fig. 48.2).

The biopsy specimen shown in Fig. 48.2 revealed intimal hyperplasia, associated with calcification of the tunica

TABLE 48.1. LABORATORY DATA ON ADMISSION AND 1 MONTH PRIOR

	Admission	One Month Prior
Sodium	137	137
Potassium	4	4.7
Chloride	92	92
Bicarbonate	32	33
Blood urea nitrogen	47	58
Creatinine	2.1	1.9
Glucose	77	198
Calcium	9.1	8.9
Phosphorus	3.7	2.2
Magnesium	2.2	2.1
Alkaline phosphatase	102	119
Calcium–phosphorous product	33.67	19.58
Parathyroid hormone	144	130

media and luminal thrombosis. These findings are consistent with calciphylaxis. Calcific uremic arteriolopathy (*calciphylaxis* was the original term coined by Hans Selye) is commonly associated with medial calcification (3–5). Intimal hyperplasia may then develop reactive to the medial calcification, resulting in narrowing of the arterial lumen (≤40 μm). This luminal narrowing predisposes to noninflammatory thrombosis and dermal necrosis.

Which of the following is/are associated with calciphylaxis?

A. Cryofibrinogenemia
B. Activated protein C and S deficiency
C. Secondary hyperparathyroidism
D. Elevated calcium phosphorus product
E. All of the above

Cryofibrinogenemia is a disorder characterized by an abnormal, circulating, cold-insoluble complex called a *cryoprecipitate*, which consists of fibrin, fibrinogen, fibrin split products with albumin, cold-insoluble globulin, factor VIII, and plasma proteins (6). Clinically, cryofibrinogenemia often manifests with thromboembolic phenomena involving skin and viscera, although it may be asymptomatic. Common clinical associations include malignancies, collagen vascular disorders, and calciphylaxis. Treatment includes plasmapheresis and fibrinolytics.

Activated protein C and S deficiency have been hypothesized to predispose to the development of calcific uremic arteriolopathy. However, these hypotheses have not been supported by several case series. Functional protein C and S deficiencies have been implicated in warfarin-associated skin necrosis, but the exact role in calcific uremic arteriolopathy is controversial.

Secondary hyperparathyroidism is commonly associated with chronic renal disease owing to a decrease in levels of 1,25 (OH)$_2$ D$_2$ and compensatory hyperparathyroidism. A series by Oh et al. demonstrated elevated parathyroid hor-

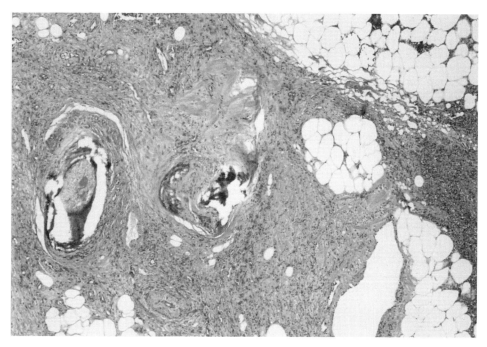

FIGURE 48.2. Skin biopsy showing intimal hyperplasia, calcification of the tunica media, and luminal thrombosis. These findings are consistent with calciphylaxis.

mone in 80% of patients (1). This may lead to elevated calcium and predispose to metastatic calcification.

Presence of an elevated calcium–phosphorus product is commonly associated with end-stage renal disease. In a study by Budisavljevic et al. (2), calcium–phosphorous product was found elevated in 33% of patients with calciphylaxis.

All the previously mentioned conditions are associated with calciphylaxis. The patient in question had chronic renal disease, associated with secondary hyperparathyroidism and an elevated calcium–phosphorus product. All these conditions predisposed her to calcific uremic arteriolopathy.

All of the following modalities are considered potential treatments of calciphylaxis except:

A. **Parathyroidectomy**
B. **Hyperbaric oxygen**
C. **Bisphosphonates**
D. **Removal of sensitizing/challenging agents**
E. **Aggressive wound management**
F. **Glucocorticoids**

Parathyroidectomy promotes wound healing and prolongs survival, and is usually advocated in patients with secondary hyperparathyroidism. A recent study by Girotto et al. randomized two groups of patients to either parathyroidectomy or medical management alone. The group that underwent parathyroidectomy had a significantly longer median survival than the group that received medical

management alone (36 versus 3 months) (7). However, as of now, the exact role of parathyroidectomy is controversial.

Hyperbaric oxygen has long been used to enhance wound healing. Podymow et al. recently reported almost complete resolution of necrotic cutaneous ulcerations with the use of hyperbaric oxygen (at 2.5 atmospheres), compared with the group treated with normobaric oxygen (8,9). This treatment modality could be advocated in the absence of hyperparathyroidism.

In a study involving a rat model, bisphosphonates prevented the induction of experimental calciphylaxis but did not seem to have an effect on the disease once it was established (10,11). The mechanism of action presumably involves abrogation of the effect of calcium that acts as a challenger in the pathogenesis of calciphylaxis. Conclusive data on humans are lacking.

Originally, Selye postulated that calciphylaxis was a condition typically involving an interaction between sensitizers and challengers. Sensitizers are usually systemic calcifying factors such as vitamin D or parathyroid hormone, and challengers are agents that precipitate calciphylaxis. Typical challengers include albumin, blood products, parenteral iron, immunosuppressive agents, and glucocorticoids. Hence removal or avoidance of the use of these agents could be advocated as part of the treatment of calciphylaxis.

Calciphylaxis carries a very high mortality—almost 80% in some series. The leading cause of mortality is overwhelming sepsis, especially in the presence of an immunocompromised state, as seen in transplant recipients. Hence, aggressive wound management, local debridement, and systemic antibiotics may be crucial in preventing mortality.

Glucocorticoids are potential "challengers" and should be avoided in uremic arteriolopathy.

CONCLUSION

The patient was aggressively treated with antibiotics and wound debridement. Toward the end of her second week in the hospital, her clinical condition improved, and she was discharged home after 16 days in the hospital.

REFERENCES

1. Oh DH, Eulau D, Tokugawa DA, et al. Five cases of calciphylaxis and a review of the literature. *J Am Acad Dermatol* 1999;40: 979–987.
2. Budisavljevic MN, Cheek D, Ploth DW. Calciphylaxis in chronic renal failure. *J Am Soc Nephrol* 1996;7:978–982.
3. Howe SC, Murray JD, Reeves RT, et al. Calciphylaxis, a poorly understood clinical syndrome: three case reports and a review of the literature. *Ann Vasc Surg* 2001;15:470–473.
4. Case records of the Massachusetts General Hospital. Weekly clinicopathological exercises. Case 31-2001. A 70-year-old woman with end-stage renal disease and cutaneous ulcers. *N Engl J Med* 2001;345:1119–1124.
5. Mathur RV, Shortland JR, el-Nahas AM. Calciphylaxis. *Postgrad Med J* 2001;77:557–561.
6. Sankarasubbaiyan S, Scott G, Holley JL. Cryofibrinogenemia: an addition to the differential diagnosis of calciphylaxis in end-stage renal disease. *Am J Kidney Dis* 1998;32:494–498.
7. Girotto JA, Harmon JW, Ratner LE, et al. Parathyroidectomy promotes wound healing and prolongs survival in patients with calciphylaxis from secondary hyperparathyroidism. *Surgery* 2001;130:645–651.
8. Podymow T, Wherrett C, Burns KD. Hyperbaric oxygen in the treatment of calciphylaxis: a case series. *Nephrol Dial Transplant* 2001;16:2176–2180.
9. Benedetto BJ, Emhoff TA. The use of hyperbaric oxygen for the management of calciphylaxis. *Curr Surg* 2001;57:507.
10. Miller S, Vernon-Roberts E, McClure J. Cutaneous calciphylactic reactions in the mouse and the rat and the effects of diphosphonates on the reaction in the rat. *J Pathol* 1984;142:7–13.
11. Rosenblum IY, Black HE, Ferrell JF. The effects of various diphosphonates on a rat model of cardiac calciphylaxis. *Calcif Tissue Res* 1977;23:151–159.

49

A HEALTHY 23-YEAR-OLD MAN WITH ACUTE MENTAL STATUS CHANGE

KEVIN J. MIKIELSKI
RICHARD A. FATICA

CASE PRESENTATION

While at work, a healthy 23-year-old man developed sudden onset of nausea, vomiting, and abdominal pain. Before leaving for work 7 hours earlier, his family stated that he was in his usual state of health. He experienced worsening symptoms while at work. When taken home by a friend 5 hours after the onset of symptoms, his family stated that he was lethargic and intermittently confused. Early the next morning, the patient was found lying unresponsive in a "pool of vomit." On presentation to another institution, his blood pressure was 126/74 mm Hg; pulse, 90 per minute; respiratory rate, 14 per minute; pulse oximetry, 94% on room air; and temperature, 37.4°C. He had no spontaneous or provoked eye opening, limb movements, or vocalization. Laboratory studies revealed sodium of 154 mmol/L, potassium of 5.1 mmol/L, chloride of 111 mmol/L, bicarbonate (HCO_3) of 7 mmol/L, blood urea nitrogen of 12 mg/dL, creatinine (Cr) of 1.1 mg/dL, glucose of 124 mg/dL, and normal liver enzymes. The calculated anion gap was 36 mmol/L. Arterial blood gas (ABG) on 2 L/min of oxygen revealed pH of 7.1, P_aCO_2 of 20 mm Hg, P_aO_2 of 154 mm Hg, HCO_3 of 7 mmol/L, and lactate of 8.4 mmol/L.

QUESTIONS/DISCUSSION

All of the following are causes of a high anion gap metabolic acidosis except:

A. Diabetic ketoacidosis
B. Methanol ingestion
C. Ethylene glycol ingestion
D. Isopropyl alcohol ingestion
E. Salicylate ingestion

Isopropyl alcohol ingestion may result in an elevated osmolal gap but is not associated with a high anion gap metabolic acidosis. All the other choices may cause high anion gap metabolic acidosis.

Complete blood count (CBC) and cerebrospinal fluid analysis were within normal limits. Computed tomography (CT) of the head without contrast was negative for any acute process. Urine and serum toxicology screens were negative. Before transfer, the patient suffered a generalized tonic–clonic seizure, for which he received intravenous lorazepam and a loading dose of fosphenytoin. He was also intubated for airway protection and started on an intravenous infusion of sodium bicarbonate. The patient was transferred to our institution for further management.

Upon arrival (approximately 9 hours after initial presentation), the patient remained unresponsive but had intact brainstem reflexes. Myoclonic jerks were also observed. Pertinent laboratory studies following transfer included HCO_3, 8 mmol/L; Cr, 2.2 mg/dL; calcium, 7.6 mg/dL; calculated anion gap of 35 mmol/L; and normal liver enzymes. ABG on arrival revealed pH of 7.21; P_aCO_2 of 21 mm Hg; P_aO_2 of 587 mm Hg; HCO_3 of 8 mmol/L on 100% FIO_2. Lactate was 9.3 mmol/L. Measured osmolality was 326 mOsm/kg, resulting in an osmolal gap of 8 mOsm/kg. Urinalysis revealed 300 mg/dL protein, no ketones, 1+ blood, and three to five red blood cells/high power field. Microscopic examination of the urine revealed many monohydrate calcium oxalate crystals. The urine did not fluoresce when examined with a Wood light. The patient became oliguric, and the creatinine rose rapidly to 4.2 mg/dL. He was subsequently started on continuous venous–venous hemodiafiltration (CVVHD) on the evening of admission.

What is the most likely diagnosis?

A. Methanol ingestion
B. Ethylene glycol ingestion
C. Ethanol ingestion
D. Salicylate ingestion
E. Alcoholic ketoacidosis

Methanol ingestion (wood alcohol) is associated with a high anion gap metabolic acidosis and central nervous system damage, including optic neuritis. An osmolal gap (>10) is usually present. However, calcium oxalate crystals are not found in the urine.

Ethanol ingestion is not associated with a high anion gap metabolic acidosis and urinary calcium oxalate crystals. An osmolal gap (>10) is usually present.

Salicylate ingestion is associated with a high anion gap metabolic acidosis, often with accompanying respiratory alkalosis. An osmolal gap and calcium oxalate crystals in the urine are not present.

Alcoholic ketoacidosis is associated with a high anion gap metabolic acidosis and may occur when chronic alcoholics abruptly cease the consumption of alcohol. It is not associated with an elevated osmolal gap or with calcium oxalate crystals in the urine. Ketones are usually detectable in the serum and urine.

Ethylene glycol ingestion is the correct answer. It is associated with a high anion gap metabolic acidosis and urinary calcium oxalate crystals. An osmolal gap is usually, but not always, present.

Ethylene glycol, methanol, paraldehyde, and acetaldehyde levels (all drawn more than 28 hours after the patient's initial complaints) were negative. Discussion with the patient's family revealed that he had not been depressed and had not discussed suicide in the previous weeks. His parents searched the house for empty antifreeze and chemical containers, but none were found. The patient worked at a bowling alley, and his boss and co-workers stated that he worked with several solvent agents.

Over the following 3 days, he regained consciousness and was extubated. He denied intentionally ingesting antifreeze or solvents as a suicide attempt. He was discharged and his renal function was supported by hemodialysis for approximately 3 months. The patient's serum creatinine eventually declined to 1.6 mg/dL. He was left without any permanent neurologic deficits.

A criminal investigation revealed that a co-worker of the patient had attempted to poison another co-worker with a solvent used at the bowling alley. The perpetrator mistakenly dumped the solvent in the patient's cola fountain drink.

Ethylene Glycol

Ethylene glycol is a sweet-tasting, viscous, nonvolatile, and colorless liquid (1). It is a polyalcohol used extensively as antifreeze and solvent in many household cleaning products. Ethylene glycol is also used in pesticides, air conditioners, brake fluid, fire extinguishers, and deicing solutions (2). Because of its accessibility, ethylene glycol is a fairly common culprit in overdoses, both in accidental ingestions and suicide attempts. Alcoholics frequently use it as an alcohol substitute because of its low cost, sweet taste, and mildly intoxicating effects.

Pharmacokinetics

Ethylene glycol is highly water-soluble and rapidly absorbed from the gastrointestinal tract. Once absorbed, it is evenly distributed to all tissues. Peak serum levels occur 1 to 4 hours following ingestion (3). The half-life is 3 to 8 hours, and elimination follows zero-order kinetics (4). Approximately 20% to 50% is excreted unchanged or as a primary metabolite in the urine (1). Ethylene glycol is a harmless chemical, but hepatic metabolism yields toxic end products (5). Alcohol dehydrogenase oxidizes ethylene glycol to glycoaldehyde. Aldehyde dehydrogenase then rapidly oxidizes glycoaldehyde to glycolic acid, which is oxidized to glyoxylic acid by lactic dehydrogenase or glycolic acid oxidase. Glyoxylic acid is converted to oxalic acid, which then rapidly binds with calcium to form calcium oxalate crystals. The crystals are then deposited in most body tissues. The conversion of glycolic to glyoxylic acid is the rate-limiting step, so the accumulation of glycolic acid is largely responsible for the metabolic acidosis that occurs with ethylene glycol poisoning. The metabolism of ethylene glycol is dependent on NAD and results in elevated levels of NADH, which facilitates the conversion of pyruvate to lactate (6). The elevated lactate level also contributes to the severity of the metabolic acidosis. The metabolites of ethylene glycol may be present in the serum for several days.

Clinical Effects

The clinical syndrome of ethylene glycol intoxication has been described as occurring in three stages. However, the signs, symptoms, and timing of each stage are highly variable. Stage 1 occurs within 30 minutes to 12 hours following ingestion and is characterized by central nervous system (CNS) involvement. Common findings include slurred speech, somnolence, ataxia, myoclonic jerks, seizures, and CNS depression. Nausea and vomiting frequently occur. Stage 2 occurs from 12 to 36 hours after ingestion and is characterized by cardiopulmonary involvement. Tachycardia, hypertension, congestive heart failure, and muscle spasms are common signs. Death most commonly occurs during this stage in untreated patients. Stage 3 occurs 24 to 72 hours following ingestion, and renal involvement is the characteristic finding. Renal failure, bone marrow suppression, and neuropathy are reported to occur during this stage (1,5,6).

The clinical effects observed following ethylene glycol ingestion result from the metabolic and toxic effects of ethylene glycol metabolites and calcium oxalate–induced tissue injury and dysfunction (1,2).

Diagnosis

The most definitive means of diagnosing ethylene glycol ingestion is the direct measurement of the serum ethylene glycol concentration (6). However, many hospital laboratories are not equipped to perform the assay. If the patient presents several hours after ingestion, ethylene glycol in the serum may be undetectable because of its rapid metabolism (3). Therefore, a presumptive diagnosis must be made based on clinical presentation and laboratory studies. The presence of a high anion gap metabolic acidosis should alert the physician to the possibility of ethylene glycol ingestion. A high anion gap metabolic acidosis is present in most cases and is secondary to the metabolites and not to ethylene glycol itself (3). Lactic acidosis is a late finding in ethylene glycol ingestion (1). An osmolal gap of more than 10 is also suggestive of ethylene glycol ingestion. The osmolal gap is secondary to ethylene glycol itself but may be absent in some cases of ethylene glycol ingestion (6). The absence of an osmolal gap is a common finding in patients presenting late following ingestion (2). An osmolal gap may also be present in cases of other alcohol ingestions, including ethanol, methanol, and isopropyl alcohol (6).

Hypocalcemia may also be present because ethylene glycol is metabolized to calcium oxalate (6). Urinalysis reveals proteinuria and hematuria in approximately 50% of cases (1). Calcium oxalate crystals may be seen on microscopic examination of the urine in 30% to 50% of cases (1,6). The presence of needle-shaped (monohydrate) or envelope-shaped (dihydrate) calcium oxalate crystals may be extremely helpful in establishing the presumptive diagnosis (Fig. 49.1) (6). Fluorescence of the urine under a Wood lamp supports ethylene glycol ingestion in the form of antifreeze because fluorescein is added to most commercial antifreeze products (4). Acute renal failure usually occurs and is thought to be secondary to multiple factors, including acute tubular necrosis (6), renal parenchymal toxicity, and obstruction of the renal medulla by calcium oxalate crystals (2).

Treatment

Following initial assessment, stabilization of the airway, breathing, and circulation is the first priority. Because of the

prolonged time required to obtain the results of the serum ethylene glycol assay, empiric treatment should be promptly initiated based on the history, physical examination, and laboratory results. Administration of syrup of ipecac and activated charcoal have not been shown to be beneficial because of the rapid absorption of ethylene glycol (5). Most sources recommend intravenous administration of sodium bicarbonate, which will increase urine output, treat the metabolic acidosis, and aid in the urinary excretion of ethylene glycol (2). Hemodialysis is utilized to enhance the elimination of ethylene glycol and its water-soluble metabolites (5). The metabolites of ethylene glycol are extremely toxic and cause the majority of metabolic derangements and organ dysfunction that result from ingestion. Therefore, the most important step in management is inhibition of ethylene glycol metabolism (1).

Through which of the following enzymes does ethanol and fomepizole competitively inhibit the metabolism of ethylene glycol?

A. **Alcohol reductase**
B. **Alcohol dehydrogenase**
C. **Lactic dehydrogenase**
D. **Aldehyde dehydrogenase**

Ethanol and fomepizole are potent inhibitors of alcohol dehydrogenase. Ethanol has greater affinity for alcohol dehydrogenase than ethylene glycol does. Ethanol may be administered orally, but the intravenous form is recommended. Inebriation is a major side effect of ethanol administration. Worsening CNS depression may occur, which can interfere with the evaluation of the clinical status of the patient. Fomepizole (4-methylpyrazole) also inhibits alcohol dehydrogenase and is available in intravenous form (7). Inebriation is not a side effect (7). Fomepizole is the only treatment approved by the Food and Drug Administration for ethylene glycol poisoning (6). Thiamine, folate, and pyridoxine should also be administered because they

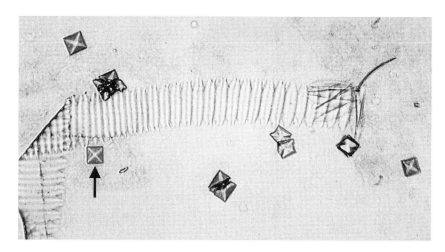

FIGURE 49.1. Urine sediment demonstrating dihydrate calcium oxalate crystals (*arrow*).

are cofactors in the pathway of ethylene glycol metabolism (3,4).

Prognosis

Limited data are available regarding the recovery and long-term prognosis of patients who suffer ethylene glycol poisoning. Recovery and long-term prognosis are favorable if patients survive the initial metabolic derangements and toxic effects (1). Very few patients with ethylene glycol–induced acute renal failure require chronic hemodialysis or renal transplant (2). Psychiatric care is essential for those patients whose ingestion was a suicide attempt.

CONCLUSION

Ethylene glycol ingestion is potentially fatal and needs to be recognized quickly. The presence of a high anion gap metabolic acidosis, elevated osmolal gap (>10), and urinary calcium oxalate crystals are highly suggestive of ethylene glycol poisoning. Treatment should be rapidly initiated based on a presumptive diagnosis. Treatment should not be delayed while waiting for the results of the serum ethylene glycol concentration.

REFERENCES

1. Egbert PA, Abraham K. Ethylene glycol intoxication: pathophysiology, diagnosis, and emergency management. *ANNA J* 1999;26: 295–300.
2. Davis DP, Bramwell KJ, Hamilton RS, et al. Ethylene glycol poisoning: case report of a record-high level and a review. *J Emerg Med* 1997;15:653–667.
3. De Chazal I, Houghton B, Frock J. The "sweet killer." Can you recognize the symptoms of ethylene glycol poisoning? *Postgrad Med* 1999;106:221–230.
4. Albertson TE. Plenty to fear from toxic alcohols. *Crit Care Med* 1999;27:2834–2836.
5. Zimmerman HE, Burkhart KK, Donovan JW. Ethylene glycol and methanol poisoning: diagnosis and treatment. *J Emerg Nurs* 1999; 25:116–120.
6. Brent J. Current management of ethylene glycol poisoning. *Drugs* 2001;61:979–988.
7. Brent J, McMartin K, Phillips S, et al. Fomepizole for the treatment of ethylene glycol poisoning. Methylpyrazole for Toxic Alcohols Study Group. *N Engl J Med* 1999;340:832–838.

50

A 77-YEAR-OLD MAN WITH ALTERED MENTAL STATUS

ANDREA WANG-GILLAM
JOHN KEVIN HIX
SAUL NURKO

CASE PRESENTATION

A 77-year-old man was transferred to our institution with altered mental status and acute renal failure. Two months earlier, the patient underwent a left total hip arthroplasty. His postoperative course was complicated by a wound infection with methicillin-resistant *Staphylococcus aureus* (MRSA) and vancomycin-sensitive *Enterococcus* that required removal of his hip prosthesis and placement of an antibiotic-impregnated cement spacer. He received approximately 4 weeks of intravenous vancomycin and gentamicin before being rehospitalized with *Pseudomonas* urosepsis. He developed worsening azotemia, and gentamicin was switched to cefepime.

Four days into his hospitalization at the outside institution, the patient was transferred to the intensive care unit (ICU) because of deteriorating respiratory status and non-oliguric renal failure. At that time, he was fully oriented and able to follow verbal commands. Laboratory data included sodium of 144 mmol/L, blood urea nitrogen of 66 mg/dL, and creatinine of 4.5 mg/dL. (Creatinine was 1.1 mg/dL 2 weeks prior.) On the second day in the ICU, the patient's respiratory status improved with diuresis, and his oxygen saturation remained above 95% on 4 L of oxygen per minute. Because of diminished oral intake, the patient was placed on 50 mL/hr of half-normal saline with 5% dextrose and 40 milliequivalents (mEq) of potassium chloride. On the fourth day in the ICU, the patient became unarousable, with chorealike movements of the arms and constant lip smacking.

The patient's past medical history was significant for hypertension, a prior stroke without residual weakness, diabetes mellitus, osteoarthritis, and hyperlipidemia. He underwent a St. Jude aortic valve replacement 20 years prior for aortic stenosis and was on long-term warfarin. Medications on transfer included famotidine, cefepime, subcutaneous heparin, intravenous narcotics as needed, and tube feedings.

Upon arrival at our institution, vital signs included a temperature of 37.5°C, blood pressure of 116/58 mm Hg, pulse of 71 beats per minute, respiratory rate of 18 per minute, and oxygen saturation of 98% on 5 L oxygen per minute via nasal cannula. The patient was unresponsive to verbal or tactile stimuli, with constant lip smacking and arm movements. His oropharynx was dry, and inspection of the neck did not reveal jugular venous distension. Examination of the chest was notable for decreased breath sounds at the bases without rales. Cardiac and abdominal examinations were unremarkable. Neurologic examination did not reveal any evidence of posturing. Deep tendon reflexes were 2+ throughout. There was 2+ pitting edema in the lower extremities and a stage 2 pressure ulcer over the sacrum.

Laboratory data obtained 1 day before transfer revealed sodium of 158 mmol/L, potassium of 4.4 mmol/L, chloride of 113 mmol/L, bicarbonate of 32 mmol/L, blood urea nitrogen of 90 mg/dL, creatinine of 5.2 mg/dL, glucose of 223 mg/dL, and serum osmolality of 353 mOsm/kg. Complete blood count showed a white blood cell count of 16.7 K/μL with 84% neutrophils, hemoglobin of 11.4 g/dL, and platelet count of 584 K/μL. Blood and urine cultures did not reveal any growth. An electrocardiogram revealed normal sinus rhythm without acute changes, and a chest x-ray did not reveal any infiltrate or edema.

QUESTIONS/DISCUSSION

Which of the following is a possible cause of this patient's altered mental status?

A. Infection
B. Central nervous system (CNS) event
C. Hypernatremia
D. Famotidine
E. All of the above

In a patient with multiple medical problems and a prolonged hospitalization, it is often challenging to diagnose the cause or causes of altered mental status. Therefore, on initial assessment, all the preceding should be considered possible causes of this patient's altered mental status.

Infection: In this case, leukocytosis suggested the possibility of either a nosocomial infection, such as pneumonia, or an unresolved infection, such as a persistent urinary tract infection. Although this patient's blood and urine cultures were negative upon transfer and chest radiography did not reveal evidence of pneumonia, the possibility of an infection, including one involving the prosthetic joint, should still be considered in this patient.

CNS events such as a stroke or seizure are possible in this setting. The patient's change in mental status was quite sudden. With his history of prior stroke, hypertension, and diabetes, a new stroke could have occurred. While the new onset of chorea-like arm movements and lip smacking without an obvious focal neurologic deficit were less suggestive of stroke, new-onset seizures remain a possibility.

Medications can frequently cause delirium in hospitalized patients, especially older patients. Since this patient had received famotidine and narcotics, both of which can cause delirium, medications need to be considered a possibility.

Hypernatremia is defined as serum sodium greater than 145 mmol/L with an osmolality greater than 290 mOsm/kg. This patient's sodium rapidly increased from 144 mmol/L to 158 mmol/L, with a serum osmolality of 353 mOsm/kg. In addition, the development of hypernatremia appeared to correlate with the onset of the patient's delirium. Therefore, altered mental status secondary to hypernatremia needs to be strongly considered in this case.

Case Continued: Computed tomography (CT) of the head did not reveal any acute ischemic changes or hemorrhage, and an electroencephalogram (EEG) did not reveal any epileptiform activity. Cardiac enzymes were negative. Urine sodium was 45 mmol/L, and urine osmolality was 435 mOsm/kg. Plain films of the left hip did not show evidence of osteomyelitis. Renal ultrasound did not show any evidence of hydronephrosis. All medications were discontinued. Blood and urine cultures remained negative. Since the patient's mental status had not improved at this point, hypernatremia was thought to be the most likely cause of his altered mental status.

Hypernatremia can affect all hospitalized patients. Populations at greatest risk for developing hypernatremia include patients receiving tube feeds or parenteral nutrition, patients without access to free water, patients with already altered mental status, patients at the extremes of age, and patients receiving osmotic diuretics (1). The clinical manifestations of hypernatremia can include irritability, restlessness, muscle twitching, hyperreflexia, seizure, and coma. The development of these signs and symptoms often correlate with the severity of hypernatremia. Hypernatremia has been reported to carry a mortality rate of 40% to 55%. Factors correlating with an increased risk of mortality include the magnitude of hypernatremia, the rapidity of onset, and the mechanism of hypernatremia (2).

What type of hypernatremia does this patient have?

A. **Hypervolemic hypernatremia**
B. **Euvolemic hypernatremia**
C. **Hypovolemic hypernatremia**

Hypernatremia can result from either water loss or sodium retention. When assessing a patient with hypernatremia, clinicians should estimate total body volume and then place the patient into one of three categories based on his or her total body sodium and water.

Hypervolemic hypernatremia is the least common form of hypernatremia. Both total body sodium and water increase, but the increase in sodium exceeds the increase in total body water. This form of hypernatremia usually results from excess infusion of hypertonic solution, such as 3% sodium chloride (NaCl) or sodium bicarbonate. Patients generally display signs of volume overload, such as jugular venous distension and pulmonary edema, although they may not demonstrate evidence of weight gain and peripheral edema.

Euvolemic hypernatremia reflects normal total body sodium with decreased total body water. In euvolemic hypernatremia, the loss of free water without an accompanying loss of sodium can occur without overt signs of intravascular volume contraction. Water loss can occur from either renal or extrarenal sources. Renal water losses occur due to underproduction of antidiuretic hormone (ADH) in the hypothalamus (central diabetes insipidus), diminished responsiveness to ADH within the kidney (nephrogenic diabetes insipidus), or loss of water while excreting hypertonic urine (osmotic diuretics). These conditions disrupt the ability of the kidneys to conserve water maximally. Extrarenal causes of water loss include situations of increased insensible losses (excess sweating or burns) and gastrointestinal losses, particularly in patients in whom losses are replaced with hypertonic solutions or tube feeds.

Patients with *hypovolemic hypernatremia* lose both total body water and sodium, but lose more free water. Clinical features in this setting include decreased skin turgor, decreased capillary refill, and dry oral mucosa. More sensitive signs of volume depletion include flat neck veins and orthostatic hypotension. Hypotension and tachycardia can also signify severe volume depletion. Patients with hypovolemic hypernatremia typically suffer fluid losses from either the kidneys or gastrointestinal tract. Renal causes of fluid loss include medications, especially loop diuretics, the polyuric phase of acute tubular necrosis, and postobstructive diuresis. Common gastrointestinal causes include vomiting and enterocutaneous fistulas (3). These patients may also develop other electrolyte abnormalities, including hypokalemia and hypercalcemia. In this case, the patient had hypovolemic hypernatremia without signs of circulatory compromise.

Which of the following is the most likely contributing factor in the development of this patient's hypernatremia?

A. Impaired thirst mechanism
B. Hypertonic infusion of saline
C. Diabetes insipidus
D. Acute renal failure
E. A and D

Hypernatremia results from either water losses or sodium retention. An *impaired thirst mechanism* can develop with aging or primary hypodipsia, which is an uncommon condition. Although these patients have appropriate stimuli when they develop a hypertonic state, they do not appropriately sense thirst. A diminished thirst mechanism can result from the destruction of the hypothalamic thirst center by metastatic tumors, granulomatous disease, vascular disease, and trauma (4). Hypodipsic hypernatremia develops most often in the geriatric population, as changes associated with aging appear to decrease the sensitivity to thirst stimuli. The elderly may develop a deficit involving an opioid-dependent mechanism that helps generate the motivation to drink (5). This patient could have had age-associated impairment in his thirst response. Furthermore, while in the hospital, the patient likely had impaired access to free water. Clinicians need to assess the adequacy of water replacement in patients who struggle to access free water on their own.

Hypertonic infusion of saline is the most common iatrogenic form of hypernatremia. Patients who receive hypertonic solutions, such as 3% normal saline or sodium bicarbonate infusions, are prone to developing hypernatremia. Hypernatremia can also result when patients receive isotonic saline without adequate free water replacement of daily hypotonic insensible losses.

Diabetes insipidus (DI) is characterized by a lack of production of ADH (central DI) or a lack of response to ADH (nephrogenic DI), both of which result in dilute urine, polyuria, and polydipsia. A urine osmolality of less than 200 mOsm/kg in the setting of serum hyperosmolality typically represents some form of diabetes insipidus, which can be further differentiated by response to exogenous ADH. Since central DI results from a defect in ADH production or secretion, administration of exogenous ADH will promptly restore the ability of the kidneys to concentrate urine (at least a 50% increase in urine osmolality) and result in a reduced urine volume. Central DI develops due to destruction of the neurohypophysis as a result of head trauma, granulomatous disease, CNS tumors, cerebrovascular disease, infection, or idiopathic causes (6). Nephrogenic DI results from resistance to the action of ADH; therefore, exogenous administration of ADH will seldom produce a

significant change in urine osmolality or volume. Etiologies of nephrogenic DI include congenital causes, medications (lithium, amphotericin B), chronic tubulointerstitial diseases, and electrolyte disorders. In either form of diabetes insipidus, the combination of dilute urine and polyuria leads to hypernatremia. With urine sodium of 45 mmol/L and osmolality of 435 mOsm/kg, this patient's hypernatremia is unlikely to be due to DI.

Acute renal failure by itself does not typically produce hypernatremia. Renal dysfunction does impair the kidney's ability to concentrate urine maximally both by tubular dysfunction and by resistance to the effects of ADH. However, these changes are typically counterbalanced by a reduction in total urine output. Therefore, in the absence of polyuria, serum osmolality often remains within normal limits.

This patient presented with a complex picture, including acute renal failure, hypovolemia, hypernatremia, and altered mental status. The primary physiologic defenses against hypernatremia and hypovolemia are to increase free water and volume intake and to minimize urinary excretion of water and sodium so as to restore isotonicity and euvolemia. In this case, the patient's medical condition prohibited his access to free water, while the acute renal failure resulted in a diminished ability to concentrate the urine. The patient likely developed hypernatremia due to a lack of access to free water and volume depletion in the setting of renal failure. Therefore, choice E is the correct answer.

Treatment of hypernatremia requires understanding that an overly conservative approach to lowering serum osmolality can cause ongoing morbidity and an overly aggressive approach to lowering serum osmolality can cause cerebral edema, neurologic damage, and death. Although definitive trials are lacking, current recommendations favor lowering the serum sodium concentration at a rate of no faster than 12 mmol/L over 24 hours, unless the patient has ongoing life-threatening symptoms attributable to hypernatremia.

Two crucial factors in the management of hypernatremia are the volume status and the rate at which hypernatremia developed. *Volume assessment* needs to occur before instituting free water replacement. In the setting of volume depletion, normal saline is an appropriate initial intravenous fluid to restore intravascular volume. In contrast, a hypervolemic state should be treated with diuretics. In the presence of renal failure and volume overload, dialysis may be an appropriate option. After euvolemia has been achieved, treatment geared specifically toward free water replacement should be initiated.

Calculation of free water deficit: The following formula is commonly used to calculate the free water deficit: water deficit = total body water × (plasma sodium − 140)/140. The total body water equals 60% of lean body mass in kg in men and 50% of lean body mass in women (6). Since this patient weighed 70 kg, his total body water was approximately 42 L. With a sodium concentration of 158 mmol/L, the calculated free water deficit was 5.4 L. This calculation estimates the deficit at the time the laboratory values are measured and does not account for maintenance free water and ongoing losses.

Choice of fluid replacement: Several types of solutions can be used to treat hypernatremia, including free water, 5% dextrose with free water, one-quarter normal saline, and one-half normal saline. Free water can be administered orally or through a feeding tube. Other fluids can be given only intravenously, and both routes are frequently utilized to achieve optimal correction of sodium.

The *infusion rate of fluids* depends on the rate at which the hypernatremia developed. Hypernatremia causes dehydration of neurons. The initial hypertonicity of neurons is partially compensated for by a shift of electrolytes into the brain cells within a few hours of the development of hypernatremia (rapid adaptation). This mechanism creates a gradient that favors the entry of water back into the neurons. Normalization of cerebral volume then occurs over several days as a result of the intracellular accumulation of organic solutes (slow adaptation) (7). These intracellular accumulations allow the central nervous system to adapt to the hypernatremia. From a clinical perspective, if hypernatremia is corrected too quickly, the intracellular environment may remain hyperosmolar, which favors continued entry of free water into the cells and could cause cellular edema, damage, and/or rupture. Therefore, in a patient who develops hypernatremia over a few hours, sodium should not be corrected any faster than at a rate of 1 mmol/L/hr. If a patient develops hypernatremia over a few days, then serum sodium should not be corrected any faster than 0.5 mmol/L/hr. Generally, half of the free water deficit should be replaced in the initial 12 to 24 hours, with the rest of the water deficit replaced over the next 1 to 2 days (5). Both mental status and serum sodium should be monitored carefully during fluid replacement. If mental status deteriorates, fluid infusion should be stopped promptly to assess for cerebral edema.

For patients with hypernatremia due to diabetes insipidus, desmopressin is effective for only central DI. Amiloride has been reported to be useful in the setting of lithium-induced nephrogenic DI (1). Accepted treatment for all forms of symptomatic nephrogenic DI includes thiazide diuretics and a low-sodium, low-protein diet.

CONCLUSION

In this patient with a free water deficit of 5 L, 2.5 L of free water was administered in the first 24 hours, both through a nasogastric tube and intravenously as one half normal saline. The following day, the serum sodium decreased to 149 mmol/L. As the serum sodium returned to normal with adequate free water replacement, the patient returned to his baseline mental status on the third day of admission. The patient's renal function steadily improved, ultimately returning to his baseline.

REFERENCES

1. Kumar S, Berl T. Sodium. *Lancet* 1998;352:220–228.
2. Long CA, Marin P, Bayer AJ, et al. Hypernatremia in an adult inpatient population. *Postgrad Med J* 1991;67:643–645.
3. Fried LF, Palevsky PM. Hyponatremia and hypernatremia. *Med Clin North Am* 1997;81:585–609.
4. Kugler JP, Hustead T. Hyponatremia and hypernatremia in the elderly. *Am Fam Physician* 2000;61:3623–3630.
5. Beck LH. Changes in renal function with aging. *Clin Geriatr Med* 1998;14:199–209.
6. Singer GG. Fluid and electrolyte management. In: Ahya SN, Flood K, Paranjothi S, eds. *The Washington manual of medical therapeutics,* 30th ed. Philadephia: Lippincott Williams & Wilkins, 2001:43–75.
7. Adrogue HJ, Madias NE. Hypernatremia. *N Engl J Med* 2000; 342:1493–1499.

51

NAUSEA, VOMITING, AND CONFUSION IN A 74-YEAR-OLD WOMAN

ROHTASHAV DHIR
NATALIE G. CORREIA

CASE PRESENTATION

A 74-year-old woman presented to the emergency department (ED) with 1 day of nausea and vomiting. Several hours before presentation, she developed confusion and slurred speech. In the ED, she experienced a generalized tonic–clonic seizure, which lasted less than 15 seconds. Her past medical history was significant for a left-sided stroke 1 year before presentation, hypertension, diet-controlled diabetes mellitus, hyperthyroidism, and anxiety disorder. Her medications on presentation included triamterene/hydrochlorothiazide (triamterene/HCTZ), olanzapine, propylthiouracil, warfarin, enalapril, and estrogen.

On physical examination, the patient was thin and anxious looking, oriented only to person. Her temperature was 36.9°C; blood pressure, 199/96 mm Hg; pulse, 95 beats per minute; and respiratory rate, 22 per minute. Her skin turgor was normal; oral mucosa was moist. There was no meningismus. Reflexes were normal bilaterally. She was moving her upper and lower extremities spontaneously. Further neurologic examination could not be performed because of her inability to follow commands. The remainder of the physical examination was unremarkable.

QUESTIONS/DISCUSSION

Which of the following is least likely to be the cause of the patient's symptoms?

A. Stroke
B. Dementia
C. Infection
D. Medication toxicity
E. Metabolic causes

Stroke is the most commonly identified cause of seizures in the elderly, accounting for up to 33% of cases in one series (1). Cerebral cortical involvement appears to be the most important risk factor for the development of seizure following stroke. Lacunar infarcts are generally not associated with seizures (2). Hemorrhagic strokes are more likely than ischemic strokes to result in seizures. Even though most stroke-associated seizures are focal, secondarily generalized seizures are not uncommon, occurring in up to 28% of cases (3). Therefore, the generalized seizure this patient experienced could be due to a stroke. This patient's history of hypertension and diabetes heightens the suspicion for an ischemic cerebrovascular event.

Neurodegenerative disorders occur commonly in the elderly, accounting for up to 10% of seizures in this population (1). Seizures associated with Alzheimer dementia are usually generalized tonic–clonic and not difficult to control. The sudden onset of acute mental status changes in this patient makes dementia an unlikely cause of her symptoms.

Central nervous system (CNS) infection remains an important consideration in this patient. The absence of fever does not rule out infection, as 5% to 6% of patients with bacterial meningitis can present without fever (4).

The elderly are particularly susceptible to the toxic effects of medications. Some factors implicated are changes in volume of distribution, altered drug elimination and receptor sensitivity, existing co-morbid illness, and polypharmacy (5). Medications most commonly implicated in the development of delirium include neuroleptic agents, narcotics, anticholinergic medications, nonsteroidal antiinflammatory drugs, and benzodiazepines.

A variety of metabolic and electrolyte disorders can produce acute mental status changes and seizures in the elderly. Disturbances involving sodium, magnesium, and calcium need to be considered. Motor seizures have been documented with hyperglycemia (6). Thyrotoxicosis can also present with delirium and seizures. These conditions are important considerations in this patient, given her history of hyperthyroidism and diabetes.

The patient's initial laboratory studies were significant for sodium (112 mmol/L), potassium (4.1 mmol/L), blood urea nitrogen (BUN) (9 mg/dL), creatinine (0.9 mg/dL), glucose (223 mg/dL), thyroid stimulating hormone (0.23 μU/mL). Serum osmolality was calculated to be 239 mOsm/kg using the formula (2 × sodium) + (glucose/18) + (BUN/2.8). Urine osmolality was measured as 378 mOsm/kg, and urine sodium was 51 mmol/L. Computed tomography of the brain without contrast did not reveal an acute bleed. Cerebrospinal fluid analysis following lumbar puncture did not show any evidence of infection. A chest x-ray did not show any abnormalities.

Based on the presentation and laboratory data, the patient's symptoms were thought to be due to severe hyponatremia.

In hyponatremia, the osmotic pressure gradient leads to the movement of water into brain cells and the development of cerebral edema, which results in the neurologic symptoms of hyponatremia. Gradual onset of hyponatremia enables the brain to adapt to minimize brain swelling. Rapid development of hyponatremia precludes such an adaptation. Therefore, clinical manifestations of hyponatremia relate not only to the serum concentration but also to the rapidity with which hyponatremia develops. Severe hyponatremia may present with headache, nausea, vomiting, muscle cramps, lethargy, confusion, muscle twitching, convulsions, coma, and respiratory arrest.

When assessing hyponatremic patients, clinicians should differentiate hyponatremia into hypo-, iso-, or hypertonic hyponatremia based on the serum osmolality. Hyponatremia associated with normal tonicity is observed in extreme hyperlipidemia or hyperproteinemia and is a consequence of using flame emission spectrometry to measure sodium concentration (pseudohyponatremia).

Hypertonic hyponatremia occurs as a result of the accumulation of osmotically active nonelectrolyte solutes. These solutes cause water to move into the extracellular spaces, which causes dilution of the serum sodium concentration. This is commonly seen in hyperglycemia. Sodium concentration falls by approximately 1.6 mmol/L for every 100 mg/dL increase in blood glucose.

Most hyponatremia occurs in the setting of hypotonicity. Hypotonic hyponatremia should be classified according to the volume status of the patient as euvolemic, hypovolemic, or hypervolemic hyponatremia. A physical examination focused on the presence of orthostasis, dry mucous membranes, edema, jugular venous distension, ascites, and pulmonary edema can provide an estimate of volume status.

Urine osmolality may be helpful in assessing the etiology of hyponatremia. If the urine osmolality is < 100 mOsm/L, the patient is excreting appropriately diluted urine and an evaluation for primary polydipsia should be performed (7,8). In other cases of hypotonic hyponatremia, urine sodium measurement in conjunction with volume status assessment can help delineate the cause of hyponatremia (Fig. 51.1).

Which of the following statements about the syndrome of inappropriate antidiuretic hormone (SIADH) is false?

A. SIADH is the most common cause of hyponatremia in hospitalized patients.
B. Common causes are malignancies, pulmonary disease, and central nervous system (CNS) disorders.
C. SIADH may be induced by medications.
D. The urine is "inappropriately" concentrated (>100 mOsm/kg), given the state of hypotonicity (effective osmolality < 270 mOsm/kg).
E. SIADH is usually associated with high serum uric acid levels.

SIADH represents a state of continued vasopressin release in the presence of increased total body water and decreased total body sodium. ADH levels are abnormal in relation to plasma osmolality. The urine remains concentrated, leading to less than maximally diluted urine (i.e., urine osmolality > 100 mOsm/kg). SIADH is the most common cause of hyponatremia in hospitalized patients, accounting for one-quarter of the cases in one series (9). Cancers cause ectopic production of ADH, which may lead to the development of SIADH. CNS disorders, including tumor, infection, trauma, and stroke, may stimulate excessive ADH release. Numerous medications can cause SIADH by stimulating ADH release or potentiating its effects. SIADH is a diagnosis of exclusion. In particular, hypothyroidism and glucocorticoid deficiency should be excluded before diagnosing SIADH. Uric acid levels in SIADH are often low. Treatment for SIADH typically focuses on fluid restriction. In resistant cases, demeclocycline may be used to antagonize the action of ADH.

On further questioning, it was revealed that the patient was started on triamterene/HCTZ for control of hypertension 2 weeks before presentation. This medication was thought to be the most likely cause of this patient's hyponatremia.

Most cases of diuretic-induced hyponatremia occur within 2 weeks of starting treatment, with small elderly women at greatest risk. Thiazide diuretics are implicated more often than other classes of diuretics. Hyponatremia is thought to develop due to an excessive natriuretic effect of thiazides coupled with ADH release in response to diuretic-induced hypovolemia. Diuretic-induced potassium loss in the urine leading to the movement of sodium into cells may also contribute to hyponatremia (10,11). Even though volume depletion appears to be important in the genesis of diuretic-induced hyponatremia, most patients appear euvolemic on presentation (12).

Which of the following is true about the therapy for hyponatremia in this patient?

A. Rapid correction with hypertonic saline is indicated.

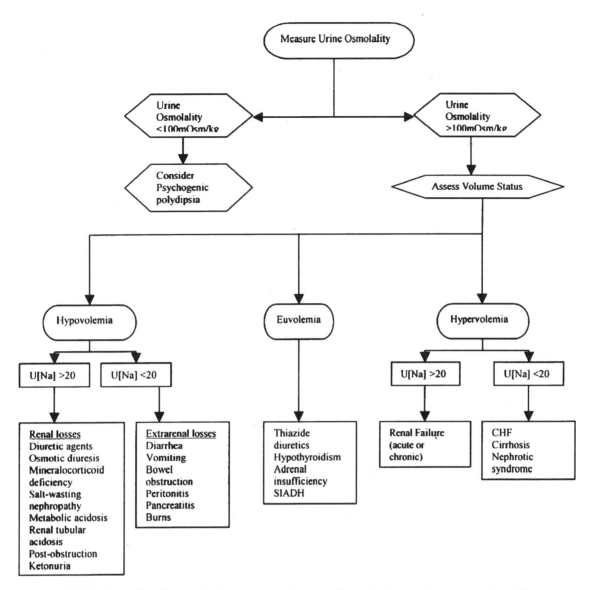

FIGURE 51.1. Algorithm outlining the approach to a patient with hypotonic hyponatremia. *CHF*, congestive heart failure; *SIADH*, syndrome of inappropriate antidiuretic hormone.

B. **Slow correction with isotonic saline is indicated.**
C. **Water restriction only is the appropriate therapeutic strategy.**
D. **Aggressive therapy should be continued until sodium reaches normal range.**
E. **Diuretics should be avoided in this patient during therapy.**

Acute-onset hyponatremia carries a high risk of permanent neurological sequelae from cerebral edema and requires rapid correction, especially in the presence of neurologic symptoms. Patients with chronic hyponatremia develop adaptive mechanisms in brain cells, which result in the immediate loss of cerebral extracellular fluid followed by the loss of potassium and organic solutes from brain cells. These mechanisms decrease intracerebral osmolality and prevent the development of brain edema. Rapid correction of hyponatremia in chronic cases can cause excessive loss of cerebral water from previously adapted brain cells, leading to osmotic demyelination. Therefore, if the duration of onset of hyponatremia is unknown, the rate and magnitude of correction should be sufficient to reverse manifestations of hypotonicity, without posing a risk of osmotic demyelination by too rapid correction.

Patients with hyponatremia in the setting of severe volume depletion can often be treated with isotonic saline. As volume is repleted, the stimulus for ADH production will cease, and the body will rapidly excrete dilute urine, result-

TABLE 51.1. CALCULATIONS FOR RATE OF SODIUM INFUSION

Estimated change in serum sodium (by infusing 1 L of infusate)	= (Infusate Na+) − (Serum Na+) / Total body water + 1
Total body water	= 0.6 × body weight [Male]
	0.5 × body weight [Female]
Rate of infusion	= Targeted change in serum Na / Estimated change in serum Na

ing in resolution of the hyponatremia. Correction with hypertonic saline is required in patients with serious neurologic manifestations of hyponatremia. Loop diuretics, such as furosemide, are often combined with hypertonic saline to limit treatment-induced expansion of extracellular fluid volume, which may precipitate congestive heart failure (CHF). The optimal rate of sodium correction is debatable; however, in symptomatic patients, it is reasonable to increase the sodium at a rate of 1 to 2 mmol/L/hr for up to 4 hours (13). In patients with less severe symptoms or with chronic hyponatremia, the correction rate should be approximately 0.5 mmol/L/hr. Symptoms may resolve with relatively small increases in sodium concentration; therefore, complete correction is not required.

Once the target sodium level and the desired rate of correction have been determined, the rate of infusion of the fluid of choice can be calculated by the formula presented in Table 51.1 (13). Rapid correction of sodium can be stopped once life-threatening symptoms have resolved or a sodium concentration of 120 to 130 mmol/L is achieved. Complete correction is usually unnecessary.

Treatment of hyponatremia in hypervolemic states requires attention to the underlying disorder. For instance, in patients with CHF, optimization of cardiac output by decreasing the afterload and increasing cardiac contractility helps resolve the hyponatremia.

CONCLUSION

Because of this patient's severe neurologic symptoms, she was initially treated with infusion of hypertonic saline (3%). The patient's total body water was estimated to be 30 L, based on her weight of 60 kg (Table 51.1). Since 3% saline contains 513 mmol/L of sodium, the change in serum sodium with the infusion of 1 L of 3% saline was estimated to be 12.9 mmol/L. The initial target was to increase the serum sodium by 2 mmol/L/hr up to 120 mmol/L. Since the patient's ini-

tial sodium was 112 mmol/L, the targeted change in serum sodium was 8 mmol/L over 4 hours. Based on the formula in Table 51.1, the infusion rate was calculated to be 155 mL/hr (2 mmol/hr divided by 12.9 mmol/L).

After 4 hours of hypertonic saline, the infusion was stopped, and the sodium was measured to be 122 mmol/L. The patient did not have further seizure activity, and her mental status improved. Triamterene/HCTZ was discontinued, and metoprolol was started for treatment of her hypertension. Upon discharge 5 days later, the patient's sodium was 136 mmol/L, and her mental status was back to baseline.

REFERENCES

1. Hauser WA. Seizure disorders: the changes with age. *Epilepsia* 1992;33(Suppl 4):S6–S14.
2. Thomas RJ. Seizures and epilepsy in the elderly. *Arch Intern Med* 1997;157:605–617.
3. Silverman IE, Restrepo L, Matthews GC. Poststroke seizures. *Arch Neurol* 2002;59:195–201.
4. Hsu SS, Kim HS. Meningococcal meningitis presenting as stroke in an afebrile adult. *Ann Emerg Med* 1998;32:620–623.
5. Harper CM, Newton PA, Walsh JR. Drug-induced illness in the elderly. *Postgrad Med* 1989;86:245–256.
6. Brick JF, Gutrecht JA, Ringel RA. Reflex epilepsy and nonketotic hyperglycemia in the elderly: a specific neuroendocrine syndrome. *Neurology* 1989;39:394–399.
7. Fall PJ. Hyponatremia and hypernatremia: a systematic approach to causes and their correction. *Postgrad Med* 2000;107:75–82.
8. Kugler JP, Hustead T. Hyponatremia and hypernatremia in the elderly. *Am Fam Physician* 2000;61:3623–3630.
9. Kumar S, Berl T. Sodium. *Lancet* 1998;352:220–228.
10. Smith DM, McKenna K, Thompson CJ. Hyponatraemia. *Clin Endocrinol* 2000;52:667–678.
11. Sonnenblick M, Friedlander Y, Rosin AJ. Diuretic-induced severe hyponatremia. Review and analysis of 129 reported patients. *Chest* 1993;103:601–606.
12. Spital A. Diuretic-induced hyponatremia. *Am J Nephrol* 1999;19:447–452.
13. Adrogue HJ, Madias NE. Hyponatremia. *N Engl J Med* 2000;342:1581–1589.

52

A 33-YEAR-OLD WOMAN WITH CHEST PAIN AND SHORTNESS OF BREATH

JONATHAN A. RAPP
MICHAEL BAYTION
YASSER M. BHAT
AMIR K. JAFFER

CASE PRESENTATION

A 33-year-old black woman presented to the emergency room with 2 days of chest pain and 2 weeks of worsening shortness of breath. She rated her chest pain as 8 out of 10 in intensity and described it as "pressurelike." The pain was retrosternal, nonradiating, and constant. The pain was worse with exertion and was not relieved with rest. The patient stated that she usually experienced shortness of breath when climbing two flights of stairs, but during the 2 weeks before presentation was having dyspnea with minimal exertion. Over this same time, she also noted the onset of two-pillow orthopnea and paroxysmal nocturnal dyspnea. In addition, the patient noted increasing frequency of bifrontal headaches. She denied visual changes, weakness, numbness, tingling, syncope, dysuria, or hematuria. Her review of systems was otherwise negative.

The patient had a 10-year history of uncontrolled hypertension and was noncompliant with her medications. She experienced a transient ischemic attack several months before this presentation. One year earlier, she was diagnosed with asthma; she had never required intubation and had never undergone pulmonary function testing.

Upon presentation, her prescribed medications included metoprolol, furosemide, amlodipine, aspirin, potassium, and fluticasone and albuterol inhalers. Family history was significant for her mother developing congestive heart failure and coronary artery disease while in her 20s and her maternal grandmother requiring coronary artery bypass surgery in her 60s. She denied the use of tobacco, alcohol, or illicit drugs.

Physical examination revealed a blood pressure of 210/150 mm Hg in both arms, pulse of 88 beats per minute, respiratory rate of 16 per minute, and temperature of 37.2°C. She was alert and oriented to person, place, and time. Funduscopic examination revealed papilledema. There was no jugular venous distension. Cardiac examination revealed regular rate and rhythm, without murmurs, gallops, or rubs. Pulmonary examination revealed mild bibasilar rales. Her abdomen was soft and nondistended, with mild left-lower-quadrant tenderness. There was no organomegaly, bowel sounds were normal, and peritoneal signs were absent. There were no abdominal bruits. Neurologic examination was nonfocal. There was no clubbing, cyanosis, or peripheral edema. Distal pulses were normal bilaterally.

QUESTIONS/DISCUSSION

Which of the following tests is/are appropriate in the initial evaluation of this patient's symptoms?

A. **Electrocardiogram**
B. **Urine toxicology screen**
C. **Chest radiograph**
D. **Serum creatinine**
E. **All of the above**

All these tests are appropriate to evaluate this patient's hypertension. Patients with uncontrolled hypertension and findings such as papilledema and heart failure that represent potential sequelae of uncontrolled hypertension need to undergo a prompt evaluation to determine potential etiologies and the presence of potential complications from uncontrolled hypertension.

Despite the patient's age, her presentation of chest pain and progressive dyspnea with a strong family history of coronary artery disease requires an evaluation for an acute coronary syndrome. Therefore, an electrocardiogram (ECG) is indicated. In this case, the ECG demonstrated left ventricular hypertrophy and new T-wave inversions in leads V4 to V6, consistent with possible coronary ischemia. Initial cardiac enzymes were within normal limits.

A urine toxicology screen is also indicated in this patient. Clinicians need to consider abuse of illicit drugs such as cocaine or amphetamines in young adults who present with severe hypertension. This consideration should be pursued even if the patient denies drug use because the history may be unreliable. Urine toxicology screen was negative in this patient. Since this woman was of child-bearing age, urine β-human chorionic gonadotropin (β-hCG) was performed, which was negative.

A chest x-ray is appropriate in this patient to evaluate for the presence of heart failure and findings suggestive of aortic dissection. Patients with accelerated hypertension are at increased risk for developing left ventricular dysfunction and congestive heart failure. Chest x-ray can assess for the presence of cardiomegaly and pulmonary edema. Patients with uncontrolled hypertension are also at increased risk for aortic dissection. Although the chest x-ray is not diagnostic for aortic dissection, the presence of superior mediastinal widening in the setting of uncontrolled hypertension and chest pain is suggestive of a dissection of the ascending aorta. If clinical suspicion for an aortic dissection is high, computed tomography or magnetic resonance imaging should be performed. In this patient, a chest x-ray revealed cardiomegaly and bilateral lower lobe infiltrates consistent with pulmonary edema. There were no pleural effusions. These findings were thought to be most consistent with congestive heart failure (CHF) in the setting of accelerated hypertension and myocardial ischemia. Her heart failure was further evaluated with a transthoracic echocardiogram that showed left ventricular hypertrophy (LVH), normal left ventricular function, and no valvular abnormalities.

Serum creatinine is also appropriate in the initial evaluation of this patient with marked hypertension and papilledema. Patients with evidence suggestive of end-organ damage (i.e., papilledema) due to uncontrolled hypertension should have their renal function assessed. These patients are at risk for developing acute renal failure as a result of the uncontrolled hypertension. This patient's blood urea nitrogen and creatinine were 26 mg/dL and 2.3 mg/dL, respectively. These figures were elevated from her normal baseline values. A urinalysis showed trace blood and no protein.

Considering the patient's uncontrolled hypertension and evidence of end-organ damage—namely, papilledema, LVH, CHF, and renal failure—the patient's presentation was thought to be most consistent with malignant hypertension, a true hypertensive emergency (1,2). Malignant hypertension is defined clinically by severe hypertension in conjunction with retinal hemorrhages and exudates (3,4). A complete ophthalmologic examination confirmed the presence of these findings. This patient had evidence of retinal, renal, and cardiac involvement due to uncontrolled hypertension.

The mechanism of malignant hypertension is unknown, but severe blood pressure elevation is thought to be a critical factor. When blood pressure reaches a certain critical level, vascular walls, including those of the endothelium,

become mechanically damaged. The normal endothelial response to elevated blood pressure includes the secretion of nitric oxide and prostacyclin; when the endothelium is damaged, this mechanism fails (5–10). Furthermore, the protection provided by vascular autoregulation, which causes vessels in the eye, brain, and kidney to constrict in the presence of high blood pressure, is lost. The end result is extremely high blood pressure that is transmitted to distal arterioles and capillaries. These events produce end-organ damage (11).

Which of the following is/are potential sequelae of malignant hypertension?

A. **Hemorrhagic and lacunar strokes**
B. **Microangiopathic hemolytic anemia**
C. **Myocardial infarction**
D. **Transient blindness**
E. **All of the above**

Malignant hypertension produces end-organ damage to multiple organ systems, most notably the eyes, brain, heart, and kidneys. Ophthalmologic sequelae include retinal hemorrhages, exudates, and papilledema. The central nervous system, including the brainstem, can also be affected. As mean cerebral arterial pressure approaches 180 mm Hg, cerebrovascular autoregulation begins to fail, which disrupts the blood–brain barrier and leads to microhemorrhages, ischemia, cerebral edema, and ultimately, hypertensive encephalopathy. Neurologic symptoms associated with malignant hypertension include an acute or subacute onset of headache, lethargy, confusion, visual disturbances (including transient blindness), and seizures (focal or generalized). If untreated, hypertensive encephalopathy can progress to coma or even death. Magnetic resonance imaging of patients with hypertensive encephalopathy demonstrates lesions predominantly in the white matter of the parietooccipital region of the brain (11).

The excessive afterload associated with severe hypertension increases left ventricular wall stress and myocardial oxygen demand. Left ventricular hypertrophy, myocardial ischemia, and heart failure may result (1). Approximately 30% of patients with malignant hypertension present with heart failure and pulmonary edema (12). Aortic dissection is another potentially life-threatening cardiovascular complication of malignant hypertension. Mortality rates from this complication remain exceedingly high (11).

Malignant hypertension can cause rapidly progressive acute renal failure. Urinalysis often reveals proteinuria, pyuria, and hematuria. In a patient with malignant hypertension, hematuria in the absence of primary renal parenchymal disease is strongly suggestive of malignant hypertension (13,14).

Many patients with malignant hypertension also have evidence of microangiopathic hemolytic anemia. All the preceding choices are potential sequelae of malignant hypertension.

Among patients with malignant hypertension, approximately 80% will die within 2 years if untreated. The 5-year survival rate is 74% (15,16). The leading causes of death are renal failure, stroke, myocardial infarction, and heart failure (17).

All of the following medications are appropriate in the treatment of malignant hypertension except:

A. Sodium nitroprusside
B. Intravenous labetalol
C. Fenoldopam
D. Nifedipine
E. Nitroglycerin
F. Nicardipine

In treating patients with malignant hypertension, it is critical that both hypertension and its secondary effects be treated appropriately. Medications used in this situation should have a rapid onset of action and should be easy to titrate. Therefore, oral agents should be avoided. Several parenteral antihypertensive agents are available to treat malignant hypertension. Sodium nitroprusside, an intravenous arterial and venous dilator, is commonly used for immediate blood pressure control. It acts within seconds and is easy to titrate. Its afterload-reducing properties also make nitroprusside appropriate for use in patients with congestive heart failure due to malignant hypertension. Sodium nitroprusside should only be administered in an intensive care unit and should be accompanied by continuous intraarterial blood pressure monitoring. Because of possible cyanide toxicity, prolonged use of the drug is not recommended (11,18).

Intravenous labetalol is also frequently used in the treatment of malignant hypertension. It blocks both α- and β-adrenergic receptors and can be given as an intravenous bolus or infusion (19). It acts within 5 to 10 minutes, and its effects last between 2 and 6 hours. The major side effects of labetalol include nausea, vomiting, bronchospasm, and heart block (11).

Therapy for patients with malignant hypertension and concomitant renal dysfunction is controversial. Nitroprusside has typically been used in this situation, but the dopamine-1 receptor agonist, fenoldopam, is a potentially favorable alternative. Fenoldopam produces vasodilatation of the splanchnic, coronary, and renal vascular beds. It has a half-life of 7 to 9 minutes in the blood and lacks toxic metabolites. Notable side effects include headaches, dizziness, flushing, and excessive hypotension. The Food and Drug Administration has approved fenoldopam for 48-hour management of hypertensive emergencies (20).

Intravenous nitrates, such as nitroglycerin, are particularly beneficial in the setting of hypertension with left ventricular failure or myocardial ischemia. Nitrates decrease left ventricular preload and increase coronary perfusion. They act within 1 to 3 minutes, and the effects last 5 to 15 minutes. Adverse effects include headache and vomiting (9).

Nicardipine is a calcium channel blocker that can be given orally or intravenously. It is a potent arteriolar dilator and is excellent in reducing severe hypertension (20). It acts within 5 to 10 minutes, with its effects lasting for up to 4 hours. Side effects include reflex tachycardia and flushing (9,20,21).

Short-acting nifedipine is not an appropriate selection for a patient with malignant hypertension. This drug is not available as an intravenous preparation and has the potential to precipitously drop blood pressure and worsen cardiac ischemia by a coronary steal phenomenon.

The goal of initial treatment of malignant hypertension is a reduction in diastolic blood pressure to approximately 100 mm Hg within 2 to 6 hours. The maximum initial drop in mean arterial pressure should not exceed 25% (9,18). More aggressive blood pressure lowering does not benefit the patient and actually puts the patient at risk for developing ischemic symptoms (22,23). Once adequate control is obtained, oral therapy can be initiated with the goal of maintaining a diastolic pressure of 85 to 90 mm Hg over the subsequent 2 to 3 months (24).

Hospital Course

This patient was treated with intravenous labetalol and nitroglycerin, which lowered her blood pressure to the target range within 6 hours of admission. She also received intravenous furosemide for pulmonary edema. On her second hospital day, her blood pressure was 138/90 mm Hg; she was started on therapy with clonidine, oral labetalol, and captopril.

Given the severity of this patient's hypertension, an evaluation for secondary causes of hypertension, including pheochromocytoma, hyperaldosteronism, and renal artery stenosis, was performed. A 24-hour urine collection for catecholamines, metanephrines, and vanillylmandelic acid was normal. Serum renin and aldosterone levels were normal, and a renal ultrasound revealed no evidence of renal artery stenosis.

The patient was discharged home with close follow-up with her primary care physician as well as an outpatient cardiac stress test.

CONCLUSION

Patients who present with uncontrolled hypertension need to be evaluated promptly to rule out evidence of end-organ damage and other life-threatening emergencies, such as aortic dissection. The combination of severe hypertension and papilledema confirms the diagnosis of malignant hypertension, which is a medical emergency requiring aggressive treatment to avoid potentially fatal complications. Several intravenous medications are available to assist in appropriate blood pressure reduction. Clinicians also need to recognize that an excessive initial reduction in blood pressure can cause significant morbidity.

REFERENCES

1. The sixth report of the Joint National Committee on prevention, detection, evaluation, and treatment of high blood pressure. *Arch Intern Med* 1997;157:2413–2446.
2. Furchgott RF, Zawadzki JV. The obligatory role of endothelial cells in the relaxation of arterial smooth muscle by acetylcholine. *Nature* 1980;288:373–376.
3. Ahmed ME, Walker JM, Beevers DG, et al. Lack of difference between malignant and accelerated hypertension. *Br Med J* 1986;292:235–237.
4. McGregor E, Isles CG, Jay JL, et al. Retinal changes in malignant hypertension. *Br Med J* 1986;292:233–234.
5. Nolan CR. Malignant hypertension and other hypertensive crises. In: Schrier RW, ed. *Diseases of the kidney and urinary tract,* 7th ed. Philadelphia: Lippincott Williams & Wilkins, 2001: 1513–1592.
6. Okada M, Matsumori A, Ono K, et al. Cyclic stretch upregulates production of interleukin-8 and monocyte chemotactic and activating factor/monocyte chemoattractant protein-1 in human endothelial cells. *Arterioscler Thromb Vasc Biol* 1998;18:894–901.
7. Funakoshi Y, Ichiki T, Ito K, et al. Induction of interleukin-6 expression by angiotensin II in rat vascular smooth muscle cells. *Hypertension* 1999;34:118–125.
8. Touyz RM, Milne FJ. Alterations in intracellular cations and cell membrane ATPase activity in patients with malignant hypertension. *J Hypertens* 1995;13:867–874.
9. MacArthur H, Warner TD, Wood EG, et al. Endothelin-1 release from endothelial cells in culture is elevated both acutely and chronically by short periods of mechanical stretch. *Biochem Biophys Res Commun* 1994;200:395–400.
10. Verhaar MC, Beutler JJ, Gaillard CA, et al. Progressive vascular damage in hypertension is associated with increased levels of circulating P-selectin. *J Hypertens* 1998;16:45–50.
11. Vaughan CJ, Delanty N. Hypertensive emergencies. *Lancet* 2000;356:411–417.
12. Isles CG. Hypertensive emergencies. In: Swales JD, ed. *Textbook of hypertension.* Oxford: Blackwell Scientific Publications, 1994: 1233–1248.
13. Schottstaedt MF, Sokolow M. The natural history and course of hypertension with papilledema (malignant hypertension). *Am Heart J* 1953;45:331–362.
14. Pickering GW. *High blood pressure,* 2nd ed. New York: Grune & Stratton, 1968.
15. Keith NM, Wagener HP, Barker NW. Some different types of essential hypertension: their course and prognosis. *Am J Med Sci* 1939;197:332–343.
16. Leishman AW. Hypertension: treated and untreated; a study of 400 cases. *Br Med J* 1959;1:1361–1368.
17. Lip GY, Beevers M, Beevers DG. Complications and survival of 315 patients with malignant-phase hypertension. *J Hypertens* 1995;13:915–924.
18. Kaplan NM. Hypertensive crises. In: Kaplan NM. *Kaplan's clinical hypertension,* 8th ed. Baltimore: Williams & Wilkins, 2002: 339–356.
19. Atkin SH, Jaker MA, Beaty P, et al. Oral labetalol versus oral clonidine in the emergency treatment of severe hypertension. *Am J Med Sci* 1992;303:9–15.
20. Elliott WJ. Hypertensive emergencies. *Crit Care Clin* 2001;17: 435–451.
21. Neutel JM, Smith DH, Wallin D, et al. A comparison of intravenous nicardipine and sodium nitroprusside in the immediate treatment of severe hypertension. *Am J Hypertens* 1994;7: 623–628.
22. Ledingham JG, Rajagopalan B. Cerebral complications in the treatment of accelerated hypertension. *Q J Med* 1979;48:25–41.
23. Haas DC, Streeten DH, Kim RC, et al. Death from cerebral hypoperfusion during nitroprusside treatment of acute angiotensin-dependent hypertension. *Am J Med* 1983;75:1071–1076.
24. Woods JW, Blythe WB. Management of malignant hypertension complicated by renal insufficiency. *N Engl J Med* 1967;277: 57–61.

53

A 65-YEAR-OLD MAN WITH DYSPNEA AND OLIGURIA

MICHAEL B. DAVIDSON
ALAN WONG
MARTIN J. SCHREIBER, JR.

CASE PRESENTATION

A 65-year-old man with chronic lymphocytic leukemia (CLL) presented to the emergency department with a 1-day history of increasing shortness of breath, chest pain, dizziness, and decreased urine output. He also noted bilateral lower-extremity swelling and fatigue but denied headaches, palpitations, nausea, vomiting, or cough. Eight hours before presentation, the patient took an extra dose of 80 mg of furosemide without any significant diuresis.

Two days before the onset of symptoms, the patient received induction chemotherapy for CLL with cyclophosphamide, vincristine, and prednisone. A bone marrow biopsy just before the initiation of chemotherapy showed probable Richter transformation to small lymphocytic lymphoma.

The patient's past medical history was otherwise significant for chronic renal insufficiency secondary to hypertension with a baseline creatinine of 2.5 mg/dL, ischemic cardiomyopathy with an estimated ejection fraction of 20%, chronic atrial fibrillation, and gout. His medications upon presentation included allopurinol 100 mg once a day, prednisone 60 mg once a day, furosemide, digoxin, atenolol, amiodarone, hydralazine, warfarin, and potassium. He was not using any over-the-counter or herbal medications. He was a 50-pack-year smoker, having quit 3 years earlier.

Physical examination revealed a thin, ill-appearing man in mild respiratory distress. He was afebrile, with a heart rate of 66 beats per minute, respiratory rate of 28 per minute, blood pressure of 110/66 mm Hg, and pulse oximetry of 96% on 4 L of oxygen by nasal cannula. The patient was awake, alert, and appropriately oriented. Oral mucosa was moist without any lesions. Jugular venous pressure was elevated 18 cm above the right atrium. Bilateral submandibular and posterior cervical adenopathy, as well as right axillary adenopathy, was present, with the largest nodes approximately 2 × 2 cm. This lymphadenopathy had been present for approximately 2 months. Cardiac examination revealed the presence of a third heart sound, without murmurs or pericardial rub. Pulmonary examination revealed bibasilar crackles. Examination of the abdomen was significant for splenomegaly. There was 1+ bilateral lower-extremity edema. Neurologic examination was nonfocal.

Admission laboratory studies were notable for potassium of 7.5 mmol/L, bicarbonate of 10 mmol/L, blood urea nitrogen (BUN) of 145 mg/dL, and creatinine of 4.2 mg/dL. Other significant findings included calcium of 6.8 mg/dL, phosphorus of 14.6 mg/dL, and uric acid of 17.3 mg/dL. Complete blood count revealed a white blood cell count of 270 K/μL, hemoglobin of 8.6 g/dL, and platelet count of 100 K/μL. Two days earlier, his white cell count was 199 K/μL, and uric acid was 12.1 mg/dL. Cardiac enzymes were negative. Arterial blood gas on 4 L of oxygen revealed a pH of 7.27, P_{CO_2} of 18 mm Hg, P_{O_2} of 104 mm Hg, and bicarbonate of 8 mmol/L. Urinalysis showed hyaline casts, without evidence of proteinuria or hematuria. Renal ultrasound revealed no evidence of hydronephrosis. An electrocardiogram (ECG) showed normal sinus rhythm, first-degree atrioventricular block, a complete left bundle branch block, and symmetrically peaked T waves in all leads. Except for the peaked T waves, none of the ECG findings were new. Chest x-ray revealed cardiomegaly and prominent pulmonary vasculature.

QUESTIONS/DISCUSSION

Which of the following is the most likely cause of this patient's presentation?

A. **Acute tumor lysis syndrome (ATLS)**
B. **Prerenal azotemia**
C. **Acute coronary syndrome**

D. Progressive chronic renal insufficiency

Acute tumor lysis syndrome (ATLS) is an oncologic emergency characterized by rapid release of cellular contents into the systemic circulation. It results in inadequate renal excretion and buffering capacity and is associated with acute renal failure and metabolic acidosis. In this case, ATLS is the likely diagnosis for several reasons. This patient's history of malignancy in conjunction with his constellation of metabolic abnormalities at presentation are classic for ATLS. In particular, the marked hyperphosphatemia and hyperuricemia, combined with acute renal failure and metabolic acidosis, make ATLS the most likely diagnosis in this case.

Although the patient's BUN-to-creatinine ratio is consistent with prerenal azotemia, it is unlikely, as the sole diagnosis in this case due to the concomitant metabolic disturbances, including hyperkalemia and hyperphosphatemia.

Since this patient with known ischemic cardiomyopathy presented in congestive heart failure, an acute coronary syndrome needs to be considered in the differential diagnosis. However, the patient did not have acute ECG changes, except for the presence of peaked T waves, which was consistent with his new hyperkalemia. Furthermore, the patient had negative cardiac enzymes after more than 24 hours of symptoms. An acute coronary syndrome also would fail to explain the severe metabolic derangements seen in this patient.

Although progressive chronic renal insufficiency (CRI) can by itself produce many of the laboratory abnormalities seen in this case, the acuity of this patient's presentation makes progressive chronic renal insufficiency a less likely cause of this patient's presentation. In addition, this patient's degree of hyperphosphatemia and hyperuricemia would be very unusual in association with progressive CRI.

Acute tumor lysis syndrome (ATLS) was initially described in association with acute leukemia and lymphoma (1). Although initially believed to occur only following chemotherapy, ATLS has been shown to occur spontaneously in a variety of tumor types (2–4). Spontaneous ATLS has been associated with both solid and hematologic malignancies. Although occurring most commonly in the setting of Burkitt lymphoma, acute lymphoblastic leukemia, or other high-grade lymphomas, ATLS has occurred in many tumor types, including chronic leukemia, breast cancer, ovarian cancer, multiple myeloma, and small cell lung cancer (5–10).

The pathophysiology of ATLS involves the release of intracellular contents of neoplastic cells into the extracellular space. This release occurs due to massive lysis of tumor cells upon treatment with chemotherapeutic agents or it can occur spontaneously (5). Although ATLS has developed with nearly all classes of chemotherapeutic agents, it has occurred more frequently with certain agents, such as corticosteroids and rituximab (5). The etiology for the association between certain agents and ATLS has not been established. In ATLS, renal excretory mechanisms are overwhelmed, which can cause potentially life-threatening electrolyte and metabolic abnormalities. Renal failure in ATLS results from uric acid nephropathy. Although uric acid is highly soluble in plasma, it precipitates into uric acid crystals upon exposure to acidic urine. Precipitation of crystals occurs in the renal tubules, which causes acute tubular necrosis (1).

Which of the following metabolic abnormalities is consistent with ATLS?

A. Hyperphosphatemia
B. Hyperkalemia
C. Hypocalcemia
D. Hyperuricemia
E. All of the above

The metabolic hallmarks of ATLS are hyperphosphatemia, hypocalcemia, hyperkalemia, and hyperuricemia (5). Hyperkalemia is the first abnormality to occur in the course of the syndrome (11). Lysis of malignant cells results in leakage of intracellular potassium into the intravascular space. In addition, the acidemia caused by hyperuricemia and renal failure leads to a further shift of intracellular potassium into the extracellular space by nonlysed cells. Hyperkalemia can occur within 6 to 72 hours after the initiation of treatment (11). A potassium value greater than 6.0 mmol/L is often regarded as the threshold to intervene to lower potassium, as elevation to this degree can quickly lead to cardiac membrane destabilization (11).

Hyperphosphatemia is the next electrolyte abnormality to occur, usually developing 24 to 48 hours following the initiation of chemotherapy. Hyperphosphatemia likely results because malignant hematologic cells are thought to contain up to four times more intracellular phosphate than mature lymphoid cells (11). Phosphorus levels greater than 10.0 mg/dL are routinely encountered in ATLS and lead to subsequent hypocalcemia. When elevated, free serum phosphorus tends to bind calcium avidly, which produces hypocalcemia. Hypocalcemia itself usually does not warrant treatment unless accompanied by neuromuscular irritability.

Hyperuricemia is the last of the metabolic abnormalities to occur in ATLS. Hyperuricemia develops 48 to 72 hours following initiation of treatment (11). It results from high nucleic acid turnover in malignant cells and the subsequent release of these products into the intravascular space. Deposition of insoluble uric acid causes the acute tubular necrosis and renal failure seen in ATLS (11).

All of the following treatments are potentially appropriate for ATLS except:

A. Hemodialysis
B. Urine alkalinization
C. Allopurinol

D. Hydration

E. Oral calcium carbonate supplementation

Treatments for ATLS are based on the metabolic abnormalities that result from the lysis of malignant cells and renal failure. As with all patients, acute hyperkalemia in ATLS needs to be managed aggressively. Hyperkalemia results when intravascular potassium levels increase faster than the rate of excretion (12). In ATLS, the combination of cellular lysis, subsequent release of intracellular contents, and acute renal failure with the resultant decrease in renal excretion of potassium all contribute to the development of hyperkalemia.

The three main goals of treatment for acute hyperkalemia are stabilization of the cardiac membrane, intracellular shifting of potassium, and removal of potassium. Stabilization of the cardiac membrane is achieved with the infusion of 10% calcium gluconate solution over several minutes. Calcium gluconate prevents life-threatening cardiac arrhythmias that are associated with hyperkalemic depolarization. Since the action of calcium gluconate is short-lived, it may need to be given every 30 minutes if ECG changes persist.

Intracellular shifting of potassium is accomplished with regular insulin, usually 10 to 20 U as an intravenous bolus, concomitantly with 25 to 50 g of glucose to prevent hypoglycemia. Isotonic sodium bicarbonate can also be used to reduce metabolic acidosis and shift potassium intracellularly. However, sodium bicarbonate should be administered judiciously in patients with acute renal failure since the sodium load is not optimally excreted and can result in inappropriate volume expansion. Inhaled β-2 agonists may also be useful for inducing an intracellular shift of potassium (13).

Potassium can be removed from the body by several methods. Resins, such as sodium polystyrene sulfate, allow cation exchange of sodium for potassium in the gastrointestinal tract and induce the subsequent excretion of potassium from the gastrointestinal tract. Typical dosing is 25 to 50 g orally in a 100-mL 20% sorbitol solution or in an enema with 50 g in 50 mL of 70% sorbitol and 150 mL water (13). Diuretics facilitate the renal excretion of potassium and can be advantageous in acute renal failure to promote urine output (5).

Since resins are typically effective over the course of hours, faster methods of potassium removal, such as dialysis, often need to be considered, especially when patients have ECG changes. Dialysis is the most effective and rapid way to remove potassium. It is appropriate in circumstances of life-threatening hyperkalemia when potassium levels cannot be adequately controlled or lowered with less aggressive measures. Patients with ATLS should undergo hemodialysis because it decreases uric acid and potassium levels more quickly and effectively than does peritoneal dialysis (5).

Hyperuricemia is treated by facilitating excretion, preventing urine crystallization, inhibiting production, and converting uric acid to more soluble forms. Uric acid secretion can be aided by establishing adequate urine flow, which is considered a urine output of at least 3 L/day (14).

Alkalinization of the urine, ideally to a pH greater than 7.0, helps to solubilize uric acid, which is approximately 98% solubilized at physiologic pH (15). However, the administration of sodium bicarbonate carries the risk of inducing urinary calcium phosphate crystallization and volume overload in patients with acute renal failure (5).

Allopurinol is a xanthine oxidase inhibitor that has long been a treatment for hyperuricemia. The last step in the formation of uric acid is dependent on xanthine oxidase; therefore, allopurinol acts to inhibit uric acid production. Doses of 300 to 800 mg/day are appropriate for ATLS. However, allopurinol has some disadvantages that need to be considered before initiating therapy. Since allopurinol does not acutely decrease serum uric acid levels, decreases in uric acid levels are not typically seen for 2 to 3 days when using only allopurinol. Allopurinol also has the potential for significant drug interactions through its inhibition of the cytochrome P450 system. Allopurinol can increase levels of xanthine, a uric acid precursor that is less soluble in urine than uric acid and can cause renal failure. Intravenous allopurinol was found to be efficacious in open-label studies, but large randomized clinical trials have not been performed (16).

Hyperphosphatemia and hypocalcemia are managed by phosphate binders, such as aluminum hydroxide or aluminum carbonate. Hypocalcemia will resolve with treatment of the hyperphosphatemia. While calcium gluconate is appropriate to treat hyperkalemia, oral calcium carbonate supplementation should not be administered because metastatic calcifications can develop (14).

Which of the following is associated with the development of acute tumor lysis syndrome?

A. Preexisting renal insufficiency

B. Large tumor burden with abdominal involvement

C. Treatment with corticosteroids

D. All of the above

As described earlier, certain malignancies are more frequently associated with ATLS. However, additional risk factors associated with the development of ATLS have been identified. Patients considered at increased risk for ATLS should receive prophylaxis to prevent the development of the syndrome.

The most important patients to identify before treatment are those with preexisting renal insufficiency. Since ATLS involves the inability of the kidneys to excrete the products of cell lysis, patients with diminished baseline glomerular filtration rates are more likely to develop acute renal failure. Hyperkalemia and hyperphosphatemia are especially likely to be troublesome in these patients. Patients with preexisting chronic renal insufficiency often have preexisting hypocalcemia, which can be exacerbated by ATLS (11).

Patients with a high tumor burden have been found to have an increased risk for ATLS. In addition, patients with abdominal involvement of their malignancy seem to have a predisposition for developing ATLS.

As chemotherapeutic interventions have become increasingly effective, a potential consequence is the development of massive tumor lysis and ATLS, especially in tumors that are very sensitive to chemotherapy (5). Although ATLS has been associated with multiple interventions, a strong correlation has been made with corticosteroids and more recently with rituximab, an anti-CD20 monoclonal antibody (5).

Elevated LDH levels have been associated with very aggressive and undifferentiated leukemias and lymphomas. Although not directly correlated with the development of ATLS, high pretreatment LDH is more common than normal or low LDH levels in patients with ATLS (11). Other identified predisposing features include male gender, age less than 25, volume depletion, acidic urine, and concentrated urine (5).

Prevention is unquestionably the most effective strategy in the treatment and management of tumor lysis syndrome. Identification of patients with potential risk factors for ATLS is important in selecting those who should receive prophylactic treatment. Maintenance of adequate hydration, eliminating phosphorus and potassium supplementation, and avoiding nephrotoxins are also important. Alkalinization of urine before chemotherapy in high-risk patients is appropriate, and allopurinol, at a dose of 200 to 400 mg/m^2/day, should be administered the day before therapy. Prophylactic treatment of ATLS has been advocated as cost-effective (17,18).

Case Conclusion

The patient was acutely dialyzed on admission due to his hyperkalemia with ECG changes, hyperuricemia, fluid overload unresponsive to diuresis, and acidosis. The patient was given intravenous fluids with sodium bicarbonate to alkalinize his urine. The hyperkalemia was initially treated with intravenous calcium gluconate, insulin, and glucose, followed by hemodialysis. Following a second hemodialysis, the patient's renal failure improved and his urine output increased. Allopurinol 800 mg daily was administered following the initial dialysis. Upon discharge, his potassium, phosphorus, and uric acid had normalized, and his creatinine had returned to his baseline of 2.5 mg/dL. The patient was discharged home with follow-up scheduled with his oncologist.

CONCLUSION

Acute tumor lysis syndrome is a true oncologic emergency that is likely to increase in frequency as chemotherapeutic interventions advance. Recognizing patients who are at increased risk of developing ATLS and providing appropriate

prophylaxis are essential in the management of ATLS. Patients with only modest preexisting renal insufficiency are prone to potentially catastrophic metabolic derangements with ATLS. When patients develop ATLS, the potentially severe metabolic derangements pose the greatest danger to patients. Profound hyperkalemia can quickly develop following cell lysis, and delay in its treatment can lead to cardiac decompensation and death. Clinicians need to monitor these patients very carefully to prevent life-threatening complications.

REFERENCES

1. Kjellstrand CM, Cambell DC 2nd, von Hartitzsch B, et al. Hyperuricemic acute renal failure. *Arch Intern Med* 1974;133: 349–359.
2. Feld J, Mehta H, Burkes RL. Acute spontaneous tumor lysis syndrome in adenocarcinoma of the lung: a case report. *Am J Clin Oncol* 2000;23:491–493.
3. Sklarin NT, Markham M. Spontaneous recurrent tumor lysis syndrome in breast cancer. *Am J Clin Oncol* 1995;18:71–73.
4. Jasek AM, Day HJ. Acute spontaneous tumor lysis syndrome. *Am J Hematol* 1994;47:129–131.
5. Jeha S. Tumor lysis syndrome. *Semin Hematol* 2001;38(4 Suppl 10):4–8.
6. Trendle MC, Tefferi A. Tumor lysis syndrome after treatment of chronic lymphocytic leukemia with cladribine. *N Engl J Med* 1994;330:1090.
7. Drakos P, Bar-Ziv J, Catane R. Tumor lysis syndrome in nonhematologic malignancies. Report of a case and review of the literature. *Am J Clin Oncol* 1994;17:502–505.
8. Bilgrami SF, Fallon BG. Tumor lysis syndrome after combination chemotherapy for ovarian cancer. *Med Pediatr Oncol* 1993;21: 521–524.
9. Fassas AB, Desikan KR, Siegel D, et al. Tumour lysis syndrome complicating high-dose treatment in patients with multiple myeloma. *Br J Haematol* 1999;105:938–941.
10. Sewani HH, Rabatin JT. Acute tumor lysis syndrome in a patient with mixed small cell and non–small cell tumor. *Mayo Clin Proc* 2002;77:722–728.
11. Flombaum CD. Metabolic emergencies in the cancer patient. *Semin Oncol* 2000;27:322–334.
12. Kokko JP. Disturbances in potassium balance. In: Goldman L, Bennett JC, eds. *Cecil textbook of medicine,* 21st ed. Philadelphia: WB Saunders, 2000:553–558.
13. Singer GG, Brenner BM. Fluid and electrolyte disturbances. In: Braunwald E, Fauci AS, Kasper DL, et al., eds. *Harrison's principles of internal medicine,* 15th ed. New York: McGraw-Hill, 2001: 271–283.
14. Sallan S. Management of acute tumor lysis syndrome. *Semin Oncol* 2001;28(2 Suppl 5):9–12.
15. Lorigan PC, Woodings PL, Morgenstern GR, et al. Tumour lysis syndrome, case report and review of the literature. *Ann Oncol* 1996;7:631–636.
16. Feusner J, Farber MS. Role of intravenous allopurinol in the management of acute tumor lysis syndrome. *Semin Oncol* 2001; 28(2 Suppl 5):13–18.
17. Pui CH, Mahmoud HH, Wiley JM, et al. Recombinant urate oxidase for the prophylaxis or treatment of hyperuricemia in patients with leukemia or lymphoma. *J Clin Oncol* 2001;19: 697–704.
18. Farber MS. Pharmacoeconomic considerations in the management of acute tumor lysis syndrome. *Semin Oncol* 2001;28(2 Suppl 5):19–22.

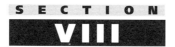

PULMONARY AND CRITICAL CARE MEDICINE

54

A 61-YEAR-OLD MAN WITH SHORTNESS OF BREATH AFTER MYOCARDIAL INFARCTION

JASON M. GUARDINO
SUSAN J. REHM
PETER J. MAZZONE

CASE PRESENTATION

A 61-year-old man awoke with crushing chest pain and came to the emergency department 5 hours later. He described his pain as substernal pressure without radiation. He noted mild shortness of breath. There was no nausea, vomiting, or diaphoresis. He had a history of non–insulin-dependent diabetes mellitus, dyslipidemia, and a three-vessel coronary artery bypass graft 10 years earlier. He smoked and drank heavily for many years but had quit 15 years earlier. An electrocardiogram showed changes consistent with an acute ST-elevation inferior myocardial infarction. His troponin I was 18.6 ng/mL (normal, 0 to 1.49 ng/mL). The next day, the patient underwent a cardiac catheterization with angioplasty for one occluded vein graft. After an uncomplicated postoperative course, he was released from the hospital.

Several days later, the patient returned to the hospital with vague complaints of chest discomfort. His troponin I was 1.04 ng/mL. The patient was hypotensive on presentation and cardiogenic shock was suspected, given his recent cardiac history. An intraaortic balloon pump was placed, and the patient was transferred to our institution for further management.

The patient arrived alert and oriented without any chest pain, but he required a nonrebreather mask with 100% oxygen to maintain his oxygen saturation above 92%. The patient denied any shortness of breath and conversed without difficulty. Physical examination revealed a well-developed man in no acute distress. His temperature was 38.9°C, blood pressure was 110/70 mm Hg, pulse was 89 beats per minute, and respiratory rate was 16 per minute. Cardiac examination revealed a regular rate and rhythm, without murmurs or gallops. Examination of the lungs was remarkable for fine bibasilar crackles. There was no jugular venous distension or hepatosplenomegaly. Peripheral edema was absent.

Further investigation with a Swan–Ganz catheter demonstrated a pulmonary artery occlusive pressure (PAOP) [i.e., pulmonary capillary wedge pressure (PCWP)] of 13 mm Hg (normal range, <13 mm Hg) and a cardiac index (CI) of 3.0 (normal range, 2.6 to 4.2 L/min/m^2). His balloon pump was discontinued.

Over the next 10 to 14 hours, the patient became progressively short of breath, and endotracheal intubation was required because of progressive hypoxia. His chest x-ray demonstrated extensive bilateral infiltrates (Fig. 54.1). An

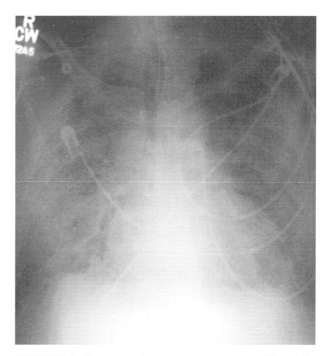

FIGURE 54.1. Chest x-ray demonstrating extensive diffuse bilateral infiltrates.

arterial blood gas (ABG) after 1 hour of mechanical ventilation on 100% oxygen demonstrated a pH of 7.45, P_aCO_2 of 40 mm Hg, P_aO_2 of 53 mm Hg, and bicarbonate (HCO_3) of 27 mmol/L. Swan–Ganz catheter readings continued to demonstrate a normal PAOP and CI several hours after intubation.

QUESTIONS/DISCUSSION

This patient has cardiogenic pulmonary edema.

A. True
B. False

Cardiogenic pulmonary edema develops as a result of increased pulmonary venous and capillary pressures, thereby resulting in congestion of the pulmonary vasculature. This increased intravascular pressure produces a net gain of fluid into the interstitium, and edema develops. Common causes of cardiogenic pulmonary edema include left ventricular dysfunction and valvular heart disease.

Noncardiogenic pulmonary edema is associated with pulmonary congestion caused by an imbalance of hydrostatic and oncotic pressures due to a mechanism other than elevated pulmonary venous and capillary pressures. There are several causes of noncardiogenic pulmonary edema. Hypoalbuminemia, leading to a decrease in the oncotic pressure needed to maintain adequate intravascular volume, can contribute to edema formation. Lymphatic insufficiency can lead to both generalized and pulmonary edema. Although its pathophysiology is not fully understood, neurogenic pulmonary edema develops due to a lung vasculature permeability abnormality and may or may not involve a hydrostatic insult (1).

Noncardiogenic pulmonary edema can also manifest as acute lung injury and/or acute respiratory distress syndrome. This patient's PAOP was not suggestive of elevated left atrial pressure. In addition, he did not have jugular venous distension or other signs of right heart failure, which is often precipitated by left heart failure. His blood pressure continued to stay within normal limits. Seventy-two hours later, his PAOP and CI remained within normal limits. This patient did not have findings suggestive of cardiogenic pulmonary edema. The acute respiratory distress syndrome, this patient's diagnosis, is a devastating clinical syndrome that is characterized as a progressive clinical, histopathologic, and radiographic syndrome.

All of the following are criteria for the acute respiratory distress syndrome except:

A. Acute onset
B. Bilateral radiographic infiltrates
C. No clinical evidence of elevated left atrial pressure or a PCWP of ≤ 18 mm Hg

D. A ratio of the partial pressure of arterial oxygen to the fraction of inspired oxygen (P_aO_2/F_iO_2) ≤ 300 mm Hg, regardless of the level of positive end-expiratory pressure (PEEP)

When "adult respiratory distress syndrome" was recognized to affect people of all ages, including infants, the preferred term became *acute respiratory distress syndrome* (ARDS). Both acute lung injury (ALI) and ARDS can be thought of as:

■ The clinical condition of acute onset of hypoxemia refractory to oxygen supplementation.
■ The physiologic process of noncardiogenic pulmonary edema.
■ The pathologic process of diffuse alveolar damage with persistent inflammation and increased vascular permeability, leading to pulmonary edema. In its later stages, it may lead to fibrosing alveolitis and a further decrease in pulmonary compliance.

The 1994 American–European Consensus Conference on ARDS issued the criteria that are accepted today by both clinicians and researchers (Table 54.1) (2,3). In essence, ARDS represents the most significant form of ALI, with a greater degree of ventilation–perfusion mismatch than is observed with ALI.

This patient's P_aO_2 was 53 mm Hg, and he required 100% oxygen via mechanical ventilation (F_iO_2 of 1.0). His P_aO_2/F_iO_2 ratio was 53. He met the four criteria and was

TABLE 54.1. ESTABLISHED CRITERIA FROM THE AMERICAN–EUROPEAN CONSENSUS CONFERENCE ON ACUTE RESPIRATORY DISTRESS SYNDROME (ARDS)

Acute Lung Injury (ALI)
Acute onset
Widespread bilateral radiographic infiltrates seen on frontal view
No clinical evidence of elevated left atrial pressure or, if measured, a pulmonary capillary wedge pressure of ≤18 mm Hg
A ratio of the partial pressure of arterial oxygen to the fraction of inspired oxygen (P_aO_2/F_iO_2) ≤300 mm Hg, regardless of the level of positive end-expiratory pressure (PEEP). The P_aO_2 is measured in mm Hg and the F_iO_2 is expressed as a value between 0.21 and 1.00

Acute Respiratory Distress Syndrome
The definition of ARDS is the same as ALI except that the hypoxia is worse, requiring a P_aO_2/F_iO_2 ratio ≤200 mm Hg, regardless of the level of PEEP.

Adapted from Bernard GR, Artigas A, Brigham KL, et al. The American–European consensus conference on ARDS. Definitions, mechanisms, relevant outcomes, and clinical trial coordination. *Am J Respir Crit Care Med* 1994;149:818–824.

diagnosed with ARDS. As illustrated in Table 54.1, choice D is consistent with ALI rather than ARDS.

Clinical Disorders Associated with Acute Respiratory Distress Syndrome

ARDS can develop within 4 to 48 hours of the initial insult and can last from days to weeks (4). Heart failure and ARDS are often difficult to distinguish both clinically and radiographically. If one cannot clinically distinguish cardiogenic from noncardiogenic pulmonary edema, a Swan–Ganz catheter can help differentiate the two. There are more than 60 causes of ARDS. Direct or indirect injury to the lung parenchyma can cause ARDS (Table 54.2). A prior history of chronic tobacco or alcohol abuse in critically ill patients can significantly increase the risk of developing ARDS (5,6).

Which of the following is the most common clinical disorder associated with ARDS?

A. Pneumonia
B. Inhalation injury
C. Sepsis syndrome
D. Blood transfusions
E. Pancreatitis

The most common disorder associated with ARDS is sepsis (4). It should be strongly considered in any patient with ARDS who has a fever, clinical manifestations of shock, or a history suggestive of infection. Blood, urine, and sputum cultures should be obtained. Additionally, if routine cultures fail to establish the diagnosis, the presence of

TABLE 54.2. CLINICAL DISORDERS ASSOCIATED WITH ACUTE RESPIRATORY DISTRESS SYNDROME

Direct Lung Injury	Indirect Lung Injury
Pneumonia (nosocomial, community, aspiration)	Sepsis
Inhalation injury (chlorine gas, smoke, high F$_i$O$_2$)	Multiple transfusions
Lung or bone marrow transplant	Drug overdose
Pulmonary contusion	Venous air embolism
Trauma	Neurologic event (seizure, intracranial bleed)
Near drowning	Pancreatitis
	Disseminated intravascular coagulation
	Cardiopulmonary bypass

Adapted from Bernard GR, Artigas A, Brigham KL, et al. The American–European consensus conference on ARDS: definitions, mechanisms, relevant outcomes, and clinical trial coordination. *Am J Respir Crit Care Med* 1994;149:818–824; and from Ware LB, Matthay MA. The acute respiratory distress syndrome. *N Engl J Med* 2000;342:1334–1349.

pathogens such as *Legionella, Mycoplasma, Mycobacteria* species, and fungi should be sought in the appropriate clinical setting.

Pneumonia is a common cause of ARDS in nonhospitalized and hospitalized patients (7). Given the diffuse radiographic abnormalities in ARDS, pneumonia is often difficult to diagnose in these patients. Community-acquired pneumonia is most often caused by *Streptococcus pneumoniae, Legionella pneumophila, Mycoplasma pneumoniae, Haemophilus influenzae, Chlamydia pneumoniae, Moraxella catarrhalis,* and respiratory viruses (8). Hospitalized patients are at risk of nosocomial pneumonias caused by *Pseudomonas aeruginosa, Serratia marcescens, Enterobacter* species, and *Staphylococcus aureus.* One-third of hospitalized patients who are diagnosed with aspiration pneumonia develop ARDS (9,10).

Inhalation of substances such as chlorine gas, smoke, and concentrated oxygen can lead to the development of ARDS. High oxygen concentrations damage lung parenchyma by forming toxic oxygen radicals (11). Effective ventilator strategies include reducing oxygen to nontoxic levels, which are thought to be less than 50% to 60%, as soon as possible.

Transfusion of more than 15 U of packed red blood cells may be a risk factor for development of ARDS (4). Whether there is direct injury to the lung is debated. The blood products may induce an antigen–antibody reaction involving human leukocyte antigen (HLA) and granulocyte antigens that causes transfusion-related acute lung injury. Transfusions of packed red blood cells, fresh-frozen plasma, and platelets have all been associated with ARDS. Testing the blood product for antibodies against the patient's white blood cells can help to confirm the diagnosis (12).

Several drugs or overdoses are known to be associated with ARDS (13). These include aspirin, morphine, cocaine, opioids, nitrofurantoin, phenothiazines, tricyclic antidepressants, protamine, chemotherapeutic agents, and contrast dye.

Venous air embolism is a less common cause of ARDS and often occurs during operating room procedures or when a central venous catheter is unintentionally left open to air. The mechanism is thought to involve activated leukocyte production and the release of toxic oxygen moieties and superoxide anions (14).

Pancreatitis-associated ARDS is probably related to digestive enzymes released from the damaged pancreas. These enzymes cause destruction of phospholipid-based surfactant and the lipid components of the endothelial and epithelial cell membranes (15).

Which of the following is/are appropriate management strategies for patients with ARDS?

A. Mechanical ventilation
B. Nutritional support
C. Prophylaxis against venous thromboembolism
D. All of the above

The most important step in the treatment of ARDS is identifying and treating the underlying cause. Although that is not always possible, supportive treatments are crucial in all cases of ARDS.

Mechanical ventilation remains the mainstay of treatment in most patients diagnosed with ARDS. Goals of mechanical ventilation include supporting oxygenation, decreasing the work of breathing, and avoiding complications (3,16). Deciding between volume-controlled ventilation (VCV) and pressure-controlled ventilation (PCV) modes depends mainly on the clinician's comfort and familiarity with each system, as the appropriate method of ventilation has been controversial since ARDS was first described. Determining appropriate ventilatory settings that will achieve the goals of mechanical ventilation while minimizing complications, such as barotrauma and nosocomial pneumonia, can be very challenging (17). In addition, sedation and paralysis are often required to improve tolerance of mechanical ventilation.

Ventilation at traditional tidal volumes (10 to 15 mL/kg of predicted body weight) may promote further lung injury. Despite chest radiograph findings, ARDS is a nonuniform injury, and large tidal volumes may distend uninjured alveoli capable of gas exchange. In a multicenter randomized trial of 861 patients, mechanical ventilation with lower tidal volumes of 6 mL/kg resulted in a 22% decrease in mortality (18). Positive end-expiratory pressure (PEEP) is used to improve oxygenation by recruiting atelectatic lung tissue. However, selecting the correct amount of PEEP is difficult because of the nonuniformity of injury. While PEEP can recruit nonfunctioning lung tissue, it may distend aerated areas. This could cause ventilator-associated lung injury (19). Studies comparing relatively high PEEP settings to relatively low levels are ongoing.

Failure to diagnose an infection in a critically ill patient can be fatal. However, inappropriate empiric treatment with antibiotics can lead to resistant organisms. If an infectious diagnosis is made, antibiotics should be implemented to cover the most common organisms of that particular disease. The antibiotic and its dosage should be tailored to each patient's hepatic and/or renal function, as well as the susceptibility of a specific organism, if available.

Nutrition in ARDS patients is crucial because they are in a catabolic state (20). As with any patient, if the gastrointestinal tract is functional, it should be used. Advantages of enteral nutrition include fewer line-related infections, gastric buffering to decrease the risk of ulcer, and preservation of the gut mucosa, which may decrease the risk of bacteremia due to enteric pathogens.

Because of prolonged immobility of patients on ventilators, clinicians need to use appropriate prophylaxis against venous thromboembolism. Patients who cannot receive heparin should receive pneumatic compression stockings.

Novel treatment strategies of ARDS include surfactant therapy, inhaled nitric oxide, corticosteroids, prone position

ventilation and partial liquid ventilation. Surfactant is known to decrease surface tension among alveoli, thereby protecting the alveoli from collapse. In a randomized, placebo-controlled trial of 725 ARDS patients, aerosolized surfactant did not have a significant effect on mortality, length of stay in the intensive care unit, or duration of mechanical ventilation (21). Critics of this study attribute the results to suboptimal delivery of surfactant as well as the nature of the synthetic surfactant. Newer preparations of surfactant contain recombinant proteins and are being studied (22).

Nitric oxide, a small lipophilic compound with a short duration of action, acts by relaxing endothelium. Since it has limited availability when bound to hemoglobin, it may have local benefit as an aerosol in lung tissue, which would decrease systemic side effects. However, the results of a 1998 randomized, placebo-controlled trial of 177 patients showed no significant difference in mortality (23). Currently, inhaled nitric oxide is not recommended for routine treatment in ARDS patients.

Because of the inflammatory nature of lung injury in ALI and ARDS, there has been interest in antiinflammatory agents, particularly corticosteroids, as a treatment for ARDS. However, previous studies have not shown a significant benefit for corticosteroids when given at the onset of ARDS (24). The NIH Adult Respiratory Distress Syndrome Network is conducting a multicenter randomized trial on the use of corticosteroids. Current studies are focusing on treating the late, fibrosing alveolitis phase of the disease.

Most patients with ARDS have increased partial pressure of oxygen when changed from a supine to a prone position during mechanical ventilation. Although the exact mechanism is not clear, the increase may be attributed to a more even distribution of ventilation and an improvement in ventilation and perfusion mismatch (19). Although short-term prone ventilation may improve oxygenation, no mortality benefit has been proved (25). Studies of longer periods of prone positioning are forthcoming.

Partial liquid ventilation refers to partially filling the lungs with liquid perflubron. Perflubron is a perfluorocarbon that has high oxygen and carbon dioxide solubility and a low surface tension. Filling the airways with perflubron provides liquid lung inflation, recruits atelectatic tissue, reduces surface tension, provides a reservoir in which oxygen and carbon dioxide can be exchanged, and washes out inflammatory debris (26). Current studies are under way to determine the doses and possible mortality benefit of partial liquid ventilation.

Mortality rates with ARDS have traditionally been greater than 50% to 60% (27). However, in recent years, the rate has declined to approximately 30% to 40% (23,28). The improvement in overall mortality is probably related to a multitude of factors, including a better understanding of mechanical ventilation and more aggressive supportive care (23,29). Although ALI and ARDS resolve completely in some patients, others progress to fibrosing alveolitis with persistent hypoxia, increased alveolar dead space, and continued decrease in pulmonary compliance (22).

CONCLUSION

The cause of ARDS in this patient, like so many others, was not clearly identified. Four days after his original admission to the hospital, one of two blood cultures grew *Streptococcus viridans,* a likely contaminant. On the second day of admission, he received ampicillin/sulbactam and ciprofloxacin for persistent fevers. After transfer to our institution, all blood cultures, respiratory cultures, urine cultures, and viral direct fluorescence antigen (DFA) panels remained negative. *Legionella* and *Mycoplasma* serologies were also negative. Presumably, his ARDS was caused by pneumonia (nosocomial or aspiration) and/or sepsis syndrome. The prompt initiation of empiric antibiotics may account for his consistently negative cultures and hemodynamic stability. Three days after being intubated, the patient failed extubation; however, he was successfully extubated 2 days later. The patient recovered and was discharged after an 11-day hospitalization. His chest x-ray on discharge revealed significant resolution of the diffuse infiltrates (Fig. 54.2).

Clinicians need to consider multiple etiologies in patients who present with hypoxia and evidence of diffuse

pulmonary infiltrates and pulmonary edema. Although many of these patients will have cardiogenic pulmonary edema, noncardiogenic causes need to be considered. ARDS is one process that presents similarly to cardiogenic pulmonary edema but has a considerably different management approach.

REFERENCES

1. Colice GL, Matthay MA, Bass E, et al. Neurogenic pulmonary edema. *Am Rev Respir Dis* 1984;130:941–948.
2. Bernard GR, Artigas A, Brigham KL, et al. The American–European consensus conference on ARDS: definitions, mechanisms, relevant outcomes, and clinical trial coordination. *Am J Respir Crit Care Med* 1994;149:818–824.
3. Artigas A, Bernard GR, Carlet J, et al. The American–European Consensus Conference on ARDS, part 2: ventilatory, pharmacologic, supportive therapy, study design strategies, and issues related to recovery and remodeling. Acute respiratory distress syndrome. *Am J Respir Crit Care Med* 1998;157:1332–1347.
4. Hudson LD, Milberg JA, Anardi D, et al. Clinical risks for development of the acute respiratory distress syndrome. *Am J Respir Crit Care Med* 1995;151:293–301.
5. Moss M, Bucher B, Moore FA, et al. The role of chronic alcohol abuse in the development of acute respiratory distress syndrome in adults. *JAMA* 1996;275:50–54.
6. Iribarren C, Jacobs DR Jr, Sidney S, et al. Cigarette smoking, alcohol consumption, and risk of ARDS: a 15-year cohort study in managed care setting. *Chest* 2000;117:163–168.
7. Mannes GP, Boersma WG, Baur CH, et al. Adult respiratory distress syndrome (ARDS) due to bacteraemic pneumococcal pneumonia. *Eur Respir J* 1991;4:503–504.
8. Bartlett JG, Dowell SF, Mandell LA, et al. Practice guidelines for the management of community-acquired pneumonia in adults. Infectious Diseases Society of America. *Clin Infect Dis* 2000; 31:347–382.
9. Fowler AA, Hamman RF, Good JT, et al. Adult respiratory distress syndrome: risk with common predispositions. *Ann Intern Med* 1983;98:593–597.
10. Tietjen PA, Kaner RJ, Quinn CE. Aspiration emergencies. *Clin Chest Med* 1994;15:117–135.
11. Freeman BA, Crapo JD. Hyperoxia increases oxygen radical production in rat lungs and lung mitochondria. *J Biol Chem* 1981; 256:10986–10992.
12. Florell SR, Velasco SE, Fine PG. Perioperative recognition, management, and pathologic diagnosis of transfusion-related acute lung injury. *Anesthesiology* 1994;81:508–510.
13. Parsons PE. Respiratory failure as a result of drugs, overdoses, and poisonings. *Clin Chest Med* 1994;15:93–102.
14. Clark MC, Flick MR. Permeability pulmonary edema caused by venous air embolism. *Am Rev Respir Dis* 1984;129:633–635.
15. Basran GS, Ramasubramanian R, Verma R. Intrathoracic complications of acute pancreatitis. *Br J Dis Chest* 1987;81:326–331.
16. Kollef MH, Schuster DP. The acute respiratory distress syndrome. *N Engl J Med* 1995;332:27–37.
17. Esteban A, Alia I, Gordo F, et al. Prospective randomized trial comparing pressure-controlled ventilation and volume-controlled ventilation in ARDS. *Chest* 2000;117:1690–1696.
18. Ventilation with lower tidal volumes as compared with traditional tidal volumes for acute lung injury and the acute respiratory distress syndrome. *N Engl J Med* 2000;342:1301–1308.
19. Tobin MJ. Advances in mechanical ventilation. *N Engl J Med* 2001;344:1986–1996.

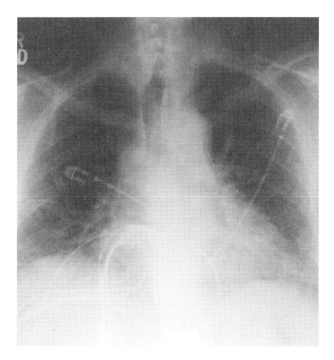

FIGURE 54.2. Chest x-ray demonstrating resolution of diffuse bilateral infiltrates after aggressive treatment for acute respiratory distress syndrome.

20. Cerra FB, Benitez MR, Blackburn GL, et al. Applied nutrition in ICU patients. *Chest* 1997;111:769–778.

21. Anzueto A, Baughman RP, Gantipalli KK, et al. Aerosolized surfactant in adults with sepsis-induced acute respiratory distress syndrome. *N Engl J Med* 1996;334:1417–1421.

22. Ware LB, Matthay MA. The acute respiratory distress syndrome. *N Engl J Med* 2000;342:1334–1349.

23. Dellinger RP, Zimmerman JL, Taylor RW, et al. Effects of inhaled nitric oxide in patients with acute respiratory distress syndrome: results of a randomized phase II trial. *Crit Care Med* 1998;26:15–23.

24. Bernard GR, Luce JM, Sprung CL, et al. High-dose corticosteroids in patients with the adult respiratory distress syndrome. *N Engl J Med* 1987;317:1565–1570.

25. Gattinoni L, Tognoni G, Pesenti A, et al. Effect of prone positioning on the survival of patients with acute respiratory failure. *N Engl J Med* 2001;345:568–573.

26. Verbrugge SJ, Lachmann B. Partial liquid ventilation. *Eur Respir J* 1997;10:1937–1939.

27. Ashbaugh DG, Bigelow DB, Petty TL, et al. Acute respiratory distress in adults. *Lancet* 1967;2:319–323.

28. Milberg JA, Davis DR, Steinberg KP, et al. Improved survival of patients with acute respiratory distress syndrome (ARDS): 1983–1993. *JAMA* 1995;273:306–309.

29. Abel SJ, Finney SJ, Brett SJ, et al. Reduced mortality in association with acute respiratory distress syndrome (ARDS). *Thorax* 1998;53:292–294.

55

A 48-YEAR-OLD WOMAN WITH POSTOPERATIVE SHORTNESS OF BREATH

SARKIS B. BAGHDASARIAN
RONY M. ABOU-JAWDE
FRANK MICHOTA

CASE PRESENTATION

A 48-year-old woman was transferred to the emergency room from a nearby ambulatory surgery center for further evaluation of persistent postoperative shortness of breath of 12 hours duration. Earlier that day, the patient underwent right shoulder arthroscopy with subacromial decompression, distal clavicle resection, and biceps tenotomy. The procedure was performed under general anesthesia following an interscalene block. Endotracheal intubation was uneventful. No significant blood loss or change in vital signs was reported during surgery. She was extubated without difficulty but began complaining of shortness of breath as soon as she woke up from general anesthesia. She required 5 L of oxygen by nasal cannula to achieve an oxygen saturation greater than 92%. The patient received several treatments with nebulized beta-agonists and racemic epinephrine in the recovery room without improvement. The shortness of breath was not associated with chest pain, diaphoresis, nausea, vomiting, cough, or wheezing. She denied any breathing difficulty associated with her daily activities prior to surgery.

The patient's past medical history was notable for mild asthma. She had never required hospitalization or emergency room care for asthma. She denied any history of cardiac disease or prior venous thromboembolism (VTE). Additional past medical history included chronic low back pain, right shoulder osteoarthritis, and bicipital tendinitis. Her only previous surgery was an uncomplicated tubal ligation under regional anesthesia. Her medications included fluticasone, albuterol, gabapentin, cyclobenzaprine, and acetaminophen. She did not smoke, drink alcohol, or use illicit drugs. Family history was negative for cardiopulmonary disease or adverse reactions to anesthesia.

QUESTIONS/DISCUSSION

Which of the following is the most likely cause of this patient's postoperative shortness of breath?

A. Pulmonary embolism
B. Myocardial infarction
C. Aspiration
D. Pneumothorax
E. Reactive airway disease/asthma

Shortness of breath in this woman should be analyzed in the context of possible precipitating factors, her age, and comorbidities. Pulmonary embolism (PE) always needs to be considered in the setting of postoperative shortness of breath. Surgical patients are at increased risk for VTE due to the venous stasis effects of anesthesia and endothelial damage caused by the surgery itself (1). This patient had two additional independent risk factors for VTE: age greater than 40 and obesity (2). However, arthroscopy is considered a low-risk procedure for causing VTE, with short operating times and limited tissue damage. Since this patient's overall risk for VTE was likely low to moderate, the likelihood for clinical pulmonary embolism would be less than 2% (3).

Myocardial infarction is another important cause of postoperative shortness of breath, as it carries a 50% mortality rate (4). However, postoperative myocardial infarction is far less common than reversible myocardial ischemia (5). In both settings, the shortness of breath represents increased left ventricular end-diastolic pressure with concomitant pulmonary edema. However, this patient had no identifiable risk factors for coronary artery disease or evidence of increased cardiac work, making myocardial infarction an unlikely explanation of this patient's shortness of breath.

Aspiration is a documented complication of general anesthesia. However, the timing of this patient's symptoms is not consistent with occult aspiration with infection. Furthermore, there was no history of postoperative emesis or complications associated with intubation that would raise suspicion for gross aspiration with chemical pneumonitis.

Pneumothorax has also been reported as an uncommon complication of interscalene block, with a prevalence of 0.2% (6). However, the most likely etiology for this patient's shortness of breath is reactive airway disease due to her known history of asthma. Patients with preexisting pulmonary disease are more prone to developing postoperative pulmonary complications (7). Early studies have demonstrated that patients with asthma have a higher incidence of postoperative pulmonary complications compared to controls (24% versus 6%) (8). There were many potential triggers for bronchospasm in this patient, including the inhalation anesthetic, microscopic aspiration, and use of intravenous narcotics.

Physical examination revealed an obese woman who was breathing comfortably on 4 L of oxygen via nasal cannula. Vital signs included a temperature of 35.7°C, heart rate of 80 beats per minute, blood pressure of 126/78 mm Hg, and respiratory rate of 24 per minute. Her peak expiratory flow rate was 145 mL/sec. The patient weighed 123 kg. The neck was supple without jugular venous distension, carotid bruits, or adenopathy. Pulmonary examination revealed decreased breath sounds throughout with bronchial sounds and tympany in the right base. There were no rales, rhonchi, or wheezing. Cardiac and abdominal examinations were normal. There was no peripheral edema. She was fully alert and oriented, clearly responded to questions, and followed commands. She did not have any voluntary movement of her right upper extremity, with 1/5 proximal and distal strength. The remainder of her neurologic examination was normal.

Initial laboratory data included white blood cell count of 10.7 K/μL, hemoglobin of 11.3 g/dL (11.0 g/dL prior to surgery), and platelet count of 236 K/μL. Troponin T was less than 0.01 ng/mL. Arterial blood gas on 4 L nasal cannula revealed a pH of 7.39, P_{CO_2} of 39 mm Hg, P_{O_2} of 74 mm Hg, and bicarbonate of 23 mmol/L. An electrocardiogram revealed normal sinus rhythm without acute changes. Figure 55.1 shows this patient's portable chest x-ray.

Given the results of the initial investigations, which of the following is the most appropriate next step?

A. Computed tomography (CT scan) of the chest
B. Duplex ultrasonography of all limbs
C. Pulmonary function tests
D. Electromyogram (EMG)
E. No further testing is indicated

This patient's history, physical examination, and laboratory findings are all consistent with new hemidiaphrag-

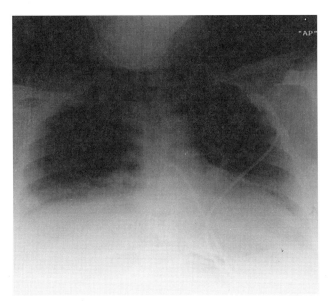

FIGURE 55.1. Chest x-ray demonstrating elevation of the right hemidiaphragm, without evidence of pneumothorax, edema, or infiltrates. The findings were consistent with new hemidiaphragmatic paralysis.

matic paralysis. Given the strong likelihood for hemidiaphragmatic paralysis, no further testing is indicated at this point. The chest x-ray demonstrated elevation of the right hemidiaphragm, without evidence of pneumothorax, edema, or infiltrates. In the setting of an interscalene regional block, the incidence of phrenic nerve (C3–C5) paralysis is virtually 100% due to the proximity of the phrenic nerve to the brachial plexus (9). Phrenic nerve paralysis is not prevented by digital pressure and occurs with a variety of local anesthetics and doses. However, it is not usually associated with significant symptoms because otherwise healthy individuals can compensate by using accessory and intercostal muscles with increased respiratory efforts. Tidal volume, minute volume, and P_aCO_2 are typically normal. However, P_aO_2 is often decreased due to atelectasis and ventilation–perfusion mismatch. Diaphragmatic paralysis may simulate restrictive lung disease on pulmonary function testing (PFT) with reduced forced expiratory volume in 1 second (FEV_1), reduced forced vital capacity (FVC), and an unchanged FEV_1/FVC ratio. The significant respiratory symptoms in this patient are likely due to the combination of her asthma, obesity, new hemidiaphragmatic paresis, and atelectasis.

Which of the following is the most appropriate conclusion about this patient's condition?

A. Her symptoms will not resolve until she loses weight.
B. She will now require home oxygen therapy.
C. Intermittent positive pressure breathing treatments will be needed indefinitely.

D. Transfer to an acute rehabilitation center will improve her chances of recovery.

E. None of the above.

The correct answer is E, none of the above. The main mechanism for this hemidiaphragmatic paresis is transient phrenic nerve block. Complete resolution of symptoms is expected in a time frame that correlates with the pharmacologic properties of the anesthetics used. Permanent symptoms are very uncommon, with only two reports in the literature of persistent phrenic nerve paralysis following interscalene regional block (10,11). In these cases, the mechanism for the injury was postulated to be due to ischemia, mechanical damage, or severe chemical neurotoxicity.

Case Conclusion

This patient was treated with supplemental oxygen, β-agonist nebulizers, and incentive spirometry. Her respiratory status steadily improved during her 2-day hospital stay. Peak expiratory flow increased to 375 mL/sec, and she was soon comfortable on room air. A repeat chest x-ray showed improvement in the right hemidiaphragm. On follow-up 5 days after her operation, she was comfortable with daily activities. Her lung examination and right-upper-extremity strength were normal.

CONCLUSION

The differential diagnosis for postoperative shortness of breath is broad and includes etiologies that carry significant morbidity and mortality. This case represents a reversible cause for postoperative shortness of breath, which might have been predicted upon preoperative assessment. Because of the almost 100% certainty of phrenic nerve involvement with an interscalene regional block, it is essential to consider the effect of this anesthetic approach on existing cardiopulmonary disease (asthma, chronic obstructive pulmonary disease, cardiac disease, or obesity) or abnormal neurologic function (vocal cord or diaphragmatic paralysis).

REFERENCES

1. Risk of and prophylaxis for venous thromboembolism in hospital patients. Thromboembolic Risk Factors (THRIFT) Consensus Group. *BMJ* 1992;305:567–574.
2. Heit JA, Silverstein MD, Mohr DN, et al. Risk factors for deep vein thrombosis and pulmonary embolism: a population-based case-control study. *Arch Intern Med* 2000;160:809–815.
3. Geerts WH, Heit JA, Clagett GP, et al. Prevention of venous thromboembolism. *Chest* 2001;119(1 Suppl):132S–175S.
4. Ashton CM. Perioperative myocardial infarction with noncardiac surgery. *Am J Med Sci* 1994;308:41–48.
5. Michota F, Frost S. Perioperative care of the hospitalized patient. *Med Clin North Am* 2002;86:1–18.
6. Borgeat A, Ekatodramis G, Kalberer F, et al. Acute and nonacute complications associated with interscalene block and shoulder surgery: a prospective study. *Anesthesiology* 2001;95:875–880.
7. Smetana GW. Preoperative pulmonary evaluation. *N Engl J Med* 1999;340:937–944.
8. Gold MI, Helrich M. A study of complications related to anesthesia in asthmatic patients. *Anesth Analg* 1963;42:238–293.
9. Urmey WF, Talts KH, Sharrock NE. One hundred percent incidence of hemidiaphragmatic paresis associated with interscalene brachial plexus anesthesia as diagnosed by ultrasonography. *Anesth Analg* 1991;72:498–503.
10. Robaux S, Bouaziz H, Boisseau N, et al. Persistent phrenic nerve paralysis following interscalene brachial plexus block. *Anesthesiology* 2001;95:1519–1521.
11. Bashein G, Robertson HT, Kennedy WF Jr. Persistent phrenic nerve paresis following interscalene brachial plexus block. *Anesthesiology* 1985;63:102–104.

56

A 56-YEAR-OLD WOMAN WITH INCREASING DYSPNEA AND COUGH

ALAN WONG
SHAUN D. FROST

CASE PRESENTATION

A 56-year-old woman presented with 3 days of increasing shortness of breath, low-grade fever, and cough productive of thick yellow sputum. Before the onset of these symptoms, she had noted a mild nonproductive cough, exertional dyspnea, and fatigue. These symptoms dated back 3 months, at which time the patient had developed an upper respiratory infection. A chest radiograph at that time was normal, and she had been treated with a 10-day course of amoxicillin/clavulanic acid.

She denied a history of tobacco use, night sweats, weight loss, diarrhea, chest pain, gastrointestinal surgery or trauma, alcohol use, or dysphagia. Her past medical history was significant for a 20-year history of rheumatoid arthritis involving her proximal interphalangeal and metacarpophalangeal joints. Her symptoms had been controlled with chronic low-dose prednisone.

On physical examination, the patient had a temperature of 38.3°C, blood pressure of 126/72 mm Hg, respiratory rate of 18 per minute, and pulse oximetry of 95% on room air. She did not exhibit shortness of breath on conversation. She had good dentition and no lymphadenopathy in the submandibular, submental, cervical, axillary, or supraclavicular regions. Pulmonary examination revealed decreased breath sounds and egophony in the right lower lobe. Pain over the anterior, lateral, and posterior aspects of her right chest wall was elicited with moderate pressure. Cardiac, abdominal, and extremity examinations were unremarkable. Her joints did not exhibit significant tenderness or effusions.

A posteroanterior (PA) chest radiograph showed a large right-sided pleural effusion (Fig. 56.1).

QUESTIONS/DISCUSSION

Which of the following is least likely to cause a pleural effusion?

A. Influenza
B. Pleural involvement of rheumatoid arthritis

C. Tuberculosis
D. Bacterial pneumonia

Influenza generally presents with a sudden onset of multiple symptoms, including myalgias, fever, chills, and cough. The cough in influenza is not usually productive, and influenza does not typically produce pleural effusions (1).

Patients with rheumatoid arthritis (RA) can develop pleural effusions as a manifestation of active disease. The prevalence of pleural effusion among patients with active RA is 2% to 3% (1). However, this patient's rheumatoid arthritis had been symptomatically controlled, and her history is more consistent with an infectious etiology for her pulmonary symptoms.

Tuberculosis (TB) is an uncommon cause of pleural effusion in the United States, although it is common in many

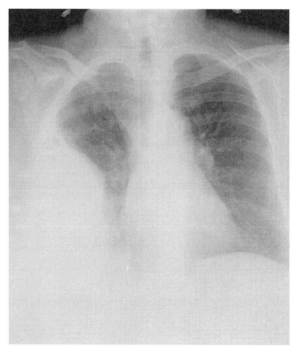

FIGURE 56.1. Posteroanterior chest x-ray showing a large right pleural effusion.

regions of the world. Patients with tuberculous pleural effusions frequently present with fever, weight loss, dyspnea, and/or pleuritic chest pain.

Bacterial pneumonia can present in a myriad of ways, depending on the patient and the organism involved. This patient is likely suffering from a bacterial pneumonia. Between 20% and 60% of patients with bacterial pneumonia develop parapneumonic effusions, and 5% to 10% of patients develop complicated parapneumonic effusions, such as an empyema, that will require surgical drainage (2). An empyema is a grossly purulent effusion. The possibility of an empyema needs to be considered in this patient with a history of unresolved pulmonary symptoms associated with a prior respiratory infection and a significant pleural effusion.

Chest radiographs can assess the presence of significant pleural effusions. Blunting of the costophrenic angle requires the presence of 200 to 500 mL of fluid. With lesser amounts of fluid, more subtle signs, such as elevation of the hemidiaphragm, may develop. If further evaluation of a potential effusion is necessary, ultrasound can often detect as little as 5 mL of fluid (2).

In the presence of a significant pleural effusion, a lateral decubitus film can help evaluate fluid viscosity. In this view, patients are placed on their side. Highly viscous fluid, such as pus, will often maintain the same position as in the upright film, while less viscous fluid will "layer out" due to gravity. This patient's decubitus film revealed that the effusion did not layer out (Fig. 56.2).

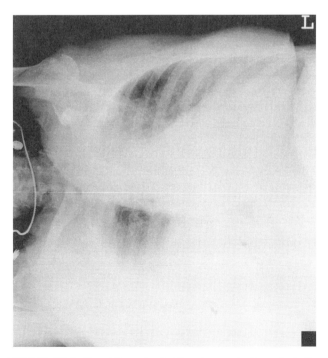

FIGURE 56.2. Decubitus chest film demonstrating that the patient's pleural effusion did not layer out. This finding increases suspicion for an empyema.

Which of the following management strategies is appropriate for this patient?

A. Admission to the hospital, with analgesics and observation
B. Admission to the hospital, with antibiotics and analgesics
C. Admission to the hospital, with a thoracentesis and antibiotics
D. Discharge for outpatient follow-up, with a prescription for analgesics

On the decubitus film, the fluid maintained much of its original configuration; it did not "layer out." This finding raises the suspicion for an empyema. Therefore, a thoracentesis to determine the nature of the fluid is the most appropriate strategy. All patients with pneumonia should be evaluated radiographically for the possibility of pleural effusion. Prompt diagnosis and treatment of empyema is imperative. In elderly patients, empyema carries a mortality of 25% to 70%; studies have shown that delays in diagnosis and treatment lead to increased length of hospitalization, morbidity, and probably mortality (3).

Evaluation of the Pleural Fluid

The visceral pleura lines the lung except at the hilum, and the parietal pleura covers the mediastinum, diaphragm, and the inner aspect of the chest wall. Normally, the space between these two continuous membranes contains approximately 5 mL of transudative fluid, but inflammatory conditions alter the permeability of the membrane to allow the influx of fluid that contains more protein (1). The utilization of biochemical testing to distinguish between exudative and transudative effusions is crucial in determining the etiology of pleural effusions. Light's criteria are the most frequently used guidelines to classify pleural effusions (4). Light's criteria classify an effusion as an exudate if *one or more* of the following apply:

1. Pleural fluid protein/serum protein greater than or equal to 0.5
2. Pleural fluid lactate dehydrogenase (LDH)/serum LDH greater than or equal to 0.6
3. Pleural fluid LDH greater than two-thirds of the normal upper limit of the serum value

The classification of a pleural effusion as an exudate or transudate assists in narrowing the differential diagnosis (Table 56.1) and guiding further treatment. When any of Light's criteria are positive, the sensitivity of an effusion being an exudate is 99%; specificity, 98%; positive predictive value, 99%; and negative predictive value, 98% (5).

When performing a thoracentesis, the fluid should be tested for pH, LDH, glucose, protein, cytology (if malignancy or esophageal rupture is suspected), Gram stain and culture, and acid-fast bacilli (if tuberculosis is suspected).

TABLE 56.1. DIFFERENTIAL DIAGNOSIS OF PLEURAL FLUID

Transudate	Congestive heart failure, cirrhosis, urinothorax, nephrotic syndrome, pulmonary embolism, hypothyroidism, peritoneal dialysis
Exudate	Collagen vascular diseases (lupus, rheumatoid arthritis), medications, gastrointestinal disease (pancreatitis, surgery, perforated esophagus), infections (bacterial, fungal, tuberculosis, viral), malignancy, pulmonary embolism, uremia

Data from Tarn AC, Lapworth R. Biochemical analysis of pleural fluid: what should we measure? *Ann Clin Biochem* 2001;38:311–322.

Simultaneous serum protein and LDH also are helpful in applying Light's criteria. Additional tests, such as amylase, may be useful, depending on the patient's clinical history.

A thoracentesis was performed on this patient. Non-bloody purulent fluid was obtained. Fluid characteristics included protein of 2.6 g/dL, glucose of less than 2 mg/dL, pH of 6.37, and LDH of 14,333 U/L. The serum LDH was 164 U/L, and serum protein was 7.2 g/dL.

Given the results of the thoracentesis, which of the following management strategies is appropriate?

A. Continue antibiotics and observation

B Insert a chest tube immediately and continue antibiotics

C. Continue antibiotics and discharge home with close follow-up

D. Discontinue antibiotics

Light has further defined the evaluation and appropriate treatment of parapneumonic effusions (6). He classified effusions into seven categories based on biochemical characteristics (pH, glucose), appearance on decubitus film, Gram stain, presence of loculations, and gross appearance. Class 1 effusions are less than 10 mm thick on a decubitus film and require no treatment. Class 6 and 7 effusions are simple and complex empyemas, respectively. Class 6 involves frank pus that is freely flowing and present in one focal location; class 7 involves frank pus with multiple loculations. Treatment for class 6 and 7 effusions includes chest tube drainage and pleural decortication as needed.

The presence of frank pus is an absolute indication for drainage of the effusion. Therefore, chest tube placement should be done and antibiotics administered as part of the treatment of an empyema. No strict guidelines exist for the treatment of empyema. Therefore, current treatment of an empyema depends on both the nature of the pleural fluid and the radiographic characteristics of the pleural effusion.

Empyema

Empyema is the presence of pus in the pleural space. The most common mechanism (about one-half of cases) of empyema is contiguous spread from a bacterial pneumonia. Empyemas may also result from surgery, trauma, rupture of the esophagus, chest tube or thoracentesis, or a subdiaphragmatic infection (2).

The most common bacterial etiologies of empyema are *Streptococcus pneumoniae, Staphylococcus aureus,* enteric Gram-negative bacilli, and anaerobes. The most common Gram-negative organisms involved are *Haemophilus influenzae, Klebsiella pneumoniae,* and *Pseudomonas aeruginosa* (2). Certain preexisting clinical conditions may predispose patients to developing certain bacterial etiologies:

■ Healthy patients most commonly have empyemas associated with *S. aureus, S. pyogenes,* and *S. pneumoniae.* While fewer patients develop pneumonia from *S. pyogenes* than from *S. pneumoniae,* the likelihood of *S. pyogenes* pneumonia developing into an empyema is considerably higher than it is for *S. pneumoniae* (3).

■ Alcoholics are predisposed to *Klebsiella* empyemas.

■ Immunocompromised patients are prone to developing Gram-negative or fungal empyemas.

■ Poor oral care and aspiration are associated with anaerobic empyemas.

■ Trauma or surgery is associated with staphylococcal empyemas.

Empyemas typically present with nonspecific symptoms. There is frequently a history of previous or ongoing pneumonia that is unresponsive to antibiotics. Associated symptoms include the presence of regional chest wall pain, unresolved cough, weight loss, and night sweats. Findings on physical examination are often consistent with the presence of an effusion. Common findings include decreased breath sounds, ipsilateral chest wall tenderness, decreased vocal and tactile fremitus, and decreased ipsilateral motion of the chest wall (Hoover sign). Compression of the lung superior to the effusion can result in findings of consolidation such as egophony and bronchial sounds (7). Therefore, a high index of suspicion is required in patients with a history of pneumonia, trauma, surgery, or esophageal rupture and nonspecific respiratory signs and symptoms.

The pathologic progression of empyema has three stages:

1. *Exudative:* This stage spans the first several days of the disease process. The pleural fluid is still free flowing but progressively becomes more protein rich, which increases its viscosity.

2. *Fibrinopurulent:* The pleural fluid becomes increasingly viscous. Fibrin deposition at this time causes the formation of fibrous networks that inhibit lung movement and, significantly, the creation of loculations within the pleural space.

3. *Organizing:* Intrapleural loculations, fibrous "peels" with fibroblast proliferation, and pus develop.

Treatment is aimed at preventing the second and third stages of empyema.

The need to treat a pleural effusion surgically is usually due to the potentially high mortality and morbidity rate of an untreated empyema and the relative safety of chest tube drainage. Administration of antibiotics alone is inappropriate management of an empyema. Therapy is aimed at effective drainage as well as effective treatment of the infection. Strictly, drainage is indicated when frank pus is obtained on the thoracentesis, and evidence supports drainage when the pH is less than 7.0, LDH is greater than 1,000 U/L, and/or glucose is less than 40 mg/dL (2,3).

Initial antibiotic selection depends on the most likely organisms, with further antibiotic selection guided by Gram stain and culture results. Monotherapy with aminoglycosides is not recommended because of their inhibition in the presence of pus and a low pH. However, aminoglycosides or ciprofloxacin may be used synergistically with a combination β-lactam/β-lactamase inhibitor for treatment of *P. aeruginosa, Enterobacter cloacae, Serratia marcescens,* and *Acinetobacter calcoaceticus* (3).

Active drainage of an empyema initially involves the use of a 22- to 34-French chest tube, although the use of percutaneous catheters for this purpose has increased in recent years. Serial chest radiographs and computed tomography of the chest can help guide further management. Fibrinolytic agents such as streptokinase and urokinase facilitate drainage by breaking up fibrin formations and decreasing effusion viscosity (2). The infusion of fibrinolytics into the pleural cavity is safe, with minimal occurrence of systemic fibrinolytic activation. If these methods are not successful, more invasive procedures such as decortication and debridement may be necessary. Video-assisted thoracoscopy is a less invasive alternative when performing less extensive decortication and debridement.

CONCLUSION

This patient's pleural fluid was found to contain *Haemophilus influenzae*. The empyema was effectively drained with a chest tube and several days of streptokinase infusions. She was discharged on home intravenous ceftriaxone, with follow-up scheduled with an infectious disease specialist.

Empyema, the presence of pus in the pleural cavity, is most commonly caused by extension of a bacterial pneumonia. Diagnosis relies on a high index of suspicion, radiographic findings, and pleural fluid analysis. Light's criteria can distinguish between transudative and exudative effusions. The need for drainage of the pleural space is made based on biochemical characteristics, Gram stain results, radiographic characteristics, and gross appearance of the pleural effusion. Frank pus, a pH of less than 7.0, LDH of greater than 1,000 U/L, or glucose of less than 40 mg/dL are consensus indications for drainage. Treatment consists of effective drainage of the empyema and appropriate antibiotics.

REFERENCES

1. Marrie TJ. Acute bronchitis and community-acquired pneumonia. In: Fishman AP, editor. *Fishman's pulmonary diseases and disorders,* 3rd ed. New York: McGraw-Hill, 1998:1985–1996.
2. Heffner JE. Infection of the pleural space. *Clin Chest Med* 1999; 20:607–622.
3. Bryant RE, Salmon CJ. Pleural empyema. *Clin Infect Dis* 1996;22: 747–764.
4. Kinasewitz GT. Transudative effusions. *Eur Respir J* 1997;10: 714–718.
5. Tarn AC, Lapworth R. Biochemical analysis of pleural fluid: What should we measure? *Ann Clin Biochem* 2001;38:311–322.
6. Light RW. A new classification of parapneumonic effusions and empyema. *Chest* 1995;108:299–301.
7. Kinasewitz GT. Pleural fluid dynamics and effusions. In: Fishman AP, ed. *Fishman's pulmonary diseases and disorders,* 3rd ed. New York: McGraw-Hill, 1998:1389–1410.

57

A 30-YEAR-OLD WOMAN WITH CYANOSIS, DYSPNEA, AND OXYGEN DESATURATION AFTER BRONCHOSCOPY

FEYROUZ T. AL-ASHKAR
PETER J. MAZZONE

CASE PRESENTATION

A 30-year-old woman with a history of acute myelogenous leukemia status post chemotherapy was admitted with a left hilar mass and a pericardial effusion. The patient underwent a left thoracotomy with hilar mass resection and a pericardial window. On postoperative day 4, the patient developed increasing shortness of breath with minimal cough. Her oxygen saturation was 95% on 3 L of oxygen by nasal cannula. Chest auscultation revealed decreased breath sounds on the left. A chest radiograph showed left lung atelectasis. A therapeutic bronchoscopy was scheduled. The patient was sedated with morphine and midazolam. Her pharynx was sprayed with benzocaine, and lidocaine gel was applied to her nasopharynx. She also received endotracheal/bronchial lidocaine. Thick secretions were suctioned throughout the left lung, after which the airway was patent. No endobronchial lesions were noted.

Toward the end of the procedure, the patient's oxygen saturation (SpO_2) dropped to 88%. She eventually required 10 L of oxygen by nonrebreather facemask to maintain a SpO_2 around 88%. The patient was awake and alert. She was mildly cyanotic and in moderate respiratory distress with a respiratory rate of 30 per minute. Her blood pressure was 116/83 mm Hg, and pulse was 120 beats per minute. Auscultation of the chest showed improved breath sounds bilaterally with mild rhonchi. Examination of the extremities did not reveal clubbing.

QUESTIONS/DISCUSSION

What is the most probable cause of this patient's persistent dyspnea, oxygen desaturation and central cyanosis?

A. Persistent mucous plugs

B. Ventilation–perfusion mismatch

C. Methemoglobinemia

D. Congenital cyanotic heart disease

All these conditions may lead to cyanosis and hypoxia. A *mucous plug* would be unlikely since the patient had undergone a bronchoscopy with suctioning of thick secretions, patent airways, and improved breath sounds on chest auscultation. Cyanosis may be seen in *cyanotic congenital heart disease* with right-to-left shunt and may either manifest during infancy and childhood or develop progressively as an adult. Sudden onset of symptoms would be unlikely, as was seen in this case. Furthermore, it is commonly associated with clubbing, which this patient did not have. In addition, the patient did not have a prior history of congenital heart disease. A *ventilation–perfusion mismatch* may have occurred as the airways had just been cleared of obstruction (thick secretions). This could paradoxically result in a mismatch between ventilation and lung perfusion. This usually corrects at least partially with inhalation of 100% oxygen. Acquired *methemoglobinemia* may present suddenly with shortness of breath, cyanosis, and decreased oxygen saturation by pulse oximetry, which is unchanged by the administration of supplemental oxygen (1). This best fits this patient's presentation.

Methemoglobin is a derivative of hemoglobin in which ferrous (Fe^{2+}) irons are oxidized to the ferric (Fe^{3+}) state (2,3). In deoxyhemoglobin, the iron moiety is in the ferrous state. When an oxidizing agent causes deoxyhemoglobin to lose an electron, deoxyhemoglobin gets transformed to the ferric state, thus becoming methemoglobin. In this state, the oxidized heme cannot transport oxygen. Methemoglobinemia represents a blood methemoglobin level greater than 1% (3). Patients typically present with shortness of breath, central cyanosis, and oxygen desaturation. Clinically, patients with methemoglobinemia have central cyanosis that is described as a chocolate color rather than a bluish discoloration (3,4). Patients typically become symptomatic with levels above 15% (3,4). Symptoms range from malaise, nausea, vomiting, and dyspnea to stupor, arrhythmia, seizure, coma, and death.

Patients with methemoglobinemia typically have pulse oximetry readings that persist in the mid-80% range, despite the administration of 100% oxygen. Pulse oximetry therefore cannot be used to assess oxygen saturation accurately (3,4). Arterial oxygen tension is not decreased. That is because oxygen tension reflects the amount of dissolved oxygen and not the oxygen molecule bound to hemoglobin (4). To determine an accurate oxygen saturation, multiple-wavelength co-oximetry should be run on an arterial blood sample. This technique measures the different forms of hemoglobin in blood and quantifies the methemoglobin level (3,4).

Case Continued: The patient was transferred to the intensive care unit. An arterial blood gas (ABG) showed a pH of 7.50, P_{CO_2} of 32 mm Hg, P_{O_2} of 338 mm Hg, total CO_2 24 of mmol/L, carboxyhemoglobin of 0, and methemoglobin (MetHgb) of 31.6%. Her methemoglobin level 4 days before this procedure was 0.3%.

Which of the following can cause methemoglobinemia?

A. **Nitroglycerin**
B. **Metoclopramide**
C. **Lidocaine**
D. **Benzocaine**
E. **All of the above**

All of these agents are potential causes of methemoglobinemia. In this case, the causative agent was benzocaine and/or lidocaine. Although uncommon, it has been reported that the topical application of benzocaine and/or lidocaine for certain procedures has led to the development of methemoglobinemia (4–7). Procedures involving esophageal or tracheal intubation, such as transesophageal echocardiography, upper endoscopy, and bronchoscopy, commonly employ topical benzocaine or lidocaine. Table 57.1 lists some of the oxidants that have been implicated in the formation of methemoglobin.

TABLE 57.1. POTENTIAL CAUSATIVE AGENTS OF METHEMOGLOBINEMIA

Chloroquine	Nitrites (including nitroglycerin and nitric oxide)
Dapsone	Phenazopyridine
Local anesthetics (benzocaine, lidocaine, prilocaine)	Phenytoin
Metoclopramide	Primaquine
Methylene blue (in high doses)	Pyridium
Naphthalene	Smoke inhalation
Nitrates	Sulfonamides
Nitric oxide	

Which of the following management st appropriate for this patient?

A. **Removal of the offending agent**
B. **Ensure airway patency**
C. **100% oxygen**
D. **Methylene blue**
E. **All of the above**

All of the preceding strategies are appropriate for this patient. Initial management should include discontinuation of the offending drug, gastric lavage, and activated charcoal. Because of enterohepatic circulation, some medications may require several doses of activated charcoal to enhance elimination. For example, dapsone requires the administration of activated charcoal every 6 hours for 4 days (4,6,8). In chronic dapsone users, cimetidine seems to diminish dapsone-induced methemoglobinemia (8). The next important measure is to maintain airway patency and hemodynamic stability. Administration of inhaled 100% oxygen is also appropriate. In cases of severe methemoglobinemia, methylene blue, as a 1 to 2 mg/kg intravenous infusion over 5 minutes, is indicated (2–4,6). A response is usually noted 30 to 60 minutes after administration; a dose may be repeated in 1 hour up to a maximum dose of 7 mg/kg (3,4,6). Exchange transfusion may be helpful in severe (more than 70%) cases of methemoglobinemia and in patients not responsive to methylene blue.

Case Continued: The patient was diagnosed with anesthetic-induced methemoglobinemia and was treated with intravenous methylene blue. A repeat ABG 2 hours later showed a pH of 7.46, P_{CO_2} of 41 mm Hg, P_{O_2} of 346 mm Hg, and a MetHgb of 18.3%. One day later, her MetHgb had fallen to 2.3%, then 1.2%. Her respiratory distress resolved completely, and her pulse oximetry was 97% on room air.

CONCLUSION

Acquired methemoglobinemia can occur after the use of certain drugs and chemicals, such as nitrites, local anesthetics, metoclopramide, aniline, nitric oxide, and dapsone. The clinical presentation, possible causative agents, and management issues need to be recognized to avoid delay in diagnosis and appropriate therapy. Although uncommon, acquired methemoglobinemia has been reported after procedures that are done on a daily basis (4–7). Failure to recognize this treatable complication results in unnecessary testing, increased morbidity, and possibly mortality.

REFERENCES

1. Braunwald E. Hypoxia and cyanosis. In: Braunwald E, Fauci AS, Kasper DL, et al, eds. *Harrison's principles of internal medicine,* 15th ed. New York: McGraw-Hill, 2001:214–216.

2. Beutler E. Methemoglobinemia and other causes of cyanosis. In: Beutler E, Lichtman MA, Coller BS, et al., eds. *Williams' hematology,* 6th ed. New York: McGraw-Hill, 2001:611–617.

3. Prchal JT, Gregg XT. Red cell enzymopathies. In: Hoffman R, Benz E Jr, Shattil SJ, et al., eds. *Hematology: basic principles and practice,* 3rd ed. Philadelphia: Churchill Livingstone, 2000:561–576.

4. Sharma VK, Haber AD. Acquired methemoglobinemia: a case report of benzocaine-induced methemoglobinemia and a review of the literature. *Clin Pulm Med* 2002;9:53–58.

5. Rodriguez LF, Smolik LM, Zbehlik AJ. Benzocaine-induced methemoglobinemia: report of a severe reaction and review of the literature. *Ann Pharmacother* 1994;28:643–649.

6. Wright RO, Lewander WJ, Woolf AD. Methemoglobinemia: etiology, pharmacology, and clinical management. *Ann Emerg Med* 1999;34:646–656.

7. Lee JS, Mendez PA, Douglass HO Jr. Unexpected cyanosis in the surgical patient. *Surg Endosc* 2000;14:595.

8. Coleman MD, Rhodes LE, Scott AK, et al. The use of cimetidine to reduce dapsone-dependent methaemoglobinemia in dermatitis herpetiformis patients. *Br J Clin Pharmacol* 1992;34:244–249.

58

A 53-YEAR-OLD MAN WITH CHEST PAIN

MAY AZEM
JAMES K. STOLLER

CASE PRESENTATION

A 53-year-old man presented to the emergency department (ED) with sudden-onset chest pain. He said the pain started when he was walking down the stairs at home. The pain was located in the left mid-axillary region. He described the pain as constant and sharp. The pain was worse with deep inspiration, and it radiated to his left arm and neck. The pain persisted for several hours, so the patient came to the ED for evaluation. He also noted mild shortness of breath, mild nausea, and a dry cough. He denied fever, chills, or diaphoresis.

His past medical history was significant for coronary artery disease, with a history of myocardial infarction 3 years prior, at which time he underwent percutaneous transluminal angioplasty (PTCA) of the right coronary artery. He had exercised regularly since his PTCA without anginal symptoms and had a negative stress test 2 years before this presentation. He also had a history of hypertension, hyperlipidemia, and nephrolithiasis. His medications on presentation included aspirin, metoprolol, atorvastatin, and ramipril. He had no history of tobacco use and drank alcohol occasionally.

Physical examination revealed an anxious-appearing man who was fully oriented. His vital signs revealed a temperature of 37.2°C, blood pressure of 109/53 mm Hg, pulse of 67 beats per minute, respiratory rate of 22 per minute, and oxygen saturation of 97% on 4 L of oxygen via nasal cannula. There was no jugular venous distension. Lungs were clear bilaterally. There was no tenderness on palpation of the chest wall. Cardiac and abdominal examinations were normal. There was no peripheral edema or calf tenderness.

QUESTIONS/DISCUSSION

Which of the following is the least likely diagnosis?

A. Acute coronary syndrome
B. Pulmonary embolus
C. Pneumonia
D. Costochondritis

The initial goal in any evaluation of new-onset chest pain is to exclude life-threatening conditions, specifically myocardial infarction, pulmonary embolus, aortic dissection, and tension pneumothorax. The history and physical examination, in conjunction with selected tests such as an electrocardiogram and chest x-ray, allow clinicians to diagnose most common causes of chest pain. One study found that using only the history and physical examination, physicians were able to differentiate nonorganic and organic causes of chest pain in 88% of patients (1).

Given this patient's history of coronary artery disease, the possibility of an acute coronary syndrome (ACS), either unstable angina or non-ST elevation myocardial infarction, needs to be considered. The age of the patient can play a role in the determination of the likelihood of an acute coronary syndrome. One study found that only 7% of patients less than 35 years of age who had chest pain were diagnosed with coronary artery disease. In contrast, the prevalence of coronary disease may exceed 50% in patients with chest pain after the age of 40 (2–5). Although this patient's pain was pleuritic and was persistent with intermittent exacerbations, an acute coronary syndrome needs to be ruled out with serial electrocardiograms and cardiac enzymes.

Pulmonary embolus (PE) also must be considered in the differential diagnosis. Although this patient did not appear to have any predisposing factors for developing PE, many features of his presentation are consistent with PE. The sudden onset of the pain, its pleuritic quality, and the patient's tachypnea and hypoxia are all findings that are concerning for the possibility of PE. Therefore, further evaluation for the presence of venous thromboembolic disease is appropriate in this case.

Patients with pneumonia caused by pyogenic organisms classically present with sudden-onset rigors followed by fever, pleuritic chest pain, and cough productive of purulent sputum. Chest pain only occurs in 30% of cases (6). However, the absence of these symptoms does not rule out

pneumonia. Moreover, a viral pneumonia
e to an atypical bacterial organism, such as
·oplasma, remains a possibility. A chest x-
.,. ....pname to evaluate for the presence of pneumonia, especially given this patient's hypoxia.

Costochondritis is the least likely diagnosis in this case.
Although costochondritis can mimic cardiac and pulmonary
causes of chest pain, patients with costochondritis typically
have reproducible pain on examination. This patient did not
have reproducible pain on examination of the chest wall.

An electrocardiogram (ECG) revealed normal sinus
rhythm without any acute changes. Two sets of cardiac
enzymes were negative. Chest x-ray did not reveal any infiltrates or effusions. The patient's electrolytes and renal function
were normal. His hemoglobin was 12.9 g/dL, and platelets
were 198 K/μL. A duplex ultrasound of the lower extremities
was negative for acute deep venous thrombosis (DVT).

Case Continued: The patient was initially treated for
unstable angina with nitroglycerin and heparin drips. His
home medications were continued. In the hospital, the
patient experienced two episodes of chest pain radiating to
the left arm and jaw along with hypotension, which was
managed with fluid boluses. Follow-up examination
revealed the presence of a new friction rub and decreased
breath sounds over the left base. Repeat chest x-ray revealed
a left lower lobe infiltrate and small bilateral effusions.

**At this point, which of the following is the most appro-
priate diagnostic test to order?**

A. **Ventilation–perfusion scan**
B. **Contrast-enhanced spiral computed tomography
(CT scan) of the chest**
C. **Pulmonary angiogram**
D. **D-dimer**
E. **Arterial blood gas**

Given the history, the new findings on physical examination, the presence of hypoxia, and the laboratory and radiographic data, the main concern at this point was pulmonary
embolism (PE). Although pneumonia remained a possibility,
the overall clinical picture was most consistent with PE. A
quick and accurate diagnosis of PE is essential, since PE is the
third most common cause of cardiovascular mortality in
North America, with an estimated incidence of 500,000
deaths per year. Pulmonary embolism is responsible for 5%
to 10% of all in-hospital deaths (7). Undiagnosed PE has a
mortality rate up to 30%; prompt diagnosis and appropriate
treatment decreases the mortality rate to approximately 8%
(7). In this case, the patient had been started on anticoagulation with heparin. However, timely diagnostic testing
remains essential to establish the diagnosis of pulmonary
embolism or an alternative diagnosis in order to avoid expos-
ing patients to unnecessary risks from anticoagulation if they
do not have venous thromboembolic disease.

Numerous diagnostic tests are available to aid in the diagnosis of PE. Given the multitude of tests, clinicians need to
recognize the information that each test provides and the
appropriate time to perform each test. Tests with the potential
to assist in the diagnosis of PE can be classified into imaging
studies, such as ventilation–perfusion scan, contrast-enhanced
spiral CT of the chest, pulmonary angiogram, venous duplex
ultrasound, venography and echocardiography, and nonimaging studies, such as arterial blood gases (ABG), ECG, and D-
dimer. Establishing an optimal strategy combining imaging
and nonimaging studies has been challenging.

For over 30 years, ventilation–perfusion (V/Q) scanning
has been the imaging study of choice to evaluate patients
with suspected PE. Its accuracy was initially evaluated in
two studies that used pulmonary angiography as the gold
standard. Both studies demonstrated that a normal perfusion lung scan essentially excludes the presence of PE and a
high-probability V/Q scan has an 85% to 90% positive predictive value for PE. However, using pulmonary angiography as the gold standard, two additional studies demonstrated that between 45% and 66% of high-probability
lung scans are falsely positive when a skilled clinician has a
low pretest probability for PE (8).

Criteria developed by the PIOPED (*Prospective Investigation of Pulmonary Embolism Diagnosis*) investigators
provided further evidence of the utility of V/Q scans. The
PIOPED data analyzed the probability of PE with low-
probability (14%), intermediate-probability (30%), and
high-probability V/Q scans (87%). Patients with high-
probability V/Q scans should be treated for PE unless there
are contraindications to anticoagulation. The designation
nondiagnostic is preferred for all scan results that are neither
normal nor high probability. Further testing is required to
exclude the diagnosis of PE in patients with nondiagnostic
scans (8). The extent to which further testing is performed
in patients with nondiagnostic scans often depends on the
clinical suspicion for thromboembolic disease. Table 58.1
demonstrates the likelihood of pulmonary embolism in the
PIOPED study based on the combination of lung scan
results and clinical probability of PE (8).

**TABLE 58.1. LIKELIHOOD OF PULMONARY
EMBOLISM BASED ON V/Q SCAN RESULT AND
CLINICAL PROBABILITY (PIOPED STUDY)**

Scan Result	Clinical Probability of Embolism (%)		
	High	Intermediate	Low
High	96	88	56
Intermediate	66	28	16
Low	40	16	4
Normal	0	6	2

Adapted from Value of the ventilation/perfusion scan in acute
pulmonary embolism. Results of the prospective investigation of
pulmonary embolism diagnosis (PIOPED). The PIOPED Investigators.
JAMA 1990;263:2753–2759.

A V/Q scan was not performed on this patient because the abnormal findings on his chest x-ray (small bilateral pleural effusions and left-lower-lobe infiltrate) would most likely lead to the scan being read as nondiagnostic.

Over the past decade, contrast-enhanced spiral CT has emerged as an alternative noninvasive imaging modality for patients with suspected PE (9,10). Spiral CT allows for direct visualization of segmental and some subsegmental arteries using a single bolus of contrast. Table 58.2 summarizes the advantages and disadvantages of spiral CT scans. A pooled analysis of five comparative studies using pulmonary angiography as the gold standard found spiral CT to be 72% sensitive and 95% specific (11). Furthermore, for central PE, the sensitivity of spiral CT increased to 94%. Three small studies have directly compared spiral CT with V/Q scanning in patients with suspected PE. These studies, which utilized pulmonary angiography as the gold standard, have favored spiral CT as the more accurate imaging procedure (10). For many of the reasons outlined previously, spiral CT is the most appropriate test to order at this point to establish a diagnosis.

Pulmonary angiography remains the gold standard for the diagnosis of PE, with sensitivity and specificity exceeding 95%. Four injections of contrast with four views should be considered the gold standard, with the order of vessel injection based on the results of ventilation–perfusion scanning. The most suspicious vascular distribution should be injected first to limit the volume of contrast administered. A positive result consists of a filling defect or sharp cutoff of small vessels (12). However, pulmonary angiography is not typically the initial diagnostic test in the evaluation of PE because of its associated morbidity and mortality (13). Mortality is reported as 0.5%, and major nonfatal morbidity is 1%. These rates are higher in patients with poor cardiopulmonary reserve before angiography. For these reasons, pulmonary angiography is not the most appropriate test at this time for this patient.

The utility of D-dimer, the degradation product of cross-linked fibrin, as a diagnostic tool for venous thromboembolic disease has been extensively studied. D-dimer is detectable at levels greater than 500 ng/mL of fibrinogen equivalent units in nearly all patients with PE. A metaanalysis of 11 studies totaling 1,337 patients demonstrated that D-dimer assays have a negative predictive value of 94%. When D-dimer was less than 500 ng/dL, the likelihood of PE was below 10%, even in cases with a pretest probability for PE as high as 55% (14). However, an elevated D-dimer is insufficient to establish the diagnosis of PE. D-dimer is nonspecific and is frequently elevated in hospitalized patients without thromboembolic disease, patients with malignancy, and patients who underwent recent surgery (15). D-dimer is not an appropriate test to establish the diagnosis of pulmonary embolism in this patient or other patients.

An arterial blood gas (ABG) can establish the presence of hypoxia, but it does not significantly assist in excluding or establishing the diagnosis of pulmonary embolus (16). Although hypoxemia or an increased alveolar-arterial gradient (A-a gradient) may suggest pulmonary embolus (PE), many other conditions can also produce these conditions. Moreover, approximately 18% of patients with PE have a partial pressure of oxygen (P_aO_2) between 85 and 105 mm Hg, and up to 6% have a normal A-a gradient (17). This patient's ABG on room air revealed pH of 7.47, P_{CO_2} 38 mm Hg, P_{O_2} of 71 mm Hg, bicarbonate of 27 mmol/L, and oxygen saturation of 96%.

A spiral CT scan showed small bilateral pleural effusions, left lower lobe atelectasis, an infarct in the anterior segment of the left lower lobe, and a wedge-shaped consolidation in the lingula, which was also consistent with an infarct (Fig. 58.1).

TABLE 58.2. ADVANTAGES AND LIMITATIONS OF SPIRAL COMPUTED TOMOGRAPHY

Advantages	Limitations
Specificity	Reader expertise required
Availablity	Expensive
Safety	Not portable
Relative rapidity of procedure	Need contrast bolus comparable to angiogram
Diagnosis of other diseases	Poor visualization of certain regions
Retrospective reconstruction	Contraindicated in renal insufficiency
Advancing technology	Contraindicated with contrast allergies

Adapted from Rathbun SW, Raskob GE, Whitsett TL. Sensitivity and specificity of helical computed tomography in the diagnosis of pulmonary embolism: a systematic review. *Ann Intern Med* 2000;132:227–232.

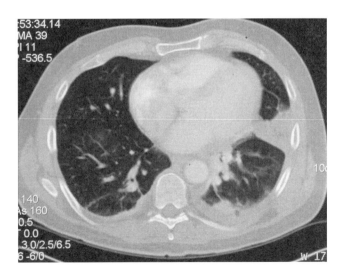

FIGURE 58.1. Spiral computed tomography of the chest demonstrating left lower lobe atelectasis, an infarct in the anterior segment of the left lower lobe, and a wedge-shaped consolidation in the lingula consistent with an infarct.

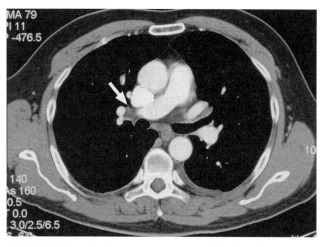

FIGURE 58.2. Spiral computed tomography of the chest (mediastinal views) demonstrating emboli in the distribution of the posterior basal segmental artery of the right lower lobe.

TABLE 58.3. INHERITED CAUSES OF THROMBOPHILIA

Factor V Leiden mutation
Prothrombin gene G20210A mutation
Protein S deficiency
Protein C deficiency
Antithrombin (ATIII) deficiency
Heparin cofactor II deficiency
Plasminogen deficiency
Dysfibrinogenemia
Factor V/XII deficiencies
Increased factor VIII coagulant activity

and P-pulmonale (increased P amplitude greater than 2.5 mVs in lead II). ECG changes may relate to hemodynamic and/or ischemic changes associated with the PE and may correlate with the severity of the PE. However, the overall utility of these findings remains limited because of their variable frequency and transient nature (19).

Recently, cardiac troponin has been recognized as an adverse prognostic factor in patients with acute pulmonary emboli. The mortality rate from PE was 44% in troponin-positive patients, as opposed to 3% in troponin-negative patients (20).

When evaluating patients with a new pulmonary embolism or deep venous thrombosis (DVT), clinicians need to consider potential underlying etiologies. Upon presentation, patients often have clinically identifiable risk factors for the development of thromboembolic disease. Underlying etiologies of DVT/PE can be broadly divided into inherited and acquired causes (Tables 58.3 and 58.4). Inherited causes of thrombophilia are present in 24% to 37% of cases, of which the most common is factor V Leiden mutation. Commonly identified risk factors in the PIOPED study included immobilization, surgery within the preceding 3 months, stroke, prior history of DVT/PE, and malignancy (8).

Not every patient with a newly diagnosed PE or DVT needs to undergo an evaluation for a hypercoagulable state.

The mediastinal views demonstrated emboli in the distribution of the posterior basal segmental artery of the right lower lobe (Fig. 58.2).

All of the following statements regarding pulmonary emboli are correct except:

A. Dyspnea is the most common presenting symptom.
B. Right bundle branch block is the most common electrocardiographic abnormality.
C. Atelectasis is the most common abnormality seen on chest x-ray.
D. Findings on ECG and/or chest x-ray are not typically diagnostic of pulmonary embolism.

Patients with pulmonary emboli present in a variety of ways, and no one particular sign or symptom is specific for PE. In PIOPED, the most common symptoms were dyspnea, which occurred in 73% of patients, pleuritic pain (65%), cough (37%), and hemoptysis (13%). The most common signs were tachypnea, which occurred in 70% of patients, rales (51%), tachycardia (30%), presence of a fourth heart sound (24%), and a prominent pulmonic component of the second heart sound (23%). Circulatory collapse was uncommon, occurring in 8% of patients (18).

Radiographic and electrocardiographic findings associated with PE are also typically nonspecific. In PIOPED, the most frequent abnormalities noted on chest x-ray were atelectasis and parenchymal abnormalities (18). Numerous studies have described a wide range of specific ECG abnormalities associated with PE, with 9% to 26% of patients having normal ECGs. The most common ECG abnormality is sinus tachycardia, which occurs in 18% to 35% of patients with pulmonary emboli. Other less commonly seen ECG changes include right bundle branch block, first-degree atrioventricular block, atrial fibrillation, atrial flutter,

TABLE 58.4 ACQUIRED CAUSES OF THROMBOPHILIA

Malignancy
Surgery
Trauma
Pregnancy
Oral contraceptives/hormone replacement therapy
Tamoxifen
Immobilization
Congestive heart failure
Hyperhomocysteinemia
Antiphospholipid antibody syndrome
Myeloproliferative disorders (Polycythemia vera, essential thrombocythemia)
Paroxysmal nocturnal hemoglobinuria

Potential indications to investigate for a hypercoagulable state include venous thromboembolism in the absence of typical risk factors, recurrent thrombotic episodes, the presence of arterial and venous thrombosis, thromboembolism at an early age (less than age 40), thrombosis at unusual sites, migratory thrombophlebitis, thromboembolic disease resistant to anticoagulation, and massive thromboembolism (21).

Clinicians should be suspicious of an underlying malignancy in patients who develop thromboembolic disease in the absence of any risk factors. One series reported a prevalence of malignancy up to 17% in patients with thromboembolic disease (22). Thromboembolic disease can be the initial presentation of pancreatic or prostate cancers; in addition, it can occur later in the course of breast, lung, uterine, or brain malignancies (23). These patients should undergo a thorough physical examination and age-appropriate cancer screening to search for an underlying neoplasm. This patient was up-to-date on his age-appropriate cancer screening.

CONCLUSION

The patient was continued on intravenous heparin and received oral anticoagulation with warfarin. His condition improved throughout the remainder of his hospitalization, with progressively lower oxygen requirements. Evaluation for a hypercoagulable state was deferred until he had completed 6 months of therapy with warfarin. The patient was discharged home off supplemental oxygen when his INR was within the target range.

REFERENCES

1. Martina B, Bucheli B, Stotz M, et al. First clinical judgment by primary care physicians distinguishes well between nonorganic and organic causes of abdominal or chest pain. *J Gen Intern Med* 1997;12:459–465.
2. Luke LC, Cusack S, Smith H, et al. Non-traumatic chest pain in young adults: a medical audit. *Arch Emerg Med* 1990;7:183–188.
3. Pryor DB, Harrell FE Jr, Lee KL, et al. Estimating the likelihood of significant coronary artery disease. *Am J Med* 1983;75:771–780.
4. Goldman L, Weinberg M, Weisberg M, et al. A computer-derived protocol to aid in the diagnosis of emergency room patients with acute chest pain. *N Engl J Med* 1982;307:588–596.
5. Lee TH, Cook EF, Weisberg M, et al. Acute chest pain in the emergency room: identification and examination of low-risk patients. *Arch Intern Med* 1985;145:65–69.
6. Marrie TJ. Community-acquired pneumonia. *Clin Infect Dis* 1994;18:501–513.
7. Rodger M, Wells PS. Diagnosis of pulmonary embolism. *Thromb Res* 2001;103:V225–V238.
8. Value of the ventilation/perfusion scan in acute pulmonary embolism: results of the prospective investigation of pulmonary embolism diagnosis (PIOPED). The PIOPED Investigators. *JAMA* 1990;263:2753–2759.
9. Remy-Jardin M, Remy J. Spiral CT angiography of the pulmonary circulation. *Radiology* 1999;212:615–636.
10. Mayo JR, Remy-Jardin M, Muller NL, et al. Pulmonary embolism: prospective comparison of spiral CT with ventilation–perfusion scintigraphy. *Radiology* 1997;205:447–452.
11. Rathbun SW, Raskob GE, Whitsett TL. Sensitivity and specificity of helical computed tomography in the diagnosis of pulmonary embolism: a systematic review. *Ann Intern Med* 2000;132:227–232.
12. Davey NC, Smith TP, Hanson MW, et al. Ventilation–perfusion lung scintigraphy as a guide for pulmonary angiography in the localization of pulmonary emboli. *Radiology* 1999;213:51–57.
13. Prologo JD, Glauser J. Variable diagnostic approach to suspected pulmonary embolism in the ED of a major academic tertiary care center. *Am J Emerg Med* 2002;20:5–9.
14. Bounameaux H, de Moerloose P, Perrier A, et al. Plasma measurement of D-dimer as diagnostic aid in suspected venous thromboembolism: an overview. *Thromb Haemost* 1994;71:1–6.
15. Guidelines on diagnosis and management of acute pulmonary embolism. Task Force on Pulmonary Embolism, European Society of Cardiology. *Eur Heart J* 2000;21:1301–1336.
16. Rodger MA, Carrier M, Jones GN, et al. Diagnostic value of arterial blood gas measurement in suspected pulmonary embolism. *Am J Respir Crit Care Med* 2000;162:2105–2108.
17. Stein PD, Terrin ML, Hales CA, et al. Clinical, laboratory, roentgenographic, and electrocardiographic findings in patients with acute pulmonary embolism and no pre-existing cardiac or pulmonary disease. *Chest* 1991;100:598–603.
18. Stein PD, Saltzman HA, Weg JG. Clinical characteristics of patients with acute pulmonary embolism. *Am J Cardiol* 1991;68:1723–1724.
19. Chan TC, Vilke GM, Pollack M, et al. Electrocardiographic manifestations: pulmonary embolism. *J Emerg Med* 2001;21:263–270.
20. Goldhaber SZ. Thrombolysis in pulmonary embolism: a debatable indication. *Thromb Haemost* 2001;86:444–451.
21. Olin, JW. Deep venous thrombosis and pulmonary emboli. In: Stoller JK, Ahmad M, Longworth DL, eds. *The Cleveland Clinic intensive review of internal medicine,* 2nd ed. Philadelphia: Lippincott Williams & Wilkins, 2000:413–427.
22. Monreal, M, Lafoz, E, Casals A, et al. Occult cancer in patients with deep venous thrombosis: a systematic approach. *Cancer* 1991;67:541–545.
23. Monreal M, Fernandez-Llamazares J, Perandreu J, et al. Occult cancer in patients with venous thromboembolism: Which patients, which cancers? *Thromb Haemost* 1997;78:1316–1318.

59

PULSELESS CARDIAC ARREST IN A 64-YEAR-OLD MAN

JOHN KEVIN HIX
DAVID V. GUGLIOTTI

CASE PRESENTATION

A 64-year-old man was brought to the emergency department after he collapsed and was found to be pulseless. He was at our institution visiting a friend at the time of the event. Cardiopulmonary resuscitation (CPR) was initiated promptly before his transfer to the emergency department (ED). According to witnesses, he was completely asymptomatic immediately before collapsing. CPR was successful in establishing a pulse, blood pressure, and spontaneous breathing. The patient was conscious, responding appropriately and able to protect his airway upon arrival in the ED.

QUESTIONS/DISCUSSION

Based on this patient's clinical presentation, which of the following is the most likely cause of his cardiac arrest?

A. **Acute asthma exacerbation/status asthmaticus**
B. **Stroke**
C. **Ventricular arrhythmia due to underlying coronary artery disease**
D. **Pulmonary embolism**
E. **Massive gastrointestinal (GI) bleed with hypotension**

Any of the preceding conditions can cause rapid clinical deterioration and result in cardiovascular collapse. However, the initial clinical presentation can help to narrow the possibilities. Even with severe asthma, a more gradual onset of pulmonary symptoms would likely have occurred before full arrest. Likewise, a GI bleed severe enough to cause circulatory collapse would have typically produced earlier symptoms. The rapidity with which the patient regained consciousness and responded appropriately makes a stroke unlikely.

Massive pulmonary embolism (PE) must be considered, as it can present with cardiovascular compromise (1). In a large single-center study, 4.5% of all outpatient cardiac arrests were due to PE (2). Thirty percent of the patients were not diagnosed with PE until autopsy. The most common symptoms present before arrest included dyspnea in 68% of patients and chest pain in 25% of patients. Approximately 70% of patients had electrocardiographic evidence of right bundle branch block, while only 8% demonstrated the frequently described $S_1Q_3T_3$ pattern.

Based on demographics alone and without further history, a ventricular arrhythmia due to underlying cardiovascular disease is the most likely cause of sudden death in this patient (3). Approximately 225,000 people per year are expected to die from coronary heart disease before reaching a hospital (3). The arrest is most often caused by an acute myocardial infarction, ischemia, or electrical disorder resulting in ventricular fibrillation or ventricular tachycardia. Arrests due to ventricular fibrillation most frequently occur in men in their 60s (3). The survival rates of such patients vary widely, and no national statistics are available. However, it is thought that the increased availability of out-of-hospital defibrillators, along with plans to make citizens taking community CPR courses familiar with their operation, should improve these survival rates. Data from casinos using automated external defibrillators (AEDs) have demonstrated that patients who were defibrillated by bystanders within 3 minutes of a witnessed collapse had a 74% survival rate (4).

Case Continued: The patient was awake and able to provide some history in the ED. He had been in his usual state of health, and, on the same day as his arrest, had driven 5 hours to visit a friend at our institution. He had complained only of mild calf pain for a few days, which he attributed to a strain from playing tennis. He reported a past medical history significant for hyperlipidemia, atrial flutter, and a left-lower-extremity deep venous thrombosis (DVT) diagnosed 3 years before. The DVT was treated with 3 months of oral anticoagulation. His medications included simvastatin, enalapril, and digoxin. He was a former smoker and drank alcohol only on occasion. The remainder of his history and review of systems was unremarkable.

Physical examination in the ED revealed a pleasant man in moderate respiratory distress. He was dyspneic with conversation and was coughing up blood during the examination. Vital signs revealed a pulse of 75 beats per minute, blood pressure of 80/60 mm Hg, and oxygen saturation of 95% on a 50% oxygen mask. Heart sounds were distant but regular. His lungs were clear. Abdomen was soft and nontender. Examination of the extremities revealed mild left calf tenderness without any edema. Neurologic examination revealed no focal deficits.

Laboratory studies revealed a troponin T of 0.01 ng/mL, sodium of 139 mmol/L, potassium of 3.7 mmol/L, chloride of 102 mmol/L, bicarbonate of 20 mmol/L, blood urea nitrogen of 14 mg/dL, creatinine of 1.1 mg/dL. Complete blood count showed white blood cell count of 12.6 K/μL, hemoglobin of 16.5 g/dL, and platelets of 215 K/μL. An arterial blood gas on 100% oxygen by mask revealed pH of 7.34, P_{CO_2} of 38 mm Hg, P_{O_2} of 145 mm Hg, and oxygen saturation of 97%.

A rhythm strip was not recorded during resuscitation efforts. An electrocardiogram (ECG) in the ED showed a heart rate of 74 beats per minute, an ectopic atrial rhythm, and an incomplete right bundle branch block. Further testing included a bedside echocardiogram, which revealed a severely dilated right ventricle (RV), severely diminished RV systolic function, 3+ tricuspid regurgitation, RV systolic pressure of 22 mm Hg, and normal left ventricular function.

These findings suggest the patient suffered a pulmonary thromboembolism. All of the following are strategies that could confirm the diagnosis except

A. **Spiral volumetric computed tomography (CT scan) of the chest**
B. **D-dimer**
C. **Pulmonary angiogram**
D. **Ventilation–perfusion scan**

Multiple studies evaluating the use of radiographic or biochemical techniques for the diagnosis of PE have incorporated clinical algorithms in an attempt to enhance the accuracy of the diagnosis. Assessing the probability of PE in an individual patient is difficult, and clinical prediction rules have met with limited success. Multiple studies have documented that information based on history and physical examination alone is insufficient to diagnose venous thromboembolism. Although a history and physical may be suggestive of PE, confirmatory tests must be done to establish the diagnosis.

Spiral volumetric CT scan (SVCT) has become an important imaging modality in the evaluation of patients with a suspected PE. Spiral CT can be performed quickly and may provide alternate diagnoses in addition to determining the presence or absence of PE. The major drawbacks of spiral CT are the need for contrast dye and the lack of sensitivity for subsegmental emboli. The sensitivity of

SVCT for central PE is high, but there is likely a lower sensitivity when evaluating subsegmental branches (5). One recent review of trials using SVCT to diagnose PE found that the reported sensitivity of SVCT ranged from 64% to 93% and the specificity ranged from 89% to 100% (6).

D-dimer has long shown promise as a noninvasive diagnostic test for venous thromboembolism. D-dimer is a degradation product of cross-linked fibrin, which is a component of venous thromboemboli as well as numerous other processes. Therefore, the finding of an elevated D-dimer is nonspecific, particularly in patients who are already hospitalized or have had recent surgery or trauma. However, a meta-analysis has suggested that a normal D-dimer level in a low risk patient may have substantial negative predictive value (7). The sensitivity of the D-dimer assay is variable, and clinicians who rely on D-dimer to guide decisions for further testing need to recognize the limitations and characteristics of the particular assay used at their institution. An elevated D-dimer is insufficient to make the diagnosis of PE.

Angiography remains the gold standard for the diagnosis of PE. A large review validated the accuracy of pulmonary angiography in establishing the presence or absence of a PE and revealed relatively low complication rates for this invasive procedure (8). The availability of pulmonary angiography is institution dependent. The risk for nephrotoxicity with the significant dye load involved must be considered in patients with underlying renal insufficiency.

Ventilation–perfusion (V/Q) scanning is among the best-studied and most widely used techniques for determining the presence of a pulmonary embolus. Most studies show a sensitivity approaching 95% for diagnosing emboli when a high-probability scan is obtained in a patient with a high pretest probability for PE (9). However, the interpretation of the test is optimal only in patients with a normal chest x-ray. Of critical importance in evaluating the results of any V/Q scan are the clinician's pretest suspicion for PE and the experience of the radiologist interpreting the scan. In a detailed analysis of V/Q scanning, Kumar noted that a high clinical suspicion raised the sensitivity of high-probability scans by almost 10%. In addition, intermediate-probability scans (the most common classification in the PIOPED study) showed the most interobserver discordance (9,10).

Case Continued: Fluid resuscitation was initiated. The patient underwent an urgent CT scan of the chest with PE protocol. The CT scan showed extensive pulmonary embolic disease, including a saddle embolus at the bifurcation of the main pulmonary artery (Fig. 59.1).

At this point, which of the following is the most appropriate management strategy for this patient?

A. **Anticoagulation with unfractionated heparin**
B. **Anticoagulation with low-molecular-weight heparin**

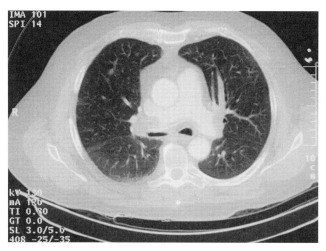

FIGURE 59.1. Spiral computed tomographic scan of the chest demonstrating extensive pulmonary embolic disease, most notably a saddle embolus at the bifurcation of the main pulmonary artery.

C. Unfractionated heparin and thrombolysis
D. Surgical thrombectomy

When assessing the risks and benefits of treatment for this patient, his hemodynamic instability needs to be considered. Although the patient could protect his airway and was fully oriented, he remained profoundly hypotensive and hypoxemic.

The initiation of anticoagulation with heparin confers a survival advantage in patients with venous thromboembolism by increasing the effectiveness of antithrombin III, which is an endogenous fibrinolytic. With heparin, antithrombin III combines more effectively with thrombin, activated factor X, activated factor IX, and other serum proteinases (11). Moreover, heparin inhibits the activation of factors V and VIII. These effects stabilize the thrombus and allow the natural endogenous fibrinolytic compounds to dissolve the thrombus. An early study revealed that patients with thromboembolism who did not receive treatment with heparin had a much higher mortality rate than those treated with heparin (12). This finding has generally been supported in subsequent studies. A minimum level of anticoagulation is needed to achieve a benefit; typically, the degree of anticoagulation is estimated by measurements of the activated partial thromboplastin time (aPTT). In general, failure to achieve a target aPTT greater than 1.5 times the control value leads to suboptimal results (11).

Most studies involving low-molecular-weight (LMW) heparins have compared these compounds to unfractionated heparin. LMW heparin preparations have shown comparable efficacy to unfractionated heparins (13). Although LMW heparin preparations are gaining acceptance in the treatment of venous thromboembolism, particularly in the outpatient setting, their inclusion in standard inpatient treatment recommendations for PE is not currently widespread in North America (14).

Thrombolytic therapy has shown mixed results in treating venous thromboembolic disease. Although early studies showed that thrombolytic agents reduce clot burden and improve physiologic parameters, they failed to demonstrate a survival advantage (15). However, later studies have shown that the use of streptokinase confers a survival advantage over heparin in the treatment of massive PE with shock (15). Subsequent studies have shown a survival advantage with thrombolytics in PE patients with either RV dysfunction or pulmonary hypertension, in the absence of shock (15). However, all the studies involving thrombolytics are either small or nonrandomized, leaving the applicability of these trials to clinical practice in question.

The available data, although limited, seem to suggest that the outcomes for patients who present with massive PE and receive thrombolytic therapy may depend on the hemodynamic stability at the time of thrombolysis. A retrospective cohort study of 153 patients who presented with massive PE and evidence of right heart failure did not find a statistically significant mortality difference between those given both thrombolytics and unfractionated heparin and those treated with heparin alone (16). However, this retrospective analysis excluded patients who presented with documented hypotension (systolic blood pressure less than 90 mm Hg), who had peripheral signs of hypoperfusion, syncope, or who needed inotropic support. However, analysis of trials that included PE patients who presented in shock has demonstrated a mortality benefit with the use of thrombolytic therapy (1,17).

Surgical thrombectomy and embolectomy has been an accepted therapy for massive PE, although there has been difficulty in studying its efficacy. The modality is utilized by a limited number of centers, and studies evaluating its efficacy have used small numbers of patients. A recent position paper suggested the use of thrombectomy in hemodynamically unstable patients with confirmed PE who have failed thrombolytic therapy (14). Embolectomy is currently regarded as a "rescue" procedure utilized in a select group of patients.

CONCLUSION

The patient was admitted to the intensive care unit (ICU). He was started on unfractionated heparin and given 100 mg of t-PA. Further work-up revealed an acute left popliteal DVT. A limited pulmonary angiogram confirmed both acute and chronic thromboembolism, as well as elevated pulmonary pressures of 42/11 mm Hg. At the time of the angiogram, the patient was clinically stable and further angiographic intervention, such as catheter-directed embolectomy, was not performed.

The patient improved during his 3-day ICU stay. His heart rate and blood pressure remained normal following thrombolysis, and his oxygenation improved to such an extent that he was saturating 95% on room air by his third hospital day. Follow-up CT of the pulmonary vasculature revealed successful lysis of the acute embolism, although evidence of bilateral thromboemboli remained, likely representing chronic disease. A repeat echocardiogram demonstrated normal right ventricular size and function, with resolution of the elevated pulmonary pressures. The patient was converted to oral anticoagulation and discharged home in good condition.

REFERENCES

1. Bailen MR, Cuadra JA, Aguayo de Hoyos E. Thrombolysis during cardiopulmonary resuscitation in fulminant pulmonary embolism: a review. *Crit Care Med* 2001;29:2211–2219.
2. Kurkciyan I, Meron G, Sterz F, et al. Pulmonary embolism as a cause of cardiac arrest: presentation and outcome. *Arch Intern Med* 2000;160:1529–1535.
3. Eisenberg MS, Mengert TJ. Cardiac resuscitation. *N Engl J Med* 2001;344:1304–1313.
4. Valenzuela TD, Roe DJ, Nichol G, et al. Outcomes of rapid defibrillation by security officers after cardiac arrest in casinos. *N Engl J Med* 2000;343:1206–1209.
5. Wolfe TR, Hartsell SC. Pulmonary embolism: making sense of the diagnostic evaluation. *Ann Emerg Med* 2001;37:504–514.
6. Garg K. CT of pulmonary thromboembolic disease. *Radiol Clin North Am* 2002;40:111–122.
7. Bounameaux H, de Moerloose P, Perrier A, et al. Plasma measurement of D-dimer as diagnostic aid in suspected venous thromboembolism: an overview. *Thromb Haemost* 1994;71:1–6.
8. Stein PD, Athanasoulis C, Alavi A, et al. Complications and validity of pulmonary angiography in acute pulmonary embolism. *Circulation* 1992;85:462–468.
9. Value of the ventilation/perfusion scan in acute pulmonary embolism. Results of the prospective investigation of pulmonary embolism diagnosis (PIOPED). The PIOPED Investigators. *JAMA* 1990;263:2753–2759.
10. Kumar AM, Parker JA. Ventilation/perfusion scintigraphy. *Emerg Med Clin North Am* 2001;19:957–973.
11. Hyers TM, Agnelli G, Hull RD, et al. Antithrombotic therapy for venous thromboembolic disease. *Chest* 1998;114(5 Suppl): 561S–578S.
12. Barritt DW, Jordan SC. Anticoagulant drugs in the treatment of pulmonary embolism: a controlled clinical trial. *Lancet* 1960;1: 1309–1312.
13. Simonneau G, Sors H, Charbonnier B, et al. A comparison of low-molecular-weight heparin with unfractionated heparin for acute pulmonary embolism. The THESEE Study Group. Tinzaparine ou Heparine Standard: Evaluations dans l'Embolie Pulmonaire. *N Engl J Med* 1997;337:663–669.
14. Hirsh J, Dalen J, Guyatt G. The sixth (2000) ACCP guidelines for antithrombotic therapy for prevention and treatment of thrombosis. American College of Chest Physicians. *Chest* 2001;119(1 Suppl):1S–2S.
15. Arcasoy SM, Kreit JW. Thrombolytic therapy of pulmonary embolism: a comprehensive review of current evidence. *Chest* 1999;115:1695–1707.
16. Hamel E, Pacouret G, Vincentelli D, et al. Thrombolysis or heparin therapy in massive pulmonary embolism with right ventricular dilation: results from a 128-patient monocenter registry. *Chest* 2001;120:120–125.
17. Ruiz-Bailen M, Aguayo de Hoyos E, Diaz-Castellanos MA. Role of thrombolysis in cardiac arrest. *Intensive Care Med* 2001; 27:438–441.

60

A 20-YEAR-OLD WOMAN WITH SHORTNESS OF BREATH

YASER ABU EL-SAMEED
RAED DWEIK

CASE PRESENTATION

A 20-year-old woman presented to the outpatient clinic after developing episodic shortness of breath, particularly on exertion. These symptoms were associated with intermittent chest pain and dry cough. Her symptoms became progressively worse over a period of 5 months.

The patient described one episode of exertional syncope. She denied any history of wheezing, urticaria, or rhinitis. There was no history of paroxysmal nocturnal dyspnea. She reported no fever, weight loss, night sweats, rash, or joint pain. She was not taking any medications and reported no drug allergies. The patient was a college student and had no industrial exposures.

QUESTIONS/DISCUSSION

Which of the following is a possible cause of this patient's symptoms?

A. Asthma
B. Sarcoidosis
C. Pulmonary hypertension
D. All of the above

Asthma is a chronic inflammatory disease of the airways characterized by reversible airway obstruction and bronchial hyperresponsiveness. Common symptoms associated with asthma include recurrent episodes of wheezing, breathlessness, chest tightness, and coughing. A variety of stimuli can provoke symptoms, including allergic, infectious, environmental, and emotional stimuli. The diagnosis is based on an appropriate clinical history and evidence of reversible airflow obstruction. Improvement in the forced expiratory volume in 1 second (FEV_1) by 12% and 200 mL or more is sufficient for diagnosis (1).

Sarcoidosis is a multisystem disorder of unknown etiology. It typically affects young adults and is more common in blacks. Sarcoidosis is characterized pathologically by noncaseating granulomas in the involved organs. It usually presents with one or more of the following: bilateral hilar adenopathy, pulmonary infiltrates, and skin and/or eye lesions. The most common presenting symptoms are cough, dyspnea, and chest pain. Cutaneous manifestations include a maculopapular eruption, lupus pernio, and erythema nodosum. The most common eye finding is anterior uveitis (2).

Pulmonary hypertension (PH) is characterized by elevated pulmonary artery pressures (mean pressure greater than 25 mm Hg at rest or greater than 30 mm Hg during exercise) (3). Pulmonary hypertension can be categorized as either primary (PPH) or secondary. Patients often present with progressive exertional dyspnea and exercise intolerance. As the disease progresses, patients may develop chest pain on exertion, presyncope, syncope, or even sudden death (4).

All the preceding diagnoses are possible causes of this patient's symptoms.

Physical examination revealed a 50-kg patient with a heart rate of 120 beats per minute and blood pressure of 100/60 mm Hg. There was no pallor, jugular venous distension, or lymphadenopathy. Cardiac examination revealed a left parasternal heave; auscultation revealed a regular heart rate and rhythm. A grade II/VI holosystolic, nonradiating murmur was heard at the lower left sternal border, and there was marked accentuation of the pulmonic component of the second heart sound (P2). The lungs were clear to auscultation. Abdominal examination did not reveal organomegaly, and there was no peripheral edema.

Which of the following conditions is associated with a loud P_2?

A. Systemic hypertension
B. Pulmonary stenosis
C. Mitral stenosis
D. Pulmonary hypertension

A loud P_2 is often found in patients with pulmonary hypertension, as high pulmonary pressures cause forceful closure of the pulmonary valve. The same principle applies to a loud aortic component of the second heart sound with systemic hypertension. Other auscultatory findings in PH include right ventricular (RV) fourth heart sound (S4) due to RV hypertrophy and a RV third heart sound due to RV failure (5). A pansystolic murmur at the lower sternal border is heard if tricuspid valve regurgitation develops. If the pulmonary valve annulus becomes dilated, an early diastolic murmur, known as a Graham–Steell murmur, can be heard due to pulmonary regurgitation (5). Patients with mitral stenosis have a loud first heart sound (S1). However, S_1 softens as the disease progresses and the valve becomes more calcific. In pulmonary stenosis, P_2 is usually soft and delayed because the valve is relatively immobile.

Case Continued: The patient's electrolytes, renal function, liver function tests, complete blood count, and coagulation tests were normal. A posteroanterior/lateral chest x-ray was unremarkable. An electrocardiogram (ECG) showed sinus tachycardia, right ventricular hypertrophy, and right axis deviation (Fig. 60.1). T-wave changes in the inferior and septal leads were present.

Based on the history, cardiac examination, and ECG findings, which of the following tests should be performed next?

A. Computed tomography (CT scan) of the chest
B. Transthoracic echocardiogram
C. Pulmonary function test (spirometry with diffusing capacity)
D. Cardiac catheterization

Since pulmonary hypertension is a distinct possibility in this patient, transthoracic echocardiography is the most appropriate initial test (5). As the findings on Doppler echocardiography only provide indirect evidence of PH, the definitive diagnosis must be made by right heart catheterization (3). Although both chest CT and pulmonary function testing can help in assessing patients with PH, neither test is diagnostic. This patient's echocardiogram showed a severely dilated right ventricle with severe dysfunction, an estimated RV systolic pressure of 82 mm Hg, and moderate pulmonary and tricuspid regurgitation. Right heart catheterization demonstrated main pulmonary artery pressure of 130/63 mm Hg, with a mean of 93 mm Hg. The systemic pressure at that time was 98/60 mm Hg, with a mean of 80 mm Hg.

Which of the following tests are appropriate as part of the evaluation for secondary causes of PH?

A. Chest CT with contrast
B. Pulmonary function test (PFT)
C. Antinuclear antibody (ANA)
D. Liver function test
E. All of the above

Once pulmonary hypertension has been confirmed, testing should be aimed at excluding potential causes of secondary PH. A variety of disease processes can produce PH, including:

■ *Primary cardiac disorders:* Mitral stenosis, severe aortic stenosis, intracardiac left-to-right shunts (e.g., ventricular septal defect), and severe congestive heart failure can cause secondary PH. Most of these disorders can be detected with echocardiography.

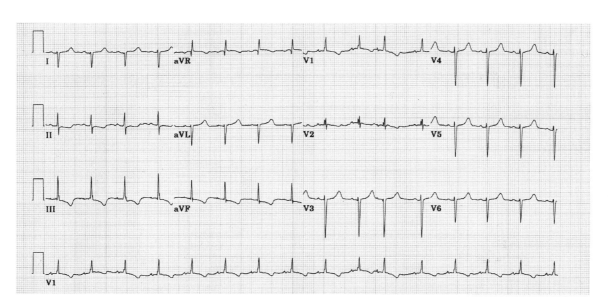

FIGURE 60.1. Electrocardiogram demonstrating sinus tachycardia, right ventricular hypertrophy, and right axis deviation. T-wave changes in the inferior and septal leads are also present.

- *Obstructive sleep apnea:* The hypoxemia these patients experience during sleep causes pulmonary vasoconstriction and subsequent PH. Overnight pulse oximetry can be used as a screening method. Definitive diagnosis requires a formal polysomnogram (5).
- *Chronic pulmonary embolism (PE):* The thromboembolic obstruction of the major pulmonary arteries due to unresolved PE is a potentially correctable cause of PH. The majority of patients with PH due to chronic PE have greater than 40% obstruction of the pulmonary vascular bed (6). Without intervention, the 5-year survival is 30% for patients with a mean pulmonary artery pressure of 40 mm Hg and 10% for patients with a mean pulmonary artery pressure of 50 mm Hg (6). Ventilation–perfusion (V/Q) scanning plays a pivotal role in determining whether PH has a thromboembolic etiology. If V/Q scanning is inconclusive in patients with suspected PE, either spiral CT scan with contrast or pulmonary angiography may be helpful.
- *Pulmonary parenchymal disorders:* Examples include emphysema and pulmonary fibrosis. These diseases result in arterial constriction or obliteration of the capillary vasculature. Pulmonary function testing and high-resolution CT scan are used to identify these disorders.
- *Connective-tissue diseases (CTD):* Scleroderma, particularly the CREST variant, is the CTD most commonly associated with PH. Prevalence varies from 2.3% to 35% in scleroderma and may approach 50% in CREST syndrome (7). PH occurs in 23% to 53% of patients with mixed CTD and 0.5% to 14% of cases of systemic lupus erythematosus (SLE). Pulmonary hypertension occurs far more infrequently in patients with rheumatoid arthritis, Sjogren syndrome, and inflammatory myositis (8–10). The prognosis for patients with CTD-related PH is typically poor. Treatment is usually similar to that utilized for primary PH, although immunosuppressive therapy may be effective in a few patients with PH secondary to SLE (11). In PH patients, ANA is an appropriate screening test for CTD.
- *Cirrhosis and portal hypertension:* Patients with pulmonary hypertension that present with thrombocytopenia and mild liver function abnormalities should be assessed for advanced liver disease (3). Patients with portal hypertension can occasionally develop pulmonary hypertension, a phenomenon called portopulmonary hypertension. Although the pathophysiology is obscure, one proposed mechanism involves the inability of the cirrhotic liver to detoxify gut-derived factors that cause adverse effects on the pulmonary epithelium (3).
- *Drugs:* Patients given appetite suppressants to treat obesity are at an increased risk of PH. The risk increases with increased duration of use, especially with fenfluramine (12). Data suggest that these patients have increased plasma serotonin levels and increased serotonin release from platelets (13,14). Serotonin has been demonstrated to cause pulmonary vasoconstriction and produce both hyperplasia and hypertrophy of pulmonary artery

smooth muscle cells (13). Nitric oxide (NO) deficiency has been postulated to be another mediator of pulmonary hypertension in these patients (15).

Table 60.1 presents a complete list of causes of PH (16). If an underlying cause is not found in a patient with PH, the disease is referred to as primary pulmonary hypertension (PPH).

TABLE 60.1. WORLD HEALTH ORGANIZATION CLASSIFICATION OF PULMONARY HYPERTENSION—1998

1. Pulmonary arterial hypertension
   1.1 Primary pulmonary hypertension
      (a) Sporadic
      (b) Familial
   1.2 Related to
      (a) Collagen vascular disease
      (b) Congenital systemic-to-pulmonary shunts
      (c) Portal hypertension
      (d) Human immunodeficiency virus infection
      (e) Drugs/toxins
         (1) Anorexigens
         (2) Other
      (f) Persistent pulmonary hypertension of the newborn
      (g) Other
2. Pulmonary venous hypertension
   2.1 Left-sided atrial or ventricular heart disease
   2.2 Left-sided valvular heart disease
   2.3 Extrinsic compression of central pulmonary veins
      (a) Fibrosing mediastinitis
      (b) Adenopathy/tumors
   2.4 Pulmonary venoocclusive disease
   2.5 Other
3. Pulmonary hypertension associated with disorders of the respiratory system and/or hypoxemia
   3.1 Chronic obstructive pulmonary disease
   3.2 Interstitial lung disease
   3.3 Sleep disordered breathing
   3.4 Alveolar hypoventilation disorders
   3.5 Chronic exposure to high altitude
   3.6 Neonatal lung disease
   3.7 Alveolar–capillary dysplasia
   3.8 Other
4. Pulmonary hypertension due to chronic thrombotic and/or embolic disease
   4.1 Thromboembolic obstruction of proximal pulmonary arteries
   4.2 Obstruction of distal pulmonary arteries
      (a) Pulmonary embolism (thrombus, tumor, ova and parasites, foreign material)
      (b) *In situ* thrombosis
      (c) Sickle cell disease
5. Pulmonary hypertension due to disorders directly affecting pulmonary vasculature
   5.1 Inflammatory
      (a) Schistosomiasis
      (b) Sarcoidosis
      (c) Other
   5.2 Pulmonary capillary hemangiomatosis

From Executive Summary from World Symposium on Primary Pulmonary Hypertension. Evian, France, September 6–10, 1998. Co-sponsored by the World Health Organization, with permission.

Case Continued: The patient's echocardiogram did not reveal any primary cardiac abnormalities. Her history and examination were not suggestive of obstructive sleep apnea. A V/Q scan was negative for thromboembolic disease. ANA was negative. Pulmonary function testing showed a mild restrictive airway disease pattern, which can be seen in patients with PH (5).

CT of the chest showed bilateral focal ground-glass opacities. These findings can be seen in patients with PH secondary to pulmonary venoocclusive disorder (PVOD), a rare disease that mostly affects children and young adults (17). The characteristic features of this disease are widespread occlusion of small pulmonary veins and venules by fibrosis and intimal proliferation associated with histologic evidence of severe PH. The triad of severe PH, radiographic evidence of pulmonary edema, and a normal wedge pressure strongly suggest the diagnosis of PVOD; however, lung biopsy is required for definitive diagnosis (17).

The patient underwent open lung wedge biopsy to evaluate for the presence of PVOD. The pathology was consistent with PPH and did not show PVOD.

Primary Pulmonary Hypertension

Primary pulmonary hypertension is defined as the presence of PH without an underlying cause. It is a rare disease, with an estimated incidence of 1 to 2 per million per year. PPH occurs more frequently in females (2.3 times) than in males. The median age at diagnosis is 36 years. Most patients survive 2 to 3 years from the time of diagnosis (5). Factors associated with survival include right atrial pressure, mean pulmonary artery pressure, and cardiac output. There seems to be a correlation between PPH and hypothyroidism; this correlation may be related to an underlying autoimmune etiology. In one cohort, 22.5% of PPH patients were found to be hypothyroid. It is recommended that patients be screened for thyroid disease at the time of diagnosis of PPH (18). Primary pulmonary hypertension can be either sporadic or familial, with familial PPH accounting for at least 6% of patients with PPH (4). In the familial form, genetic studies reveal an autosomal dominant inheritance with very low penetrance. This patient reported that her brother died at the age of 13, 2 years after being diagnosed with PPH. In addition, her aunt died from PPH a few years after diagnosis.

All of the following medications are used in the treatment of PPH except:

A. **Warfarin**
B. **Nifedipine**
C. **Digoxin**
D. **Intravenous epoprostenol**
E. **Long-acting nitrates**

The principal medical treatment of PPH involves a combination of anticoagulation and vasodilatation (19). Anticoagulation is associated with a significant improvement in survival. Digoxin improves cardiac function in patients who develop right-sided heart failure (20). Oral high-dose calcium channel blockers can improve survival by acting as vasodilators in the pulmonary circulation. All PPH patients should be given a trial of calcium channel blockers, such as nifedipine, as first-line therapy for PPH. Those patients who do not respond should be started on prostaglandin (epoprostenol) treatment (21). Intravenous infusion of prostaglandin (epoprostenol) is associated with long-term improvement in pulmonary hemodynamics and increased survival. In addition to acting as a potent pulmonary vasodilator, epoprostenol has anti–platelet aggregation effects and may facilitate pulmonary vascular remodeling. Epoprostenol needs to be administered into a central vein through a Hickman catheter. Infusion needs to be continuous with a 24-hour infusion pump because of the drug's short half-life of 2 to 3 minutes (19,21). Exogenous administration of nitric oxide (NO) by inhalation is an effective and specific therapy for PPH. Unfortunately, the cost and equipment required to administer the drug preclude its availability for practical use (21,22). Drugs under development include oral and subcutaneous prostaglandins and endothelin receptor antagonists (19). Long-acting nitrates do not have a role in the treatment of PPH. For patients who do not respond to medications or cannot tolerate them, lung or heart–lung transplant is an option (19).

CONCLUSION

Since this patient had a significant family history of PH and did not have an identifiable secondary cause for PH, she was felt to have familial primary pulmonary hypertension. She was admitted to the intensive care unit and underwent a trial of oral nifedipine, to which she did not respond. The patient was then given intravenous (IV) epoprostenol, which significantly reduced her pulmonary pressures and improved her symptoms. She was discharged home on a continuous infusion of IV epoprostenol. Upon follow-up, the patient had an improved 6-minute walk time and subjectively felt better.

REFERENCES

1. Dweik RA, Ahmad M. Diagnosis and treatment of asthma. *Resident Staff Phys* 1998;44:36–51.
2. Newman LS, Rose CS, Maier LA. Sarcoidosis. *N Engl J Med* 1997;336:1224–1234.
3. Krowka MJ. Pulmonary hypertension: diagnostics and therapeutics. *Mayo Clin Proc* 2000;75:625–630.
4. Rubin LJ. Primary pulmonary hypertension. *N Engl J Med* 1997;336:111–117.

5. Gaine SP, Rubin LJ. Primary pulmonary hypertension. *Lancet* 1998;352:719–725.
6. Fedullo PF, Auger WR, Kerr KM, et al. Chronic thromboembolic pulmonary hypertension. *N Engl J Med* 2001;345:1465–1472.
7. Minai OA, Dweik RA, Arroliga AC. Manifestations of scleroderma pulmonary disease. *Clin Chest Med* 1998;19:713–731.
8. Sullivan WD, Hurst DJ, Harmon CE, et al. A prospective evaluation emphasizing pulmonary involvement in patients with mixed connective tissue disease. *Medicine* 1984;63:92–107.
9. Alpert MA, Goldberg SH, Singsen BH, et al. Cardiovascular manifestations of mixed connective tissue disease in adults. *Circulation* 1983;68:1182–1193.
10. Quismorio FP Jr, Sharma O, Koss M, et al. Immunopathologic and clinical studies in pulmonary hypertension associated with systemic lupus erythematosus. *Semin Arthritis Rheum* 1984;13:349–359.
11. Sanchez O, Humbert M, Sitbon O, et al. Treatment of pulmonary hypertension secondary to connective tissue diseases. *Thorax* 1999;54:273–277.
12. Abenhaim L, Moride Y, Brenot F, et al. Appetite-suppressant drugs and the risk of pulmonary hypertension. International Primary Pulmonary Hypertension Study Group. *N Engl J Med* 1996;335:609–616.
13. Herve P, Launay JM, Scrobohaci ML, et al. Increased plasma serotonin in primary pulmonary hypertension. *Am J Med* 1995;99:249–254.
14. Voelkel NF. Appetite suppressants and pulmonary hypertension. *Thorax* 1997;52(Suppl 3):S63–S67.
15. Archer SL, Djaballah K, Humbert M, et al. Nitric oxide deficiency in fenfluramine- and dexfenfluramine-induced pulmonary hypertension. *Am J Respir Crit Care Med* 1998;158:1061–1067.
16. Executive summary from the World Symposium on Primary Pulmonary Hypertension. Evian, France, 1998. Co-sponsored by the World Health Organization.
17. Katz DS, Scalzetti EM, Katzenstein AL, et al. Pulmonary veno-occlusive disease presenting with thrombosis of pulmonary arteries. *Thorax* 1995;50:699–700.
18. Curnock AL, Dweik RA, Higgins BH, et al. High prevalence of hypothyroidism in patients with primary pulmonary hypertension. *Am J Med Sci* 1999;318:289–292.
19. Arroliga AC, Dweik RA, Kaneko FJ, et al. Primary pulmonary hypertension: update on pathogenesis and novel therapies. *Cleve Clin J Med* 2000;67:175–190.
20. Ozkan M, Dweik RA, Laskowski D, et al. High levels of nitric oxide in individuals with pulmonary hypertension receiving epoprostenol therapy. *Lung* 2001;179:233–243.
21. Rich S, Seidlitz M, Dodin E, et al. The short-term effects of digoxin in patients with right ventricular dysfunction from pulmonary hypertension. *Chest* 1998;114:787–792.
22. Dweik RA. The promise and reality of nitric oxide in the diagnosis and treatment of lung disease. *Cleve Clin J Med* 2001;68:486–493.

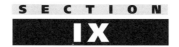

RHEUMATOLOGY

61

A 46-YEAR-OLD MAN WITH LEFT KNEE PAIN

MICHAEL J. LEE
DERRICK C. CETIN

CASE PRESENTATION

A healthy 46-year-old man presented with a 1-year history of intermittent pain of the anterior and medial aspects of the left knee. He regularly participated in basketball, running, cycling, and skiing but did not recall any antecedent trauma. The patient also noticed occasional episodes of knee swelling without redness or warmth. He also described episodes of clicking or locking of his knee that lasted for several minutes to hours. The patient did not have difficulty bearing weight or have pain going up or down stairs. The patient could not rise from a seated position with his legs crossed. The patient described morning stiffness lasting for a few minutes. He did not note any other joint symptoms or systemic complaints.

QUESTIONS/DISCUSSION

Which of following is the least likely diagnosis for this patient's knee pain?

A. **Osteoarthritis**
B. **Bursitis**
C. **Meniscal or ligamentous injury**
D. **Patellofemoral syndrome**
E. **Osgood–Schlatter disease**

More than 3 million new visits to physicians each year involve complaints of knee pain. Ten percent to 15% of all adults report symptoms involving the knee. Knee symptoms account for 3% to 5% of all physician visits (1).

Evaluation of knee pain should begin with a thorough history (1–3). The location of the pain and related factors such as radiation, duration, and joint stiffness should be elicited. Clinicians should inquire about recent trauma or other instigating events. The position of the patient and the direction of the forces at the time of an injury are critical pieces of history (1). The presence of a "pop" at the time of injury, swelling, and/or joint instability are all important pieces of information (1).

The site of initial pain can help establish a diagnosis (2). Anterior knee pain can occur with quadriceps muscle strain, large knee effusions, patellofemoral syndrome, osteoarthritis, prepatellar bursitis, patellar tendonitis, Osgood–Schlatter disease, or inflammatory arthritis. Medial knee pain can occur with osteoarthritis, anserine bursitis, medial meniscal injury, or medial collateral ligament injury or strain. Injuries to the lateral counterparts of the medial structures can cause lateral knee pain. One notable difference is the presence of focal pain over the femoral condyle with a palpable snap, which suggests iliotibial band syndrome (2).

The most common site of osteoarthritis (OA) is the knee (4). OA can occur in the medial, lateral, or patellofemoral compartments of the knee, with the medial compartment the most common site of involvement (2). Primary or idiopathic osteoarthritis is the most common type of OA and is not associated with a known predisposing factor (5). Secondary osteoarthritis is pathologically similar to primary osteoarthritis but is associated with an underlying medical cause. Underlying etiologies include trauma, diabetes mellitus, obesity, hypothyroidism, calcium pyrophosphate dihydrate deposition, avascular necrosis, Wilson disease, alcaptonuria, and acromegaly (5).

Risk factors associated with osteoarthritis include increasing age, joint trauma, repetitive joint stress, obesity, and previous inflammatory joint disease. The distal interphalangeal, proximal interphalangeal, first carpometacarpal, acromioclavicular and weight-bearing joints of the knee, hips, and spine are commonly affected. Pain is usually described as a deep ache confined to the affected joints, which become more painful with continued use and improve with rest. Morning stiffness is present but lasts for 30 minutes or less, in contrast to rheumatoid arthritis (2). Patients with rheumatoid arthritis frequently have morning stiffness for greater than an hour. Signs of active synovitis and systemic symptoms are often present. In patients with osteoarthritis, examination can reveal crepitus and bony tenderness and enlargement. Synovitis is not present. A varus deformity may be present with osteoarthritis of the medial compartment, whereas involvement of the lateral compartment may result in a valgus deformity (5). Radiographs can reveal sclerosis, osteophyte formation, and subchondral cysts. Weight-bearing films of the knees should be obtained to look for joint space narrowing, which may be missed on standard films.

Bursitis typically presents with localized tenderness over an inflamed bursal sac. Swelling and erythema may be present. Bursae are lined by the synovial membrane, which secretes and absorbs synovial fluid. The bursae lubricate the periarticular structures, including bones, muscles, ligaments, and tendons. The most common causes of bursitis are minor trauma and overuse. Other causes include crystal disease, infection or rheumatoid arthritis. In prepatellar bursitis, there is often a ballottable swelling, focal tenderness, erythema, and warmth over the lower half of the patella. Bursal aspiration can help distinguish the etiology of bursitis.

Meniscal and ligamentous injuries are most commonly caused by trauma. Medial meniscal tears are more common than lateral tears (3). Joint position at the time of injury and the direction of the incurring force determine the nature of the injury (1). A combination of angulating and rotational forces on the knee, such as a twisting of the knee with a foot planted on the ground, causes most of these injuries (1,4). Older patients are more likely to develop meniscal tears secondary to degeneration (1). Some patients may not recall an instigating event or trauma. In any meniscal injury, patients may note difficulty with weight bearing, locking of the knee, pain, or an inability to flex the knee fully. The menisci do not have pain fibers; therefore, pain is usually due to tearing and bleeding into peripheral structures in the setting of an acute injury or due to degenerative arthritis in patients with more chronic injuries (1).

Active patients from their mid-teens into the fifth decade most commonly present with acute and chronic ligamentous injuries. The anterior cruciate and medial collateral ligaments are most often involved (3). In ligamentous injuries, patients typically describe pain at the time of the initial injury, along with subsequent stiffness and fullness over the affected ligament (2). Particularly with anterior or posterior cruciate ligamentous injuries, patients recall a significant injury and describe the knee giving out or difficulty bearing weight.

Examination for ligamentous and meniscal injuries may reveal tenderness along the corresponding joint line and pain or joint instability with appropriate maneuvers (2,4). A thorough history and an appropriate examination are the most sensitive and specific tools for diagnosing a meniscal or ligamentous injury (1,3). Table 61.1 outlines the specific maneuvers used to test different structures. Plain radiographs can reveal fractures, the width of the medial and

lateral cartilage, and signs of concomitant arthritis. However, the diagnosis of ligamentous and meniscal injuries is best made by arthroscopy or magnetic resonance imaging (MRI) (3).

Patellofemoral syndrome is the most common cause of anterior knee pain. Thirty percent of athletes have complaints involving the patellofemoral joint (4). Patellofemoral syndrome is the leading cause of knee pain in patients less than 45 years of age (2). Patellofemoral syndrome can occur as a result of the following conditions:

- Patella alta develops when the patellar tendon exceeds the patella in length by greater than 1 cm (4). This condition can be diagnosed with a lateral x-ray. The increased length causes hypermobility of the patella and joint instability (4).
- Patellar subluxation describes a lateral subluxation or hypermobility of the patella (2,4). This results in the patella tracking unevenly in its groove. Physical examination can reveal a positive apprehension test. With the patient supine and the knee flexed at 30 degrees, the examiner applies lateral pressure to the patella. Pain or fear of pain with this maneuver is considered a sign of lateral patellofemoral instability (6). A sunrise view on a knee radiograph may show lateral subluxation (3).
- Chondromalacia is a pathologic condition characterized by the breakdown of cartilage. This is a histologic diagnosis made by arthroscopy. Patients may have pain without cartilage degeneration (2,4). Chondromalacia is the end result of recurrent irritation and trauma to the patella.
- Patellofemoral arthritis is arthritis of the patella, which results from repetitive trauma and stress (2).

Patellofemoral syndrome usually develops in young patients with anterior knee pain under or around the patella. Swelling is not usually present. Repetitive flexion, as occurs with climbing stairs, precipitates and exacerbates the pain. Prolonged sitting can also cause pain. A useful historical question to ask patients is if they have to shift positions or stand during an extended period of sitting (3). Examination reveals pain behind the compressed patella against the femoral groove as the leg is flexed and extended. Crepitations can be present, but an effusion or true locking of the knee is rare (6). Radiographs should be obtained to check for fracture, arthritis, osteochondritis dissecans, and other causes of pain due to repetitive trauma. A lateral view to check for patella alta and a sunrise view for lateral subluxation should be included.

Osgood–Schlatter disease is the least likely diagnosis in this patient. This condition is a common cause of knee pain in young men and women who still have intact growth plates (2). Pain develops due to inflammation of the patellar tendon at its insertion at the tibial tubercle. Patients describe gradual onset of pain at the tibial tubercle occurring with or just after activity. Examination reveals enlargement and ten-

TABLE 61.1. PHYSICAL EXAMINATION MANEUVERS IN THE ASSESSMENT OF KNEE PAIN

Physical Examination Maneuver	Description
Lachman test, anterior cruciate ligament	The patient is supine with the knee flexed 20 to 30 degrees. The examiner has one hand above the knee and the other on the proximal tibia. The hand on the tibia pulls on the lower leg. The test is considered positive if there is increased movement of the tibia.[a]
Anterior drawer test, anterior cruciate ligament	The patient is supine with the knee flexed at 90 degrees. Both hands are placed on the proximal tibia and the examiner pulls away from the patient. The test is positive when a discrete end point is not felt or if there is increased translation compared with the other leg.[a]
Lateral pivot shift test, anterior cruciate ligament	The patient is supine with the knee flexed 45 degrees. The examiner has one hand on the lateral aspect of the knee pressing medially. The other hand is supporting the base of the foot, pushing laterally. Together this causes valgus stress. The knee is straightened slowly. A positive test is a "thud" noticed at 10 to 20 degrees of knee flexion.[a]
Posterior drawer test, posterior cruciate ligament	The patient is supine with the knee flexed at 90 degrees. The knee is inspected to see if the tibia is subluxed posteriorly. A positive sign is if the subluxation can be corrected with anterior pulling of the lower leg. It is also positive if one does the opposite of the anterior drawer and there is no discrete end point with posterior translation.[a]
Apley compression test, menisci	The patient is prone and the knee is flexed at 90 degrees. The examiner's knee is over the patient's posterior thigh, with hands holding the foot. The lower leg is externally rotated, followed by downward compression of the tibia. A positive test is the generation of pain with downward compression.[a]
McMurray test, menisci	The patient is supine with knee fully flexed. The examiner places one hand on the medial aspect of the knee and the other supporting the heel. Medial pressure is applied with hand at the knee causing a valgus stress. The knee is extended while internally rotating the tibia to test the lateral meniscus. The test is done again with external rotation of the tibia to test the medial meniscus. A positive test is a "popping" and reproduction of symptoms along the joint line. Often a "locking" occurs with the inability to fully extend the knee.[a]
Varus stress test, lateral collateral ligament	The patient is supine. The examiner has one hand above the knee to stabilize it and the other at the proximal tibia, providing medial pressure. A positive test is with pain, movement of the lateral joint space, and increased medial translation as compared to the other side.[b]
Valgus stress test, medial collateral ligament	The patient is supine. The examiner has one hand above the knee to stabilize it and the other at the proximal tibia, providing lateral pressure. A positive test is with pain, movement of the medial joint space, and increased lateral translation as compared to the other side.[b]

[a]Solomon D, Simel D, Bates D, et al. The rational clinical examination. Does this patient have a torn meniscus or ligament of the knee? Value of the physical examination. *JAMA* 2001;286:1610–1620.
[b]Anderson RJ, Anderson BC. Evaluation of the patient with knee pain. UpToDate version 10.1, 2002.

derness of the tibial tubercle and its adjacent structures. Atrophy of the quadriceps may be present as a result of disuse (4).

Case Continued: On physical examination, there was no effusion, warmth, or redness at or around the knee. There was pain with passive and active flexion and extension of the knee. Medial joint line tenderness was present. The patient also had a positive McMurray test and a positive valgus stress maneuver. The patella tracked smoothly within the femoral groove, and patellar compression did not cause pain. No varus laxity was present. The Lachman and anterior and posterior drawer tests were negative.

Based on the examination, which of the following diagnoses is most likely?

A. Lateral meniscus tear
B. Medial meniscus tear
C. Anterior cruciate ligament tear
D. Lateral collateral ligament tear

The findings on examination point toward either osteoarthritis or an internal derangement of the medial aspect of the knee, either a medial meniscal or medial collateral ligament injury. The positive McMurray test and laxity with valgus stress reinforce the likelihood of an internal derangement along the medial aspect of the knee. The history of the knee "giving out" or locking is also suggestive of an internal derangement.

Examination of the knee should start with an evaluation of the function of the knee by assessing gait, squat, and the patient's ability to transfer (6). An inability to walk or bear weight could be indicative of a fracture or other serious injury and warrants radiographic evaluation.

Inspection begins with an examination of the symmetry of the knees and legs. The knee should be checked for evidence of abrasions, ecchymosis, soft tissue swelling, and quadriceps atrophy (3). The presence of an effusion is suggested by a general fullness or loss of the peripatellar grooves (1,2). An assessment of localized swelling over specific structures should also be made (1).

The knee and its surrounding structures should be palpated. Signs of an effusion include fullness with passive flexion and/or positive ballottement of the patella (1). The joint lines should be palpated for tenderness to assist in identifying an underlying irritation or internal derangement. The bursae and the lateral femoral condyle should be palpated for signs suggestive of bursitis or iliotibial band syndrome, respectively (2). The popliteal fossa should be evaluated for fullness, since a Baker cyst can cause symptoms of knee pain and, if ruptured, can result in pseudothrombophlebitis.

An assessment of range of motion includes checking for active and passive range of motion (1). Pain with both active and passive range of motion is suggestive of an articular process. Pain on only active range of motion is more consistent with a periarticular process, such as pes anserine bursitis.

The mechanical stability of the joint should be checked with varus and valgus stress, as well as anterior and posterior drawer signs. These tests assess the stability of the collateral and cruciate ligaments, respectively. Patellofemoral syndrome is assessed with reproduction of pain with pressure and movement of the patella and with the apprehension test. Additional maneuvers, such as the McMurray test and Apley compression test, can assess for a meniscal tear. A lateral pivot shift test examines the stability of the anterior cruciate ligament.

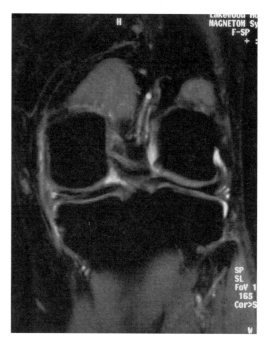

FIGURE 61.1. Magnetic resonance imaging of the left knee with a coronal view showing a torn medial meniscus.

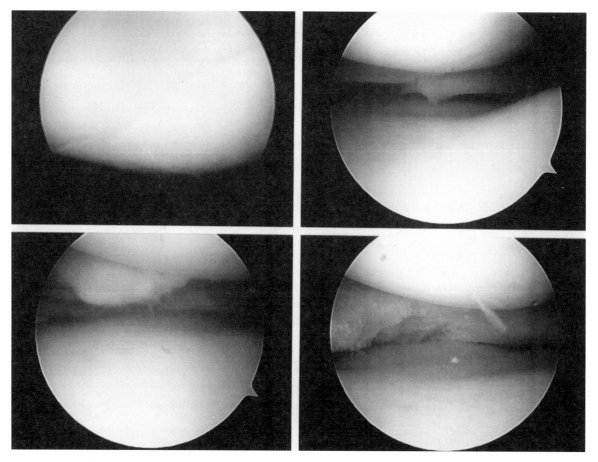

FIGURE 61.2. Pre- and postrepair arthroscopy photographs. The **lower left panel** shows the torn meniscus, and the **lower right panel** shows the meniscus after repair.

Which imaging modality has the greatest sensitivity and specificity for confirming this patient's diagnosis?

A. **Plain radiographs of the knee**
B. **Magnetic resonance imaging (MRI)**
C. **Computed tomography (CT scan)**
D. **Ultrasound**
E. **Bone scan**

MRI of the left knee revealed degenerative changes and a posterior horn meniscal tear (Fig. 61.1). MRI is the imaging technique of choice to diagnose internal derangements of the knee. In a metaanalysis, Mackenzie et al. found MRI of the menisci and cruciate ligaments to be 88% sensitive and 94% specific (7). None of the other imaging studies listed earlier are as sensitive and specific as MRI. The American College of Radiology suggests the following clinical parameters for ordering imaging of the knee following trauma (8):

- Effusion formation within 24 hours of trauma
- Palpable tenderness over the patella or head of the fibula
- Inability to walk or bear weight immediately after trauma, up to 1 week after the initial event
- Inability to completely flex the knee to 90 degrees

Follow-up

The patient underwent arthroscopic surgery to correct the meniscal tear (Fig. 61.2). Meniscal tears that cause symptoms usually require repair, especially in patients who have displaced menisci that cause the knee to lock (6). Postoperatively, the patient's pain resolved.

CONCLUSION

The assessment of the painful knee begins with a detailed and systematic history. A complete examination comprised of inspection, palpation, assessment of joint stability, range of motion, and assessment of joint function is best at diagnosing the etiology of knee pain. Specific maneuvers can suggest a diagnosis, but they are not diagnostic. MRI is very useful in diagnosing internal derangements of the knee.

REFERENCES

1. Solomon D, Simel D, Bates D, et al. The rational clinical examination. Does this patient have a torn meniscus or ligament of the knee? Value of the physical examination. *JAMA* 2001;286: 1610–1620.
2. Anderson RJ, Anderson BC. Evaluation of the patient with knee pain. UpToDate version 10.1, 2002.
3. Skinner HB, Scherger JE. Identifying structural hip and knee problems. Patient age, history, and limited examination may be all that's needed. *Postgrad Med* 1999;106:51–61.
4. Byank RP, Beatie WE. Exercise-related musculoskeletal problems. In: Barker LR, Burton JR, Zieve PD, eds. *Principles of ambulatory medicine,* 5th ed. Baltimore: Williams & Wilkins, 1999:939–949.
5. Brandt KD. Osteoarthritis. In: Braunwald E, Fauci AS, Kasper DL, et al., eds. *Harrison's principles of internal medicine,* 15th ed. New York: McGraw-Hill, 2001:1987–1994.
6. Ruffin MT 5th, Kiningham RB. Anterior knee pain: the challenge of patellofemoral syndrome. *Am Fam Physician* 1993;47:185–194.
7. Mackenzie R, Palmer CR, Lomas DJ, et al. Magnetic resonance imaging of the knee: diagnostic performance studies. *Clin Radiol* 1996;51:251–257.
8. Pavlov H, Dalinka MK, Alazraki N, et al. Acute trauma to the knee. American College of Radiology. ACR Appropriateness Criteria. *Radiology* 2000;215S:365–373.

62

A 62-YEAR-OLD WOMAN WITH LEFT HAND EDEMA

MARTIN E. LASCANO
SUSAN J. REHM

CASE PRESENTATION

A 62-year-old woman presented to the emergency department with 1 week of left hand edema and pain. Her symptoms started after returning from a 3-day trip to Minnesota. Progressive edema limited range of motion in the hand, although over-the-counter ibuprofen partially relieved her symptoms. She denied any trauma to the affected area or insect bites during her recent trip. She did notice several episodes of chills and night sweats without documented fever. She also noted mild fatigue over the same period of time during which her hand edema developed. The patient also described mild left foot erythema surrounding a chronic pressure ulcer on her second toe. She denied any associated pain in this area.

Her past medical history was significant for 20 years of type 2 diabetes mellitus complicated by retinopathy and neuropathy in the lower extremities. Six years earlier, she underwent amputation of the left hallux secondary to an ulcer that progressed to osteomyelitis. Her medical regimen included multidose subcutaneous injections of insulin, metformin, and lisinopril/hydrochlorothiazide. She denied any history of tobacco, alcohol, or illicit drug use.

Physical examination revealed an obese, ill-appearing patient who was awake, alert, and fully oriented. Vital signs included a temperature of 36.3°C, heart rate of 103 beats per minute, respiratory rate of 18 per minute, and blood pressure of 151/80 mm Hg. The oral mucosa was dry, with evidence of thrush. Neck was supple without jugular venous distension. Lungs were clear to auscultation, and cardiac examination revealed no murmurs or gallops. The abdomen was soft and nontender, without organomegaly. Examination of the left upper extremity revealed 2+ pitting edema extending distally from the mid-forearm. Range of motion in the wrist was mildly diminished, and the overlying skin was warm and dry. There was no evidence of a wrist effusion. There was an ulcerated wound on the second digit of the left foot with the distal phalanx exposed and sur-

rounded by necrotic tissue. The third toe of the right foot had changes consistent with dry gangrene. There was no lymphadenopathy. Neurologic examination was significant only for absent pinprick sensation in the feet.

Initial Hospital Course: The patient was admitted with a presumptive diagnosis of osteomyelitis of the left second toe and cellulitis of the left forearm. Blood cultures were obtained, and empiric therapy with intravenous ampicillin/sulbactam was initiated. Initial laboratory testing revealed white blood cell count of 21.4 K/µL, hemoglobin of 9.8 g/dL, hematocrit of 27.4%, and platelet count of 184 K/µL. Radiographs of the left hand revealed moderate soft-tissue swelling with normal joint spaces and no bony abnormalities. Radiographs of her feet were significant for bony erosions involving the left second toe.

Within 24 hours of admission to the hospital, the patient underwent left transmetatarsal and right third toe amputations. Postoperatively, the left forearm edema extended proximally, with evidence of diminishing range of active and passive motion and increasing pain in her wrist and fingers. A small wrist effusion could be detected. Additionally, the patient became febrile and developed shaking chills.

QUESTIONS/DISCUSSION

Which of the following is the most appropriate next diagnostic step?

A. Magnetic resonance imaging (MRI) of the wrist
B. Computed tomography (CT scan) of the wrist
C. Ultrasound of the wrist
D. Arthrocentesis with synovial fluid analysis

The first step in evaluating a patient with joint pain is identification of the structure involved. Pain arising from surrounding soft tissues and juxtaarticular bone needs to be distinguished from intraarticular pain. Arthritis is likely if

TABLE 62.1. DIFFERENTIAL DIAGNOSIS OF ARTHRITIS BASED ON PATTERN OF JOINT INVOLVEMENT

Characteristic	Involvement	Common Diagnoses
Number of joints involved	Monarticular	Trauma, septic arthritis, crystal-induced arthritis, Lyme disease
	Oligoarticular (two to four joints)	Reiter disease, psoriatic arthritis, inflammatory bowel disease
	Polyarticular (five or more joints)	Rheumatoid arthritis (RA), systemic lupus erythematosus (SLE)
Site of joint involvement	Distal interphalangeal	Osteoarthritis (OA), psoriatic arthritis (not RA)
	Metacarpophalangeal, wrists	RA, SLE (not OA)
	First metatarsophalangeal	Gout, OA

there is diminished range of motion and if active and passive movements worsen the pain. If joint motion is preserved, and there is tenderness over adjacent ligaments, tendons, or bursae, pathology in these structures should be sought. If joint pathology is suspected, the number of affected joints and the specific sites of involvement can help narrow the differential diagnosis (Table 62.1).

In this patient, the presence of a wrist effusion and decreased passive and active range of motion in the wrist favored an intraarticular process. The most likely causes of monarticular symptoms are trauma, infection, and crystal-induced disease (gout and pseudogout) (1). Since this patient did not have a history of trauma and left-hand radiographs did not show any bony abnormalities, septic arthritis and crystal-induced arthritis were thought to be the most likely diagnoses. Imaging studies such as ultrasound, CT scan, and MRI are useful in detecting early fluid collections and may help with proper needle placement for arthrocentesis (2). However, since this patient had a palpable wrist effusion, arthrocentesis should be attempted before obtaining further imaging studies.

In the evaluation of monarticular pain, the most important test is synovial fluid analysis (3). Intraarticular infections can lead to significant morbidity, including permanent loss of articular function; therefore, prompt diagnosis of intraarticular infections by synovial fluid analysis is essential.

Although synovial fluid is often sent for multiple studies, the white cell count and differential, Gram stain and cultures, and polarized light microscopy typically provide the

most information as to the etiology of an effusion (4). Based on the appearance of the fluid and the white cell count, the effusion can be characterized as inflammatory, noninflammatory, septic, or hemorrhagic (Table 62.2). Although the white cell count is not diagnostic, it can help guide further diagnostic therapy and testing. Microbiologic analysis is necessary to confirm the presence of a joint space infection. However, Gram stain and culture are positive in only 50% and 90%, respectively, of patients with nongonococcal septic arthritis (5). On polarized light microscopy, the presence of strongly negative birefringent needle-shaped crystals is diagnostic of gout, and the presence of weakly positive birefringent rhomboid crystals is characteristic of pseudogout.

Case Continued: Arthrocentesis of the left wrist was performed, obtaining 5 mL of yellowish, opaque fluid. By this time, initial blood cultures became positive for β-hemolytic group B streptococci, susceptible to all penicillins and cephalosporins. Cell count of the synovial fluid showed 181,300 white blood cells/μL with 90% neutrophils, and polarized light microscopy did not reveal any crystals. Gram stain showed Gram-positive cocci in pairs with many polymorphonuclear leukocytes (PMNs), consistent with a diagnosis of septic arthritis. The patient also developed pain and edema of her right wrist, with decreased range of motion and a palpable effusion. Arthrocentesis of the right wrist was performed, and Gram stain again showed Gram-positive cocci in pairs and many PMNs.

TABLE 62.2. SYNOVIAL FLUID ANALYSIS

Measure	Normal	Noninflammatory	Inflammatory	Septic	Hemorrhagic
Appearance	Clear	Clear, yellowish	Clear to opaque	Opaque, yellow–green	Bloody
WBC (per μL)	<200	200–2,000	2,000–10,000	>100,000	200–2,000
PMN (%)	<25	<25	>50	>75	50–75
Protein (g/dL)	1–2	1–3	3–5	3–5	4–6
Lactate dehydrogenase (compared to serum)	Very low	Very low	High	Variable	Similar
Glucose (mg/dL)	Nearly equal to serum	Nearly equal to serum	>25, lower than serum	<25, much lower than serum	Nearly equal to serum
Culture	Negative	Negative	Negative	Usually positive	Negative

PMN, polymorphonuclear leukocytes; WBC, white blood cell count.

Septic arthritis in native joints usually develops as a result of hematogenous seeding during bacteremia (5,6). Blood cultures are positive in 50% to 70% of cases of non-gonococcal bacterial arthritis. Direct inoculation secondary to instrumentation or trauma and spread from contiguous sites of infection (osteomyelitis, septic bursitis) are less common etiologies of septic arthritis (2). Once bacteria enter a closed joint space, an acute inflammatory synovitis is triggered, which promotes the influx of acute and chronic inflammatory cells. These cells release pro-inflammatory cytokines and proteolytic enzymes that lead to cartilage degradation and articular damage.

Staphylococci are the most commonly implicated bacteria in septic arthritis in adults, accounting for up to 80% of cases in patients with predisposing comorbidities, such as rheumatoid arthritis and diabetes mellitus (5). β-Hemolytic streptococci are the second most common bacterial cause of septic arthritis, with Gram-negative bacilli and pneumococcus less common causes. Among sexually active young adults and adolescents, *Neisseria gonorrhoeae* is the most commonly implicated organism (7). If untreated, gonococcal arthritis may lead to disseminated gonococcal infection (DGI) in 1% to 3% of cases (5). Clinically, patients with DGI develop migratory polyarthralgias, rash, tenosynovitis, dermatitis, and fever. The rash typically begins as multiple small papules that progress to hemorrhagic pustules. Synovial Gram stain and culture are positive in DGI in less than 25% and 50% of cases, respectively. Therefore, isolates should be sought from genitourinary sources, which yield positive cultures in 70% to 90% of patients (8).

Which of the following is/are risk factors for developing septic arthritis?

A. Prosthetic joints
B. Diabetes mellitus
C. Age greater than 60 years
D. Intravenous drug use
E. All of the above

All of the above are associated with an increased risk for developing bacterial arthritis (2,3). This patient had multiple risk factors, including advanced age, longstanding diabetes mellitus, and the presence of a remote site of infection leading to bacteremia. Clinicians also need to recognize that patients with underlying chronic joint disease, especially rheumatoid arthritis, are more prone to develop septic arthritis. Synovial fluid analysis should be performed whenever septic arthritis is suspected (5). This patient had polyarticular involvement, which occurs in 10% to 20% of cases of nongonococcal septic arthritis (9). Common predisposing factors for the development of polyarticular arthritis are rheumatoid arthritis, systemic connective-tissue disease, and sepsis.

Which of the following is the appropriate next step in this patient's management?

A. Continue intravenous antibiotics and observe
B. Arthroscopic drainage and irrigation of both wrists
C. Bilateral wrist intraarticular antibiotic irrigation
D. Start corticosteroids as adjunctive therapy

The basic principle for the treatment of any purulent collection is prompt drainage. There is controversy regarding the most appropriate method of drainage for septic arthritis. Serial aspirations are an alternative, but formal surgical drainage by arthroscopy or arthrotomy is the preferred method of treatment (10). This is especially true in smaller joints, like the wrist, that might be difficult to aspirate repeatedly. Copious irrigation and debridement of any purulent material within the joint are essential. Continuation of intravenous antibiotics tailored to the susceptibility of the organism isolated is also appropriate.

Septic arthritis is a surgical emergency, and drainage should not be delayed (10). Nongonococcal septic arthritis is potentially the most destructive form of acute arthritis. Despite the advent of better antibiotics and improved methods of articular drainage, morbidity and mortality from septic arthritis have not decreased significantly over the past few decades. Permanent joint damage occurs in 50% of cases, and mortality ranges from 10% to 16% (5).

Patients with nongonococcal septic arthritis are typically treated with intravenous antibiotic therapy for 2 to 4 weeks. In gonococcal arthritis, alternative shorter courses and oral antibiotics are often effective (5). Intraarticular antibiotic instillation is not appropriate, as it may cause chemical synovitis. Furthermore, most antibiotics have good penetration into inflamed joints (6). Animal studies have indicated that intraarticular and systemic corticosteroids could theoretically reduce the severity of articular cartilage destruction (7). However, prospective studies have not been done in humans; corticosteroids are currently not indicated for septic arthritis.

Joint immobilization is appropriate for a short period of time (1 to 3 days), but passive range of motion should be initiated as soon as possible to preserve joint mobility (2).

Case Conclusion

The patient underwent bilateral wrist arthroscopy with thorough irrigation, debridement, and extensive synovectomy. Drains were placed in both wrists, which were splinted for purposes of comfort. By postoperative day 2, the drains were removed, and the patient started a rehabilitation program with progressive improvement in range of motion. Cultures from both arthrocenteses also grew β-hemolytic group B streptococci with the same susceptibility as the initial blood cultures. Intravenous ampicillin/sulbactam was continued throughout the hospitalization, and a peripherally inserted central catheter was placed to complete a course of 4 weeks of intravenous antibiotics as an outpatient. The patient was discharged home with arrangements for home physical therapy and outpatient follow-up.

CONCLUSION

Acute monarticular arthritis is a challenging clinical entity with a broad differential diagnosis. A thorough history and physical examination can help narrow the possibilities; whenever there is suspicion for an inflammatory process, infection must be the initial working diagnosis. Arthrocentesis and synovial fluid analysis provide the most useful laboratory information to guide subsequent diagnostic testing and therapy.

Septic arthritis requires immediate intervention. The cornerstone of treatment is prompt joint drainage coupled with appropriate antibiotic therapy. Preservation of articular function should be the main goal, and all efforts should be directed toward rehabilitation of the affected joint once the inflammatory process begins to resolve.

REFERENCES

1. Sack K. Monarthritis: differential diagnosis. *Am J Med* 1997;102:30S–34S.
2. Pioro MH, Mandell BF. Septic arthritis. *Rheum Dis Clin North Am* 1997;23:239–258.
3. Goldenberg DL, Reed JI. Bacterial arthritis. *N Engl J Med* 1985;312:764–771.
4. Shmerling RH, Delbanco TL, Tosteson AN, et al. Synovial fluid tests. What should be ordered? *JAMA* 1990;264:1009–1014.
5. Goldenberg DL. Septic arthritis. *Lancet* 1998;351:197–202.
6. Carreño Perez L. Septic arthritis. *Baillieres Best Pract Res Clin Rheumatol* 1999;13:37–58.
7. Thaler SJ, Maguire JH. Infectious arthritis. In: Braunwald E, Fauci AS, Kasper DL, et al., editors. *Harrison's principles of internal medicine,* 15th ed. New York: McGraw-Hill, 2001:1998–2003.
8. O'Brien JP, Goldenberg DL, Rice PA. Disseminated gonococcal infection: a prospective analysis of 49 patients and a review of pathophysiology and immune mechanisms. *Medicine* 1983;62:395–406.
9. Dubost JJ, Fis I, Denis P, et al. Polyarticular septic arthritis. *Medicine* 1993;72:296–310.
10. Murray PM. Septic arthritis of the hand and wrist. *Hand Clin* 1998;14:579–587.

SUBJECT INDEX

Note: Page numbers followed by *f* indicate a figure; page numbers followed by *t* indicate a table.

in HIV infection, 158–159
in methemoglobinemia, 263
in pulmonary embolism, 267
Blood pressure. *See also* Hypertension;
    Hypotension
  inadequate control of, in postural
      orthostatic tachycardia syndrome,
      205–206, 206*f*
  measurement of, in extremities, in
      peripheral vascular disease, 24–25,
      25*t*
Blood smear, in thrombotic
      thrombocytopenic
      purpura–hemolytic uremic
      syndrome, 151
Blood transfusions. *See* Transfusions
Blood volume, measurement of, in vasovagal
      response, 206
Blue finger, in Buerger disease, 18–22
Blue toes, in ischemia, 18–22
Bone
  cancer metastasis to, 135–139
  demineralization of, hypocalcemia in,
      72–76
  fractures of
    in metastatic cancer, 135–139
    in multiple myeloma, 141
    in osteomalacia, 75
  metabolic disease of, hypocalcemia in,
      73–76
  metastasis to, vs. multiple myeloma, 141
  multiple myeloma effects on, 140–143
  rapid deposition into, in hungry bone
      syndrome, 65
Bone marrow
  biopsy of
    in multiple myeloma, 141
    in *Mycobacterium avium intracellulare*
        pneumonia, 186
    in pancytopenia, 145
    retroperitoneal hematoma from,
        148–150
    in thrombotic thrombocytopenic
        purpura–hemolytic uremic
        syndrome, 151
  transplantation of, in multiple myeloma,
      143
BOOP (bronchiolitis obliterans with
      organizing pneumonia), 185
Brachydactyly, hypocalcemia in, 64–68
Bradycardia, torsades de pointes in, 51
Brain
  abscess of, in systemic lupus
      erythematosus, 161–165
  biopsy of, in abscess, 163
  disorders of, syndrome of inappropriate
      antidiuretic hormone in, 236
  edema of, in hyponatremia, 236–238
  hemorrhage of
    vs. abscess, 162
    in thrombolytic therapy, 217
  imaging of, in postural orthostatic
      tachycardia syndrome, 204
  infarction of. *See* Stroke
  vitamin B$_{12}$ deficiency effects on, 209
Breath, shortness of. *See* Dyspnea
Breath sounds, in lung abscess, 175
Bronchiolitis obliterans with organizing
      pneumonia, 185

Bronchoalveolar lavage, in *Mycobacterium
      avium intracellulare* pneumonia,
      186–187
Bronchoscopy, therapeutic,
      methemoglobinemia after, 262–264
Bruits, in peripheral vascular disease, 25
Buerger disease (thromboangiitis obliterans)
  blue finger in, 18–22
  limb ischemia in, 4
Burch and Wartofsky criteria for thyroid
      storm, 81–82, 82*t*
Bursitis, of knee, vs. meniscal tear, 282
Bypass grafting
  in limb ischemia, 6
  in peripheral vascular disease, 28

C

C-reactive protein, measurement of, in
      Buerger disease, 20
Calcification, in aortic stenosis, 15–16
Calciphylaxis, 223–226
Calcium
  abnormal. *See* Hypercalcemia;
      Hypocalcemia
  malabsorption of, hypocalcemia in, 75
Calcium–phosphorus product, in
      calciphylaxis, 225
Calcium oxalate, formation of, in ethylene
      glycol poisoning, 229, 229*f*
Calf
  pain in, in peripheral vascular disease,
      23–28
  ulcer of, in ischemia, 4*f*
CALMSHAPES mnemonic, for
      hypercoagulability, 5, 5*t*
Campylobacter jejuni infections,
      Guillain–Barré syndrome after,
      201
Cancer
  vs. angioimmunoblastic
      lymphadenopathy, 132
  breast, metastasis from, to bone, 135–139
  chemotherapy for, tumor lysis syndrome
      in, 243–246
  extension of, vs. retroperitoneal
      hematoma, 148
  hypercoagulability in, limb ischemia in, 7
  liver
    vs. liver abscess, 170
    vs. sarcoidosis, 96
  lung, metastasis from, 137
  metastasis from. *See* Metastasis
  ovarian, limb ischemia in, 3–9
  vs. pyoderma gangrenosum, 212
  vs. sarcoidosis, 96
  syndrome of inappropriate antidiuretic
      hormone in, 236
  thyroid, 77–79
  of unknown primary, back pain in,
      135–139
Carcinoembryonic antigen, in cancer of
      unknown primary, 137
Carcinoma
  hepatocellular, vs. liver abscess, 170
  with neuroendocrine differentiation, in
      cancer of unknown primary, 138
  poorly differentiated, in cancer of
      unknown primary, 138
  thyroid, 77–79

Cardiac arrest
  adrenal hemorrhage in, 60
  pulseless, 270–273
Cardiac arrhythmias. *See* Arrhythmias
Cardiac tamponade, after valve repair,
      42–44
Cardiogenic pulmonary edema, vs. acute
      respiratory distress syndrome, 250
Cardiomegaly, in malignant hypertension,
      240
Cardiomyopathy
  in cocaine abuse, 29
  dilated, torsades de pointes in, 51
  hypertrophic, congestive heart failure in,
      14–15
  hypertrophic obstructive, vs. postural
      orthostatic tachycardia syndrome,
      205
  peripartum, 45–48
Cardiovascular disease, 3–56
  aortic dissection, 10–13, 35–38
  aortic stenosis, 14–17
  blue finger, 18–22
  Buerger disease, 18–22
  calciphylaxis, 223–226
  cardiac arrest in, 270–273
  cardiac tamponade, 42–44
  chest pain in, 10–13
    in aortic stenosis, 16–17
    with cocaine abuse, 29–34
    in myocardial infarction, 249–254
    after valve repair, 39–44
  congestive heart failure. *See* Congestive
      heart failure
  dyspnea in, 45–48
  endocarditis
    vs. calciphylaxis, 223–224
    prosthetic valve, 189–192
    in Whipple disease, 111
  heart palpitations, 29, 53–56, 77–79
  intermittent claudication in, 23–28
  leg pain, 23–28
  limb ischemia, 3–9
  lower-extremity edema, 14–17
  malignant hypertension, 239–242
  in Marfan syndrome, 35–38
  myocardial ischemia, with cocaine abuse,
      29–34
  peripartum cardiomyopathy, 45–48
  peripheral arterial disease, 23–28
  polymorphic ventricular tachycardia,
      49–52
  vs. postural orthostatic tachycardia
      syndrome, 204
  pulmonary embolism. *See* Pulmonary
      embolism
  pulmonary hypertension, 274–278
  in thyroid storm, 82, 82*t*
  torsades de pointes, 49–52
  ulcers in, vs. pyoderma gangrenosum,
      212
  Wolff–Parkinson–White syndrome,
      53–56
Cavernous hemangioma, of liver, vs. abscess,
      170
Cellulitis
  clostridial, vs. necrotizing cellulitis, 167
  synergistic necrotizing, of finger,
      166–169

L

Lachman test, in knee pain, 283t
Lactate dehydrogenase
    in pleural fluid, 259–260
    in thrombotic thrombocytopenic
        purpura–hemolytic uremic
        syndrome, 151–152
Lactic acidosis, in HIV infection, 157–160
Laminectomy, infection from, vs.
        endocarditis, 189
Lateral pivot shift test, in knee pain, 283t
Leg
    edema of, in myelofibrosis, 144–146
    pain in
        in bone metastasis, 135
        in hematoma, 117
        in hypocalcemia, 73–76
        in peripheral vascular disease, 23–28
        in pyoderma gangrenosum, 211–213
    spasms of, in osteomalacia, 73
    ulcers of, in calciphylaxis, 223–226
Leiomyoma, uterine, iron deficiency anemia
        in, 128–130
Leukemia
    chemotherapy for, tumor lysis syndrome
        in, 243–246
    in myelofibrosis, 146
    pancytopenia in, 145
Leukocyte(s), fecal, detection of, in diarrhea,
        in kidney transplantation, 104
Leukocyte esterase test, in urinary tract
        infections, 121–122
Leukocytosis
    in cholangitis, 93
    in liver abscess, 170
    in myelofibrosis, 146
    in postcardiac injury syndrome, 41
Ligamentous injuries, of knee, 282–284,
        283t
Light's criteria, for pleural effusion
        classification, 259–260, 260t
Lip, ulceration of, in angioimmunoblastic
        lymphadenopathy, 131
Lipomatosis, in antiretroviral therapy, 160
Livedo reticularis, of hand, in ischemia, 4f
Liver
    abscess of, 170–174
    adenoma of, vs. liver abscess, 170–171
    biopsy of
        in abscess, 171
        in ascites, 88
        in sarcoidosis, 96, 96f
    cancer of
        vs. liver abscess, 170
        vs. sarcoidosis, 96
    cirrhosis of
        edema in, vs. myelofibrosis, 144–145
        pulmonary hypertension in, 276
    dysfunction of, in antiretroviral therapy,
        159–160, 159f
    enlargement of. *See* Hepatomegaly
    focal nodular hyperplasia of, vs. abscess,
        171
    metastasis to, vs. abscess, 170
    sarcoidosis of, 97, 97t
Long QT syndrome, acquired, 49–52
Lumbar puncture, in meningitis, 181
Lung. *See also* Pneumonia; *subjects starting
        with* Pulmonary

abscess of, 175–179
acute injury of, 250–253, 250t, 251t
acute respiratory distress syndrome and,
        249–254
biopsy of, in pulmonary hypertension,
        277
cancer of, metastasis to bone, 137
edema of. *See* Pulmonary edema
empyema effects on, 260
mucous plug in, 262
parenchymal disorders of, pulmonary
        hypertension in, 276
sarcoidosis of, vs. pulmonary
        hypertension, 274
surgery on, methemoglobinemia after,
        262–264
Lupus anticoagulant, in antiphospholipid
        antibody syndrome, 7
Lymph nodes
    biopsy of, in angioimmunoblastic
        lymphadenopathy, 133
    examination of, 131–132
    sarcoidosis of, 97
Lymphadenopathy
    angioimmunoblastic, 131–134
    chemotherapy for, 243
Lymphoma
    vs. angioimmunoblastic
        lymphadenopathy, 132
    chemotherapy for, tumor lysis syndrome
        in, 243–246
    extension of, vs. retroperitoneal
        hematoma, 148–150
    vs. sarcoidosis, 96
Lymphoproliferative disease, lactic acidosis
        in, 159

M

McMurray test, in knee pain, 283, 283t
Macrocytic anemia, in vitamin B_{12}
        deficiency, 209
Macroovalocytosis, in vitamin B_{12}
        deficiency, 209, 209f
Macrophages, foamy, in Whipple disease,
        112
Magnesium, depletion of, hypocalcemia
        and, 65, 74
Magnetic resonance angiography
    in peripheral vascular disease, 25–26, 27f
    in stroke, 216
Magnetic resonance
        cholangiopancreatography, in
        cholangitis, 93
Magnetic resonance imaging
    in aortic dissection, 11
    in bone metastasis, 138, 138f
    in brain abscess, 161–163, 162f
    in liver abscess, 171
    in liver hemangioma, 170
    in malignant hypertension, 240
    in meniscal tear, 284f, 285
    in multiple myeloma, 141
    newer technologies for, 216
    in postural orthostatic tachycardia
        syndrome, 204
    in spinal cord compression, 200
    in stroke, 215–216, 219, 219f
    in thyroid nodule, 77
    in transverse myelitis, 200

Malabsorption
    hypocalcemia in, 75
    vitamin B_{12} deficiency in, 209–210
Malignancy. *See* Cancer
Malignant hypertension, 239–242
Mammography, in cancer of unknown
        primary, 137
Marfan syndrome, aortic dissection in,
        35–38
MASS phenotype, vs. Marfan syndrome, 35
Mean corpuscular volume, in vitamin B_{12}
        deficiency, 209
Mechanical ventilation
    for acute respiratory distress syndrome,
        252
    for Guillain–Barré syndrome, 202
Meckel diverticulum, bleeding in, 100
Mediastinal widening, chest, 10–11, 10f,
        11f
Medullary carcinoma, of thyroid, 79
Melena, in thrombocytopenia, 124
Meningitis
    bacterial, 180–183
    cryptococcal, 163
    differential diagnosis of, 181, 181t
    vs. hyponatremia, 235
    in systemic lupus erythematosus, 162
    vs. thyroid storm, 81
Meniscal tear, in knee, 281–285
Mental retardation, hypocalcemia in, 64–68
Mental status changes
    in adrenal insufficiency, 61
    in ethylene glycol poisoning, 227–230
    in gastrointestinal bleeding, 99
    in hyperglycemic hyperosmolar
        syndrome, 70
    in hypernatremia, 231–234
    in hyponatremia, 235–238
Mesenteric stranding, in ascites, 88, 88f
Metabolic acidosis
    anion gap, in ethylene glycol poisoning,
        227–229
    in HIV infection, 158–159
Metastasis
    to bone
        from breast cancer, 135–139
        vs. multiple myeloma, 141
    to liver, vs. abscess, 170
Methanol poisoning, vs. ethylene glycol
        poisoning, 228
Methemoglobinemia, anesthetic-induced,
        262–264
Methylmalonic acid, in vitamin B_{12}
        deficiency, 209
Microscopic polyangiitis, vs. persistent
        pneumonia, 185
Migraine headache
    dizziness in, vs. postural orthostatic
        tachycardia syndrome, 205
    vs. thyroid storm, 80–81
Mitral valve
    regurgitation of
        congestive heart failure in, 14
        murmurs in, 15
        in peripartum cardiomyopathy, 47
        repair of, chest pain after, 39–44
    stenosis of
        congestive heart failure in, 14
        murmurs in, 15